Lameness in Cattle

Editor

J.K. SHEARER

VETERINARY CLINICS OF NORTH AMERICA: FOOD ANIMAL PRACTICE

www.vetfood.theclinics.com

Consulting Editor
ROBERT A. SMITH

July 2017 • Volume 33 • Number 2

ELSEVIER

1600 John F. Kennedy Boulevard • Suite 1800 • Philadelphia, Pennsylvania, 19103-2899

http://www.vetfood.theclinics.com

VETERINARY CLINICS OF NORTH AMERICA: FOOD ANIMAL PRACTICE Volume 33, Number 2
July 2017 ISSN 0749-0720, ISBN-13: 978-0-323-53158-0

Editor: Katie Pfaff
Developmental Editor: Meredith Madeira

Veterinary Clinics of North America: Food Animal Practice (ISSN 0749-0720) is published in March, July, and November by Elsevier Inc., 360 Park Avenue South, New York, NY 10010-1710. Subscription prices are $240.00 per year (domestic individuals), $386.00 per year (domestic institutions), $100.00 per year (domestic students/residents), $265.00 per year (Canadian individuals), $509.00 per year (Canadian institutions), $335.00 per year (international individuals), $509.00 per year (international institutions), and $165.00 per year (international and Canadian students/ residents). To receive student/resident rate, orders must be accompanied by name of affiliated institution, date of term, and the signature of program/residency coordinator on institution letterhead. *Clinics* subscription prices. All prices are subject to change without notice. **POSTMASTER:** Send address changes to *Veterinary Clinics of North America*: *Food Animal Practice*, Elsevier Health Sciences Division, Subscription Customer Service, 3251 Riverport Lane, Maryland Heights, MO 63043. Customer Service (orders, claims, online, change of address): Elsevier Health Sciences Division, Subscription **Customer Service, 3251 Riverport Lane, Maryland Heights, MO 63043. Tel: 1-800-654-2452 (U.S. and Canada); 314-447-8871 (ouside U.S. and Canada). Fax: 314-447-8029. E-mail: journalscustomerservice- usa@elsevier.com (for print support); journalsonlinesupport-usa@elsevier.com (for online support).**

Reprints. For copies of 100 or more, of articles in this publication, please contact the Commercial Reprints Department, Elsevier Inc., 360 Park Avenue South, New York, NY 10010-1710. Tel.: 212-633-3874; Fax: 212-633-3820; E-mail: reprints@elsevier.com.

Veterinary Clinics of North America: Food Animal Practice is covered in *Current Contents/Agriculture, Biology and Environmental Sciences, MEDLINE/PubMed (Index Medicus), and Excerpta Medica.*

Contributors

CONSULTING EDITOR

ROBERT A. SMITH, DVM, MS
Diplomate, American Board of Veterinary Practitioners; Veterinary Research and Consulting Services, LLC, Greeley, Colorado

EDITOR

J.K. SHEARER, DVM, MS, DACAW
Diplomate, American College of Animal Welfare; Professor, Department of Veterinary Diagnostic and Production Animal Medicine, College of Veterinary Medicine, Iowa State University, Ames, Iowa

AUTHORS

DAVID E. ANDERSON, DVM, MS
Diplomate, American College of Veterinary Surgeons; Professor and Head, Department of Large Animal Clinical Sciences, College of Veterinary Medicine, University of Tennessee Institute of Agriculture, Knoxville, Tennessee

HANS BOTHE, DVM
Aurora Organic Farms, Platteville, Colorado

MICHELLE S. CALVO-LORENZO, PhD
Technical Consultant, Elanco Animal Health, Division of Eli Lilly Company, Greenfield, Indiana

JOHANN F. COETZEE, BVSc, Cert CHP, PhD
Diplomate, American College Veterinary Clinical Pharmacology; Diplomate, American College of Animal Welfare; Diplomate, European College of Animal Welfare Science, Ethics, and Law; Professor, Department of Anatomy and Physiology, College of Veterinary Medicine, Kansas State University, Manhattan, Kansas

NIGEL B. COOK, BSc, BVSc Cert, CHP, DBR, MRCVS
Professor and Chair, Department of Medical Sciences, University of Wisconsin-Madison, School of Veterinary Medicine, Madison, Wisconsin

GERARD CRAMER, DVM, DVSc
Associate Professor, Dairy Production Medicine, Veterinary Population Medicine Department, University of Minnesota, St Paul, Minnesota

ANDRÉ DESROCHERS, DMV, MS
Diplomate, American College of Veterinary Surgeons; Diplomate, European College of Bovine Health Management; Professor, Department of Clinical Sciences, Faculty of Veterinary Medicine, Université de Montréal, St-Hyacynthe, Québec, Canada

LILY N. EDWARDS-CALLAWAY, PhD
Animal Welfare Specialist, Callalily Consulting LLC, Fort Collins, CO

MARCIA I. ENDRES, DVM, MS, PhD
Professor, Department of Animal Science, University of Minnesota, St Paul, Minnesota

TEMPLE GRANDIN, PhD
Professor, Department of Animal Sciences, Colorado State University, Fort Collins, Colorado

MICHAEL D. KLEINHENZ, DVM
Graduate-Assistant Research, Department of Anatomy and Physiology, College of Veterinary Medicine, Kansas State University, Manhattan, Kansas

JOHANN KOFLER, Dr Med Vet
Diplomate, European College of Bovine Health Management; Associate Professor, Department of Farm Animals and Veterinary Public Health, Clinic for Ruminants, University of Veterinary Medicine Vienna, Veterinaerplatz, Vienna

ADAM KRULL, DVM, PhD
Veterinary Diagnostic and Production Animal Medicine, Iowa State University College of Veterinary Medicine, Ames, Iowa

DIEGO MANRIQUEZ, DVM
Department of Animal Sciences, Colorado State University, Fort Collins, Colorado

PABLO PINEDO, DVM, PhD
Department of Animal Sciences, Colorado State University, Fort Collins, Colorado

PAUL J. PLUMMER, DVM, PhD, DACVIM(LAIM), DECSRHM
Veterinary Diagnostic and Production Animal Medicine, Iowa State University College of Veterinary Medicine, Ames, Iowa

JOHN A. SCANGA, PhD
Senior Technical Consultant, Protein Product Analytics, Elanco Knowledge Solutions, Elanco Animal Health, Division of Eli Lilly Company, Greenfield, Indiana

J.K. SHEARER, DVM, MS, DACAW
Diplomate, American College of Animal Welfare; Professor, Department of Veterinary Diagnostic and Production Animal Medicine, College of Veterinary Medicine, Iowa State University, Ames, Iowa

MATTHEW L. STOCK, VMD, PhD
Diplomate, American Board of Veterinary Practitioners (Food Animal); Diplomate, American College Veterinary Clinical Pharmacology; Department of Veterinary Diagnostic and Production Animal Medicine, College of Veterinary Medicine, Iowa State University; Department of Biomedical Science, College of Veterinary Medicine, Iowa State University, Ames, Iowa

GRANT C. STODDARD, BS
PhD Student, Veterinary Population Medicine Department, University of Minnesota, St Paul, Minnesota

SAREL R. VAN AMSTEL, BVSc, MMedVet
DipMedVet; Diplomate, American College of Veterinary Internal Medicine; Professor Emeritus, Department of Large Animal Clinical Sciences, College of Veterinary Medicine, University of Tennessee Institute of Agriculture, The University of Tennessee, Knoxville, Tennessee; Professor, Department of Veterinary Diagnostic and Production Animal Medicine, College of Veterinary Medicine, Iowa State University, Ames, Iowa

DAVID C. VAN METRE, DVM
Professor, Diplomate of the American College of Veterinary Internal Medicine; Professor, Department of Clinical Sciences, College of Veterinary Medicine and Biomedical Sciences, Colorado State University, Fort Collins, Colorado

JUAN VELEZ, MS, DVM
Aurora Organic Farms, Platteville, Colorado

HELEN REBECCA WHAY, BSc(Hons), PhD, NDA
Professor, School of Veterinary Sciences, University of Bristol, Bristol, United Kingdom

Contents

The five freedoms offer a framework for discussion of lameness and its impact on the welfare of cows. Altered feeding behavior is a cause of reduced body condition, smaller digital cushion, and lameness. Providing a comfortable environment is critical to recovery and welfare. Pain associated with injury or disease of feet or legs is manifested by lameness. Pain management is an important part of therapy. In cases of severe lameness, euthanasia may be preferred. Lameness interferes with an animal's ability to exhibit natural behaviors by altering lying time, social interaction, ovarian activity and estrus intensity, and rumination behavior.

Digital dermatitis is a polybacterial disease process of dairy and beef cattle. Lesions are most commonly identified on the plantar aspect of the interdigital cleft of the hind limbs. *Treponema* spp are routinely present in large numbers of active lesions. Lesions are painful to the touch and can result in clinical lameness. The infectious nature generally results in endemic infection of cattle herds and management requires a comprehensive and integrated multipronged approach. This article provides current perspectives regarding management and treatment of digital dermatitis on dairy and beef cattle operations and provides a review for clinicians dealing with a clinical outbreak.

Bovine foot rot (BFR) is an infectious disease of the interdigital skin and subcutaneous tissues of beef and dairy cattle that occurs under a variety of management and environmental settings. The anaerobic, gram-negative bacteria Fusobacterium necrophorum, Porphyromonas levii, and Prevotella intermedia are commonly isolated from lesions. A multitude of host, agent, and environmental factors contribute to the development of BFR. Initiation of systemic antimicrobial therapy early in the course of disease commonly leads to resolution. Delays in treatment may result in extension of infection into deeper bone, synovial structures, or ligamentous structures, and the prognosis for recovery is reduced.

during the 1950s in Dutch black and white cattle. The affected claws are longer and narrower than the claw and have an inward and upward spiral rotation of the toe. Similarly, the bearing surface of the wall is displaced inward. The animal starts to bear weight on the abaxial wall surface, particularly the caudal segment, and the sole may become completely non–weight bearing. The axial wall is displaced dorsomedially and a fold develops in the wall.

VETERINARY CLINICS OF NORTH AMERICA: FOOD ANIMAL PRACTICE

THE CLINICS ARE NOW AVAILABLE ONLINE!
Access your subscription at:
www.theclinics.com

Preface

Bovine Lameness

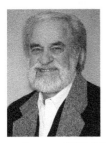

J.K. Shearer, DVM, MS
Editor

It is a distinct honor for me to serve as Guest Editor for this issue of the *Veterinary Clinics of North America: Food Animal Practice* on Bovine Lameness. As many may know, I am following in the footsteps of Dr David Anderson, who served as Guest Editor for the first issue devoted entirely to bovine lameness published in 2001. As a bovine practitioner in the 1970s, I will admit that the treatment of lameness was one of my least favorite tasks. It was hard work, sometimes dangerous, and always took longer than I felt it should; all of which created a dilemma when attempting to calculate a proper fee for the service rendered. Looking back, I am sure that I could have improved my efficiency and effectiveness had my hoof knife been sharper and had I known of the benefits an angle grinder offers when trimming feet or correcting claw lesions. I have also often thought of how much more I might have enjoyed working with lameness had I better understood its pathogenesis and better ways of treating lameness conditions. For the past 30 years, I have focused the majority of my professional life and career on bovine lameness. So much has changed since the 1970s. I credit much of my renewed enthusiasm, and most certainly, my understanding of lameness to insight I have gained from colleagues both here in North America and throughout the world.

Few diseases rival lameness in terms of cost or impact on the welfare of affected animals. Based on the work of Dr Chuck Guard from Cornell University, losses associated with a single case of clinical lameness conservatively approach $500, surpassing nearly all other disease conditions including clinical mastitis. Lameness is the manifestation of pain associated with disease or injury to the foot or proximal limb. Studies on the prevalence of lameness indicate that on average nearly one in every four animals on US dairies is affected. In recent years, the emergence of fatigue cattle syndrome and growing problems with digital dermatitis in feedlot cattle has generated a greater interest in lameness of beef cattle. Moreover, unlike many disorders for which therapeutic intervention provides prompt relief, the disability and pain associated with

Vet Clin Food Anim 33 (2017) xiii–xiv
http://dx.doi.org/10.1016/j.cvfa.2017.04.001
0749-0720/17/© 2017 Published by Elsevier Inc.

lameness often lingers for weeks despite effective treatment. Without a doubt, lameness is clearly one of the most important health and welfare issues in cattle.

Lameness is an immense subject; therefore, the greatest challenge is determining what information is likely to be most critical to the day-to-day work of veterinary practitioners. Veterinarians play a key role as advisors, and many provide specific treatment to lame cows. With this in mind, I attempted to find a balance between providing the kind of information that would assist practitioners in solving herd problems and yet still address the needs of those looking for technical information on proper foot care and treatment practices. For example, treatment options for organic dairies are quite different compared with those in conventional dairy systems. Similarly, pain management is a fundamental component of nearly all therapeutic regimens and particularly in the case of lameness; however, there are no drugs approved for analgesia in cattle. Therefore, a discussion of pain assessment and management associated with lameness has been included.

As I conclude my comments, I want to express my sincere gratitude to all who answered the call to author or coauthor an article. I am deeply indebted to each one. It is my hope that readers will find the information herein informative and useful in their day-to-day work as veterinary practitioners. I also want to acknowledge Dr Robert A. Smith, Consulting Editor, and Meredith Madeira, Developmental Editor, for their guidance and assistance during the editorial process. Finally, I want to acknowledge my wife, Leslie, the unsung hero behind all that I do, for her unwavering support.

J.K. Shearer, DVM, MS
Department of Veterinary Diagnostic
and Production Animal Medicine
Iowa State University
College of Veterinary Medicine
2436 Lloyd Vet Med Center
Ames, IA 50011-1250, USA

E-mail address:
jks@iastate.edu

The Impact of Lameness on Welfare of the Dairy Cow

Helen Rebecca Whay, PhD, NDA[a], J.K. Shearer, DVM, MS[b],*

KEYWORDS

- Lameness • Animal welfare • The five freedoms

KEY POINTS

- The five freedoms offer a useful framework for the discussion of lameness and its impact on the welfare of lame cows.
- Altered feeding behavior may be an important cause of reduced body condition, a smaller digital cushion, and lameness due to sole ulcers and white line disease.
- Providing a comfortable environment for lame cows during the post-treatment period is critical to their recovery and welfare.
- Pain associated with injury or disease of feet and/or legs is manifested by lameness. Pain management is an important part of therapy. In cases of severe lameness (SL), euthanasia may be the preferred option to end otherwise uncontrollable suffering.
- Lameness interferes with an animal's ability to exhibit natural behaviors by altering lying time, social interaction, ovarian activity and estrus intensity, and possibly rumination behavior.

INTRODUCTION

The estimated cost (in today's US dollars) of clinical lameness in dairy cattle approaches $500 per case.[1] Less finite is the actual welfare cost of a problem, such as lameness, because much of an animal's internal experience is inaccessible to humans. The welfare of animals is measured in different currencies. For example, how can the welfare consequences of a change in a cow's ability to express a normal behavior be compared with a case of severe acute mastitis? It is like comparing the price of a product in Japanese yen and US dollars without being told the conversion ratio. Regardless of the difficulty of placing a value on welfare problems, an overview of the welfare challenges experienced by lame dairy cattle is still valuable. An

The authors have nothing to disclose.
[a] School of Veterinary Sciences, University of Bristol, Langford House, Langford, Bristol, BS40 5DU, UK; [b] Department of Veterinary Diagnostic and Production Animal Medicine, College of Veterinary Medicine, Iowa State University, 2436 Lloyd Veterinary Medical Center, Ames, IA 50011, USA
* Corresponding author.
E-mail address: jks@iastate.edu

appreciation of the more subtle as well as the obvious compromises to welfare resulting from lameness is the first step in considering how to better support lame cows and minimize the impact of a problem.

A useful framework for considering the welfare impact of lameness on dairy cows is the five freedoms,[2] which suggest that a basis for provision of good animal welfare is to deliver

Freedom from hunger and thirst
Freedom from discomfort
Freedom from pain, injury, and disease
Freedom to express normal behavior
Freedom from fear and distress

To move beyond the five freedoms requires an environment where animals not only survive but also thrive, an environment where the positive experiences outnumber the negative.[3] Opportunities to improve the welfare of lame cows are abundant.

FREEDOM FROM HUNGER AND THIRST

Provisions of freedom from hunger and thirst are met by providing ready access to fresh water and a diet to maintain full health and vigor.

The impression of most veterinarians is that lameness causes cows to become thin. It is assumed that when cows become lame they lose weight because of inappetence and changes in eating behavior associated with the debilitating effects of the lameness condition. This seems logical because lameness causes pain, reducing the number of trips to the feed bunk, time spent eating, and the ability of the cow to compete for feeding space.

Alternatively, it may be that cows that become thin are more likely to become lame.[4–6] Researchers investigating the relationship between claw lesions, body condition, and thickness of the digital cushion (DC) found that the prevalence of sole ulcers and white line disease increased as thickness of the DC decreased. They also observed that thickness of the DC decreased steadily throughout lactation, reaching nadir (ie, its lowest point) at 120 days after calving. Body condition scores (BCSs) of cows were positively associated with thickness of the DC, whereby an increase in BCSs was associated with a corresponding increase in mean thickness of the DC.[4] The highest prevalence of sole ulcers occurred near peak lactation (ie, 60–100 days in milk), the point at which shrinking of the DC was approaching nadir. This is not unlike observations from other studies and supports an association with a thinner, less functional DC. The rumen acidosis-laminitis complex, the effects of hoofase or activation of metalloproteinase activity, and/or the impact of peripartum hormonal changes, however, can all be theorized as causes of these conditions in a similar time frame.[7–9] Therefore, these observations do not preclude or reduce the significance of other causative factors. Rather, they highlight lameness' complicated pathogenesis and its multifactorial causes.

It seems likely that there is some level of interaction between these 2 theories. BCS can be viewed as a proxy indicator of hunger and loss of body condition through a combination of inappetence, lack of time for eating, inability to successfully compete for food, and burning of energy as the body mounts a defense against the clinical disease of lameness. Whether hunger in dairy cattle results in an experience similar to hunger in humans is unknown, but if the term, *hunger*, is used in its broadest sense as a catch-all term for suboptimal nutrition, then hunger seems to be a problem associated with lameness.

Finally, there has been little attention to drinking behavior associated with lameness in dairy cattle; however, water is second in importance only to oxygen for sustaining life, let alone performance of dairy cattle. A clean palatable supply of water is not just a nice thing; it is an absolute requirement. During periods of heat stress, water intake increases by as much as 20% to 50% or more to support evaporative cooling losses through the skin and respiratory systems. Changes in time budget and drinking behaviors related to elevated temperatures and lameness[10] suggest that more attention to water intake and drinking behavior of lame dairy cows is warranted.

FREEDOM FROM DISCOMFORT

Provisions of the freedom from discomfort are met by providing an appropriate environment that includes shelter and a comfortable area to rest.

This freedom refers to freedom from discomfort from the environment and thus includes aspects of housing, lying area design, ventilation, light, and so forth in relation to a dairy cow's comfort. How often is it that maximizing comfort for the animals that need it most fails? Sometimes the most uncomfortable place on the farm is that area set aside for lame, sick, and convalescing animals. It is not a conscious decision but a failure to recognize what cows need when their health is compromised by disease or injury. Just as it is for humans, everything requires a little more effort when complicated by pain and/or the body is not functioning at 100%. Therefore, common sense indicates that some extra effort is needed to provide additional comforts on dairies in special needs, hospital, and foot care areas.

Lame cows are likely to have more difficulty lying down and standing up in a stall, so a hospital area or special needs barn that offers a clean, dry, and soft area for resting aids recovery because the cow can rest comfortably. A bedded pack, dry lot, or pasture (when weather permits) offers the freedom of unrestricted movement for natural lying and rising behaviors. Experience shows that poor recovery rates from lameness are less often a consequence of improper therapy; more often it is the level of comfort during the convalescent period.[11,12] Soft lying surfaces, such as sand and deep straw, offer better traction than mattresses or mats. A more secure footing surface reduces injuries and instills confidence in an animal attempting to lie down or rise up.

Studies of dairy cattle in regions where there are high temperature-humidity levels show that lying time decreases as the environment becomes hotter.[13] When a cow is standing, she is able to expose a larger amount of her body surface area for evaporative cooling (ie, the primary mode for dissipation of body heat in hot weather conditions). Cows with higher locomotion scores are less able to modify behavior to increase standing time and are less able to regulate their temperature because of lameness. Although good footing, attitude of the cow, and body condition are fundamental to the care of compromised animals, research from a UK study suggests that good nursing care alone may have the single greatest effect on improving the prognosis of disabled cattle.[14]

FREEDOM FROM PAIN, INJURY, AND DISEASE

The provisions of the freedom from pain, injury, and disease are met by the prevention or rapid diagnosis and treatment of pain, injury, and disease.

Lameness is an abnormal gait that normally results from injury, disease, or dysfunction of 1 or more feet and/or limbs. The most common cause of altered gait is pain.

Therefore, it is this freedom that most readily springs to mind when justifying why lameness is a matter of welfare concern.

The perception of pain in animals and humans is similar and occurs by way of multiple tissue receptors designed to sense mechanical or physical stimulations. These receptors are well distributed throughout the body, permitting the sensation of pleasurable as well as noxious types of stimuli. Pain associated with lameness affects primarily nociceptors. Tissue damage at the site of injury results in a barrage of impulses that travel from the site of injury to the spinal cord and ultimately the brain, which interprets them as pain. Inflammation accompanies these events and initiates the release of multiple pain mediators, inflammatory cells, and other chemical substances that contribute to the process. Peripheral nerves in the vicinity of these expanding inflammatory mediators become sensitized and spontaneously send impulses to the spinal cord and brain, thus amplifying the perception of pain. So although the original site of injury may be small, as the inflammatory process progresses, pain can be felt over a much larger area.

Hyperalgesia is an increased sensitivity to a noxious stimulus, particularly common in cattle suffering from chronic lameness disorders. It is characterized by an animal that exhibits an exaggerated reaction to pain in response to a lesser stimulus. Not only does hyperalgesia exacerbate suffering in animals with long-standing lameness but also it is difficult to treat in cattle. Lame animals generally require an extended length of time for recovery to a nonlame, pain-free state on their injured limbs. Whay and colleagues[15,16] reported significant decreases in the nociceptive threshold of lame animals, indicating hyperalgesia lasting 28 days beyond the point of detection.

The acute and chronic nature of pain in cattle associated with lameness suggests that a multimodal approach may improve the success of pain management therapies. This type of strategy includes the use of pharmaceuticals, corrective trimming, foot blocks to relieve weight bearing on injured claws, and appropriate housing during the recovery period. For example, the following might be considered: (1) use of intravenous regional or ring block anesthesia for corrective trimming and treatment of painful conditions; (2) careful and thorough corrective trimming that avoids damage to adjacent healthy corium tissues; (3) use of an orthopedic foot block applied to the healthy claw to relieve weight bearing on injured claws; (4) avoidance of topical therapies that increase discomfort and prolong recovery; (5) administration of analgesics, nonsteroidal anti-inflammatory drugs, and sedative-analgesics; and, critically, (6) comfortable housing and attentive management of lame cows during the post-treatment period.[17]

Severe Lameness

Cows with severe forms of lameness characterized by an inability or reluctance to stand or walk on the affected limb(s) suffer tremendously. Weight loss and debilitation rapidly lead to emaciation and weakness whereby affected cows may become completely nonambulatory. Causes may be associated with injuries of the proximal limb; however, more often the problem is related to a complicated claw lesion (sole ulcer or white line disease) or foot rot in which infection has migrated to the distal interphalangeal joint or other deeper structures of the foot. The misery for animals affected with these lesions is compounded by delays in diagnosis and ineffective approaches to therapy. For example, once the distal interphalangeal joint is affected or the infection has led to deep sepsis that may include tenosynovitis, antibiotic therapy is unlikely to be of value and only prolongs suffering. Treatment of these conditions may include surgery in carefully selected cases where proper follow-up can be assured, but for most cases euthanasia is the best option. These animals should not be marketed because they do not fit the criteria required for transport.

Prevalence rates for LS (4 on a 4-point scale or 5 on a 5-point scale) in North America are reported at 4.5%,[18] 6%,[19] and a range of 3.6% to a high of 8.2%.[20] In a Minnesota study of 5626 cows in 50 herds, the top quartile of herds had 15% of cows that scored as clinically lame (ie, LS $\geq$3) and 2.5% scored as severely lame (ie, LS = 5).[19] For the top 10% of herds, the overall mean prevalence of lameness (LS $\geq$3) was only 5.4%, with 1.5% scored as lame (LS = 4) and no cows scored as severely lame.[18] By comparison, 11% (summer) and 14% (winter) of cows in 30 herds (3621 cows) were scored as lame, but less than 0.2% of cows were scored as severely lame in the top quartile of herds in a Wisconsin study.[18] Based on these data it is reasonable to expect that the prevalence of SL should not exceed 1% of cows in the herd. Welfare auditing standards for prevalence of lameness on US dairy farms vary depending on whether all cows or just certain groups are evaluated. Nearly all programs, however, require that cows with SL have verifiable evidence that they are receiving treatment and that part of the therapy includes euthanasia for animals that are not making progress toward recovery.

FREEDOM TO EXPRESS NORMAL BEHAVIOR

The provisions of the freedom to express normal behavior are met by providing sufficient space, proper facilities, and the company of the animal's own kind.

Time Budgets for Lame and Nonlame Cows

Considerable research has been conducted looking at the time budget of lame and nonlame cows. A time budget describes the tasks or activities that dairy cows need to perform within a 24-hour period. A suggested time budget for normal lactating Holstein dairy cattle in free-stall housing might be (1) eating: 3 h/d to 5 h/d (9–14 meals/d); (2) resting (lying time): 12 h/d to 14 h/d; (3) social interactions: 2 h/d to 3 h/d; (4) ruminating (while standing and lying): 7 h/d to 10 h/d; (5) drinking 0.5 h/d; and time required for travel to and from the milking parlor: 2.5 h/d to 3.5 h/d.[21] Because there are only 24 hours in a day, time spent outside of the pen beyond 3.5 hours forces the cow to sacrifice time from the required behaviors of resting and feeding. This portion of the time budget is easily disturbed by management practices and grouping strategies that result in overcrowding, commingling of primiparous with multiparous cows, excessive standing time in parlor holding areas, and the maintenance of cows in lockups for extended periods of time for treatment or other purposes. The mere change from a 2 times/d to a 3 times/d milking schedule alone creates a circumstance where there is little margin for error.

The Importance of Lying Time

Cows have a strong motivation to rest,[22] so much so that they choose to rest rather than eat when necessary to recoup lost resting time. Research indicates that behavior associated with lying time or lying pattern may itself be an indicator of lameness, whereas a reduction in lying time, especially at the herd level, may be a risk factor for lameness. Although many factors influence lying time in dairy cattle, especially the lying surface and design of stalls where they are in use, it is widely held that the average dairy cow needs to rest approximately 12 hours to 14 hours per day. Data from free-stall systems show that nonlame dairy cattle are generally quite active, getting up and down to move between lying and other activities an average of 12.9 times per day, with each lying bout lasting approximately 1.2 hours.[11]

A consistent finding of lying behavior research is that lame cows spend a greater proportion of their 24-hour time budget lying down compared with nonlame cows. They seem to do this by increasing the length of their lying bouts and reducing the number of bouts, possibly so they spend less time on their feet and having to go through the process of lying and standing fewer times. Lame cows also seem to spend more time standing in proximity to a stall, often with just the front feet in the stall (a behavior referred to as perching) or standing (all 4 feet) in the stall. Some investigators speculate that this indicates that lame cows find the process of lying down in a stall more difficult and are thus hesitant to lie down. More recently evidence has emerged that shows lying behavior in the presence of lameness is influenced by the severity of the lameness, the temperature and humidity levels in the environment, and the softness of the lying surfaces in stalls.[11,12]

Cow-to-Cow Interactions and Stocking Density

Cows are social animals, preferring to be in the company of herd mates to whom they are accustomed. Observation confirms, however, that cow-to-cow interactions are not always cordial, particularly when animals are introduced to new groups. Fighting ensues soon after new animals are introduced and continues until a new hierarchy is established, which normally takes from 2 days to 4 days. During this period of adjustment, less-dominant animals are more frequently displaced from the feed manger (up to 2.5 times more often), and lying bouts and lying time may decrease by as much as 15% to 20%.[21] It is also of interest and perhaps understandable that lame cows are less likely to be the aggressors in aggressive interactions.[23] These problems also occur when younger animals are housed (in mixed groups) with older animals. Primiparous animals are normally smaller and do not compete well with their older multiparous herd mates. Research indicates that grouping primiparous cows separately from multiparous cows improves feed intake, resting time, and performance compared with maintaining animals in mixed groups.[24]

Stocking densities above 100% are common in dairies throughout the United States, in part because dairymen and bank lenders prefer higher stocking densities as a hedge on improving return on the farm's investment in facilities. On the down side, observation and research show that overcrowding increases idle standing in alleyways and reduces time spent resting, which predisposes to poorer performance and lameness. Stocking rates in excess of 120% in 4-row barns or 100% in 6-row barns are likely to have a negative impact on productivity and economic returns.[21] Animals most affected adversely by overcrowding are primiparous, lame, and subordinate cows. As stocking density increased from 100% to 113%, milk yield of younger cows decreased by approximately 4 kg/d.[25]

One of the most oft-cited studies on the effect of overcrowding and reduced lying time on the incidence of lameness is by Leonard and colleagues.[26] These researchers studied a group of heifers stocked at 200% (ie, 2 animals/stall) during the precalving and postcalving periods. Lying times averaged 7.5 h/d with a range of 2.7 h/d to 11.9 h/d. Of 7 animals characterized as having short lying times (less than 5 h/d), 4 (57%) developed clinical lameness compared with less than 10% in the medium (7 h/d) and long lying (10 h/d) groups. In addition to overcrowding, lying time is reduced by poor stall design, hard uncomfortable stall surfaces, insufficient stall bedding, large milking group sizes and slow or reduced milking parlor throughput, excessive time spent in lockups, and a preference of cows to stand (to increase evaporative cooling rates) during periods of hot weather.

Most herds move lame cows to a hospital barn or lame cow pen where they can be cared for more easily. Assuming these areas are not overcrowded, lame animals benefit from easier noncompetitive access to feed, water, and place to rest. On the contrary, housing lame cows with healthy nonlame herd mates puts the lame cows at a distinct disadvantage. High stocking rates exacerbate the problem, leading to a continued decline in performance and a lesser possibility for recovery. In the study by Hill and colleagues,[25] an increase in stocking rate from 100% to 131% resulted in a difference in milk yield between sound and lame cows of 11.8 kg/d. Investigators attributed the decrease in milk yield to the effects of high stocking density on reduced resting time and rumination activity.

Effect of Lameness on Social Behavior

Social interaction with pen mates is an important part of natural herd behavior that is frequently manifested by licking. Research suggests that although all animals within a group are licked, not all animals do the licking.[27] The effects of lameness on this and other social behaviors was studied in 10 lame and 10 nonlame cows. Researchers observed both groups of cows for 32 hours with specific attention to social and individual behaviors. They observed that lame cows were less likely to initiate aggressive interaction with herd mates compared with nonlame cows. Time spent licking or grooming pen mates was similar for lame and nonlame cows; however, lame cows were more frequently the recipients of licking. Finally, total lying time was similar between groups but lame cows spent significantly more time lying outside of the stalls. The conclusion was that lame cows have a more difficult time coping in herd environments, possibly because of pain or a feeling of weakness, and therefore avoid aggressive interaction. It was also suggested that licking may play an important role in alleviating discomfort in herd members suffering pain or illness.[23]

Effects of Lameness on Rumination Behavior

Ruminants are able to acquire nutrients from plant-based foods through fermentation in the rumen. Rumination is defined as the regurgitation of fibrous digesta from the rumen to the mouth, remastication, and reinsalivation followed by swallowing and returning of the material to the rumen.[28] Depending on diet and feeding, cows are estimated to spend approximately one-third of their day ruminating. Rumination provides similar physiologic benefits to the cow that humans obtain from deep sleep. A ruminating cow stands or lies quietly and relaxed, with her head down and eyelids lowered. Actual time spent sleeping is short in cattle, at approximately 3 h/d of non–rapid eye movement sleep and 45 min/d of rapid eye movement sleep.[29]

Rumination is an innate behavioral need and, therefore, considered an important parameter to monitor in studies involving cattle well-being. In general, lame cows make fewer visits to the feed manger, spend less total time feeding, and eat faster compared with nonlame cows. Effects of lameness on rumination activity are less clear. Rumination rates in lame animals were reduced in a UK study[10] but unaffected in another.[30] This seems to be an area in need of additional study.

Effects of Lameness on Estrous Behavior

Lameness is often associated with involuntary culling due to infertility. Specific causes seem to be both direct (ie, affecting ovarian function) and indirect (ie, associated with external factors). A Florida study by Garbarino and colleagues[31] found that lame cows had 3.5-times greater odds of delayed cyclicity compared with nonlame cows. A delay in cyclicity was also observed in cows treated for lameness that had an 18-day delay from calving to first luteal activity compared with healthy nonlame herd mates.[32] Specific mechanisms at the level of the ovary are complex and unclear, but lameness may act as a chronic stressor, thereby contributing to a reduction in progesterone concentrations prior to estrus.[32] More obvious are the effects of lameness on energy balance and weight loss associated with increased lying time and reduced dry matter intake, which have inhibitory effects on follicular development. Lameness results in reduced intensity of estrus and can contribute to ovulation failure, which is largely due to reduced preovulatory estradiol secretion and failure of the luteinizing hormone surge. Cows developing lameness within 30 days postcalving were 2.6 times more likely to develop cystic ovarian disease compared with normal cows.[33]

It is also suggested that behavioral modifications associated with lameness, such as increased lying time and reluctance to mount and ride other animals, may compromise the ability of farm staff to detect estrus.[34] Similar observations were made in a commercial herd in tropical India where researchers found that the duration of estrus and frequency of behavioral signs were analogous for lame and nonlame cows, but the intensity of behavorial signs was significantly subdued in lame cows. Researchers concluded that lameness suppressed estrus behavior and increased the difficulty of estrus detection.[35]

FREEDOM FROM FEAR AND DISTRESS

Feelings of fear and distress are not emotions unique to humans. To meet the objectives of the freedom from fear and distress, conditions and treatment that avoid mental suffering must be assured.

Human Interaction

The process of examination and treatment of lameness disorders in dairy cattle provokes fear and distress. Merely separating a lame cow from herd mates causes measurable increases in cortisol. Some of these effects can be reduced by not singling out individuals but by treating them in the presence of another cow. It is important that personnel working with cattle in any capacity have a basic understanding of their behavior. There is generally a good reason why animals do not do as humans would like or might anticipate in certain situations. Looking at these situations from the cow's perspective often provides both an explanation and solution. Personnel need to understand the natural behavior of cows and the way in which they perceive their environment. Experience shows that when they do, the animal's fear and distress are greatly reduced and cattle handling is safer, more efficient, and enjoyable.

Cows have good memories of bad experiences. Rarely is it that entry into a trim chute becomes a precursor to a pleasant experience. As a consequence, cows commonly balk at the entrance to a trimming chute. This is sometimes followed by aggressive attempts to move the cow into a chute that may include yelling, pushing, prodding, and so forth by operators that only adds to the negativity of the chute experience. Add to this the discomfort that often accompanies corrective trimming and treatment and it is not hard to see why an animal might be fearful and hesitant to enter a trim chute the next time foot care is necessary.

Some of these problems can be corrected by improving facility design and training employees in proper animal handling. For example, designing foot care areas with curved alleyways normally improves cattle flow and takes advantage of a cow's tendency to want to return from where she came. Furthermore, because cattle normally follow a lead animal, the tub design (curved alleyway) takes advantage of this natural following behavior and in large operations may improve cattle flow into the trim chute.[36,37]

Probably one of the most important ways to limit fear and distress, however, is to create an environment or culture where cattle learn to become secure and comfortable with human interaction early on in their existence. Research and observation indicate that the perception of humans by cattle is formed within the first 3 months to 4 months of life. Handling in a positive manner during the first 9 months to 12 months decreases the comfort zone between heifers and herdsmen and reduces the adverse effects of negative interactions associated with painful but necessary management procedures occurring later. This underscores the reason and need for continual training of employees in normal animal behavior and proper cattle handling.

These specific examples of an association between lameness and fear and distress are supported by limited scientific evidence; much is anecdotal and experiential. The compromises to freedoms, described previously, lead to a cow that is hyperalgesic (very probably in pain), becoming less fit, losing body condition and diminishing its energy reserves, less mobile, slower moving, and becoming behaviorally desynchronized from the rest of the herd. This increasing isolation of a herd animal from pen mates is likely to make a lame cow feel vulnerable at a most basic level — vulnerable to predation and fearful as she becomes separated from the security of the herd.

Tilt Tables Verses Stand-up–Style Chute Systems

Tilt tables are normally preferred for foot work on beef cattle because they provide better restraint for large bulls, beef cows, and feedlot cattle that are less accustomed to human contact and handling. A survey of hoof trimmers who do predominantly dairy cattle foot care and claw trimming, however, found that of 102 respondents, 53 (54%) reported using a tilt table for trimming and foot care compared with 49 (46%) who reported using a hydraulic stand-up type of chute.[38] An issue of frequent debate between users of both systems is which restraint system causes the greater degree of stress or discomfort for the cow? An Austrian study measured serum cortisol levels in cattle trimmed in either a stand-up or tilt table–style of chute. They observed that cortisol levels were elevated in both types of restraint systems. Cortisol levels were observed to be even higher than those measured in bulls after castration. These investigators also offered that the tilt table was preferable to the stand-up chute because it was their opinion that cows were quieter and better restrained on the tilt table.[39] Researchers concluded that restraint alone was a major stressor for cattle at the time of trimming and that there was no difference between the stand-up or tilt table systems in terms of stress. Similar results were observed in a study conducted on 207 dairy cows. Animals were divided into 2 groups: 1 group trimmed in a stand-up (walk-in)–style crush (chute) and a second group trimmed on a tilt table. Fecal cortisol metabolite concentrations and evasion scores (ie, avoidance behaviors based on visual observation and scoring) were significantly higher in cows trimmed in the walk-in–style (stand-up) chute compared with those trimmed on the tilt table. Researchers also observed that claw trimming procedure using the tilt table required significantly less time than trimming on the walk-in–style chute.[40]

On the contrary, an Iowa study determined that cattle were less stressed in the stand-up–style chute compared with the tilt table.[41] Researchers assessed stress levels in 66 cows (tilt table = 31 animals; stand-up = 35 animals) by counting vocalizations/cow and assessing the number of times the animal passed manure while restrained in the chute. Results demonstrated a highly significant difference in distress responses associated with the type of restraint device used; cows in the stand-up–style chute vocalized less frequently and exhibited fewer eliminatory behaviors (defecating and urinating). A UK study confirmed that the processes of restraint in a cattle crush and of lifting a foot elevated cortisol levels, regardless of whether the foot received a routine trim or treatment of a lameness-causing lesion.[15] These studies do not provide a definitive answer to the question of which type of chute causes more stress beyond saying that restraint alone induces fear and distress.

SUMMARY

By using the five freedoms as a framework for considering the welfare impact of lameness in dairy cattle, it is clear that the welfare consequences of lameness are diverse and that no freedom is left uncompromised. In the farm environment, humans have almost complete control over animals; that is, humans determine the availability of food and water, the housing conditions in which they must live, and the management practices they must endure. It is the decisions and behavior of humans (either directly or indirectly) that have the greatest influence on the welfare status of farm animals. Despite the ideals as expressed in the five freedoms and their provisions, it is not possible to "free" animals from "all" pain or distress. As 1 investigator points out, animals are designed to detect negative sensory inputs because these are necessary for survival as well animals' ability to cognitively sense external circumstances.[3] To create the conditions for animals to have "a life worth living," it is necessary to move beyond survival–critical measures. Lameness reduces an animal's quality of life, tipping it in the direction of "a life worth avoiding."[3] Humans have the ability to minimize the pain and debilitating effects of lameness in cattle through early detection, prompt treatment, and providing a comfortable housing environment during the recovery period. Facilities can be better designed to meet natural behavioral needs and create environments that prevent lameness. A better job can be done of applying what is understood about cattle behavior to reduce fear and anxiety in animals with respect to human interactions.

REFERENCES

1. Guard CL. Quantification and the associated costs of lameness on today's dairies. Proc Am Assoc Bovine Pract Proc 2006;39:144–6.
2. Farm Animal Welfare Council. Report on priorities for animal welfare, research and development. London: Farm Animal Welfare Council; 1993.
3. Mellor DJ. Updating Animal Welfare Thinking: Moving beyond the "Five Freedoms" towards "A Life Worth Living". Animals 2016;6(3):1–20.
4. Bicalho RC, Machado VS, Caixeta LS. Lameness in dairy cattle: a debilitating disease or a disease of debilitated cattle? A cross-sectional study of the prevalence of lameness and the thickness of the digital cushion. J Dairy Sci 2009;92: 3175–84.
5. Solano L, Barkema HW, Pajor EA, et al. Prevalence of lameness and associated risk factors in Canadian Holstein-Friesian cows housed in freestall barns. J Dairy Sci 2015;98:6978–91.
6. Tisdall DA, Brown WJ, Groenvelt M, et al. The relationship between body condition score and mobility score in dairy cows on four commercial UK farms. In proceedings of the 17th International Symposium and 9th International Conference on Lameness in Ruminants. Bristol (United Kingdom), August 11–14, 2013.
7. Tarlton JF, Webster AJF. A biochemical and biomechanical basis for the pathogenesis of claw horn lesions. Proc of the 12th Int Sym on Lameness in Ruminants, Orlando (FL): 2002. p. 395–8.
8. Tarlton JF, Holah DE, Evans KM, et al. Biomechanical and histopathological changes in the support structures of bovine hooves around the time of first calving. Vet J 2002;163:196–204.

9. Knott L, Tarlton JF, Craft H, et al. Effects of housing, parturition and diet change on the biochemistry and biomechanics of the support structures of the hoof of dairy heifers. Vet J 2006;174:277–87.
10. Stokes JE, Leach KE, Main DCJ, et al. The accuracy of detecting digital dermatitis in the milking parlour. Vet J 2012;193:679–84.
11. Gomez A, Cook NB. Time budgets of lactating dairy cattle in commercial freestall herds. J Dairy Sci 2010;93:5772–81.
12. Ito K, von Keyserlingk MAG, LeBlanc SJ, et al. Lying behaviour as an indicator of lameness in dairy cows. J Dairy Sci 2010;93:3553–60.
13. Cook NB, Mentink RL, Bennett TB, et al. The effect of heat stress and lameness on time budgets of lactating dairy cows. J Dairy Sci 2007;90:1674–82.
14. Chamberlain AT, Cripps PJ. Prognostic indicators for the downer cow. Proceedings of the 6th International Conference on Production Diseases in Farm Animals, Belfast, Northern Ireland. the Executive Committee; 1986. p. 32–5.
15. Whay HR. The perception and relief of pain associated with lameness in dairy cattle [PhD Thesis]. University of Bristol; 1998.
16. Whay HR, Waterman AE, Webster AJ, et al. The influence of lesion type on the duration of hyperalgesia associated with hindlimb lameness in dairy cattle. Vet J 1998;156:23–9.
17. Shearer JK, Stock ML, Van Amstel SR, et al. Assessment and management of pain associated with lameness in cattle. Vet Clin North Am Food Anim Pract 2013;29(1):135–56.
18. Cook NB. Prevalence of lameness among dairy cattle in Wisconsin as a function of housing type and stall surface. J Am Vet Med Assoc 2003;223:1324–8.
19. Espejo LA, Endres MI, Salfer JA. Prevalence of lameness in high-producing Holstein cows housed in freestall barns in Minnesota. J Dairy Sci 2006;89:3052–8.
20. von Keyserlingk MAG, Barrientos AK, Ito K, et al. Benchmarking cow comfort on North American freestall dairies: Lameness, leg injuries, lying time, facility design, and management for high-producing Holstein dairy cows. J Dairy Sci 2012;95:7399–408.
21. Grant R. Current concepts in time budgeting for dairy cattle. Grantville (PA): Penn State Dairy Cattle Nutrition Workshop; 2011. p. 101–5.
22. Jensen MB, Pedersen LJ, Munksgaard L. The effect of reward duration on demand functions for rest in dairy heifers and lying requirements as measured by demand functions. Appl Anim Behav Sci 2005;90:207–17.
23. Galindo F, Broom DM. Effects of lameness of dairy cows. J Appl Anim Welf Sci 2002;5(3):193–201.
24. Grant RJ, Albright JL. Feeding behaviour. In: D'Mello JPF, editor. Farm animal metabolism and nutrition. New York: CABI Publishing; 2000. p. 365–81.
25. Hill CT, Grant RJ, Dann HM, et al. The effect of stocking rate, parity, and lameness on the short-term behavior of dairy cattle. J Dairy Sci 2006;89(Suppl 1):304–5.
26. Leonard FC, O'Connell JM, O'Farrell KJ. Effect of overcrowding on claw health in first-calved friesian heifers. Br Vet J 1996;152:459–72.
27. Sato S. Social licking pattern and its relationships to social dominance and live weight gain in weaned calves. Appl Anim Behav Sci 1984;12:25–32.
28. Welch JG. Rumination, particle size reduction and passage from the rumen. J Anim Sci 1982;54:885–94.
29. Ternman E, Hanninen L, Pastell M, et al. Sleep in dairy cows recorded with a non-invasive EEG technique. Appl Anim Behav Sci 2012;140:25–32.

30. Thorup VM, Nielsen BL, Pierre-Emmanuel R, et al. Lameness affects cow feeding but not rumination behavior as characterized from sensor data. Front Vet Sci 2016;3:1–11.

31. Garbarino EJ, Hernandez JA, Shearer JK, et al. Effect of lameness on ovarian activity in postpartum Holstein cows. J Dairy Sci 2004;87:4123–31.

32. Petersson KJ, Strandberg E, Gustafsson H, et al. Environmental effects on progesterone profile measures of dairy cow fertility. Anim Reprod Sci 2006;91:3–4, 201–14.

33. Melendez P, Bartolome J, Archbald LF, et al. The association between lameness, ovarian cysts and fertility in lactating dairy cows. Theriogenology 2003;59: 927–37.

34. Walker SL, Smith RF, Routly JE, et al. Lameness, activity time-budgets, and estrus expression in dairy cattle. J Dairy Sci 2008;91:4552–9.

35. Sood P, Nanda AS. Effect of lameness on estrous behavior in crossbred cows. Theriogenology 2006;66:1375–80.

36. Grandin T. Improving Animal Welfare, a practical approach. 2nd edition. In: Grandin T, editior. 2015. p. 65-95.

37. Shearer JK, van Amstel SR. Manual of foot care in cattle. 2nd edition. Fort Atkinson (WI): W.D. Hoard's and Sons Company; 2013.

38. Kleinhenz K, Plummer PJ, Danielson J, et al. Survey of veterinarians and hoof trimmers on methods applied to treat claw lesions in dairy cattle. Bovine Pract 2014;48(1):47–52.

39. Stanek CH, Mostl E, Pachatz H, et al. Claw trimming, restraint methods, and stress in dairy cattle. Proceedings of the 10th International Symposium on Lameness in Ruminants. Lucerne, Switzerland, 1998. p. 13–16.

40. Pesenhofer G, Palme R, Pesenhofer RM, et al. Comparison of two methods of fixation during functional claw trimming - walk-in crush versus tilt table - in dairy cows using faecal cortisol metabolite concentrations and daily milk yield as parameters. Vet Med Austria 2006;93:288–94.

41. Spasov DS, Higginson JH, Shearer JK, et al. Investigation of bovine stress associated with tilt table and lift restraint devices for hoof trimming. 10th Annual Merck-Merial-NIH National Veterinary Scholars Symposium. Bethesda (MD), August 5–8, 2010.

Clinical Perspectives of Digital Dermatitis in Dairy and Beef Cattle

Paul J. Plummer, DVM, PhD*, Adam Krull, DVM, PhD

KEYWORDS

- Digital dermatitis • Treponema • Bovine • Lameness

KEY POINTS

- Digital dermatitis (DD) is a common disease process of the skin of both dairy and beef cattle.
- Advanced lesions are associated with clinical lameness, whereas early lesions cause local skin disease with minimal lameness.
- Topical treatment with oxytetracycline is the common therapy for advanced lesions but has a high rate of recrudescence.
- An integrated management plan that relies on a combination of topical treatment of advanced lesions coupled with footbathing to control progression of earlier lesions is the most effective strategy.

INTRODUCTION
Description of Digital Dermatitis

The first article to describe the macroscopic appearance of a large number of DD lesions was done on 10 California dairies by Read and Walker in 1998.[1] A majority of the lesions were circumscribed, erosive to papillomatous, and surrounded by a ridge of hyperkeratotic skin bearing hypertrophied hairs. These lesions were typically circular to oval, raised above the surrounding skin, and 2 cm to 6 cm in diameter. Lesions were more likely to involve the rear legs (82%) and a majority (83%) were located on the proximal border of the interdigital space. The macroscopic differences in DD lesion morphology have been described with several novel scoring systems primarily used in research settings.[2–4] The "M" scoring system and the Iowa DD scoring system both describe the macroscopic changes that take place between a normal bovine foot and an end-stage DD lesion. Although each system describes lesions slightly differently, both describe lesions in preclinical and clinical states, with lameness

The authors have nothing to disclose.
Veterinary Diagnostic and Production Animal Medicine, Iowa State University College of Veterinary Medicine, Ames, IA USA
* Corresponding author.
E-mail address: pplummer@iastate.edu

only associated with certain stages. It has also been shown that there can be dynamic macroscopic changes between these stages in as few as 7 days.[5,6]

The histopathologic changes associated with DD have been described in numerous publications,[4,7–17] with several of these studies summarizing the histopathologic changes associated with a large set of DD lesions.[4,11] DD lesions were described as having a highly proliferative epidermis, pronounced rete ridge formation, hyperplastic stratum corneum, and acanthotic stratum spinosum. Additional descriptions include lesions having zones of acute degeneration, necrosis, and focal thinning of the stratum corneum with inflammatory cell infiltration. A consistent finding is the microscopic observation of spirochetes within the lesions through the use of silver staining.

Pathophysiology and Etiology

Bovine DD was first morphologically described in 1974 at the 8th International Meeting on Diseases of Cattle in Milan, Italy,[18] but despite more than 40 years of research, the fulfillment of Koch's postulates[19] in identification of an etiologic agent has yet to be achieved. The first report of a spirochete-like, filamentous organism within DD lesions was described by Blowey and Sharp in 1988.[16] It was soon found that these organisms belong to the species *Treponema* and that became the first bacterial species cultivated and implicated in the etiology of bovine DD.[20] Even from the original report, which described 2 unique bacterial morphologies that belonged to the *Treponema* spp, the identification of multiple *Treponema* spp through visual, biochemical, immunologic, and molecular techniques has been a consistent finding.

Treponema spp have been implicated as the causative agent in DD due to their identification in DD lesions by cultivation,[21–23] fluorescence in situ hybridization (FISH),[8,22,24–30] polymerase chain reaction (PCR),[21,31–33] and metagenomics.[3,25,34,35] The nomenclature for the different types of *Treponema* spp has been constantly undergoing changes based on many of the phylotypes having yet to be cultivated. At this point, there are 4 clusters—cluster 1 (*T denticola/T pedis*–like), cluster 2 (*T phagedenis*–like), cluster 3 (*T refringens*–like), and cluster 4 (*T medium/T vincentii*–like) — that have been reported in the majority of the literature as having clinical relevance to DD.[26] Studies of DD-associated *Treponema* spp have also identified them as having the ability to cause disease by impairing the innate immune and wound repair functions of bovine macrophages.[36] Multiple immunologic studies have also found an increase in antibodies to *Treponema* spp in herds and individual cows with DD.[37,38] Despite all the evidence for *Treponema* spp as the causative agent for DD, Koch's postulates have yet to be fulfilled. Attempts to induce DD lesions with pure cultures of *Treponema* spp have largely failed to consistently induce disease with the characteristic size and severity of naturally occurring DD lesions.[39,40] Additionally, vaccinations against DD-associated *Treponema* spp have failed to decrease the incidence or severity of disease.[41] There is not enough evidence currently available to differentiate *Treponema* spp from a causative organism or merely an organism associated with clinical DD lesions.

For these reasons, numerous other organisms have been studied to determine each one's significance in causing disease. Various *Campylobacter* species as well as *Dichelobacter nodosus* have been cultured from DD lesions and from normal bovine skin.[24] Several researchers[26] have used FISH to determine the level of tissue invasion of various potential pathogens. *D nodosus* was found in 27% and 51% of DD lesions and *Fusobacterium necrophorum* was identified in DD lesions but was found to have minimal invasion in any of the DD tissues evaluated. PCR detection using species-specific primers found *D nodosus* in 100% of DD lesions but also in 60% of normal skin. Similarly, a study in beef cattle using species-specific PCR found *F necrophorum* in 44% of DD lesions but also found that 32% of healthy feet were positive for *F necrophorum*.[42] In an evaluation of the immune response of cattle and herds with and without a history of DD and found no statistical difference in reactive antibodies to *F necrophorum*[43] between cows or across herds with or without a history of DD. Conversely, cows within herds with DD were more likely to have an immune response to *Bacteroides* spp and *Porphyromonas* spp.[23,43] Viral etiologies, such as *Bovine papillomavirus*, have been proposed as a potential pathogen, but several studies have found no evidence of viral involvement.[14,33]

The use of culture-independent metagenomic techniques has provided the ability to determine the relative abundance of all bacteria within DD lesions without looking for specific targets. In a comparison of DD lesions to normal bovine skin, Yano and colleagues[34] found high numbers of *Treponema* spp and *Bacteroides* spp in DD lesions versus the normal microbiota of bovine skin consisting of *Moraxella* and *Corynebacterium*. Krull and colleagues[3] followed a series of cows for several years and obtained biopsies from DD lesions as they developed from normal skin to DD lesions; 11 families were identified as composing at least 5% of the microbiota at the various stages of lesion development. The Spirochaetaceae family increased dramatically from only 1.3% in control feet and to 69.7% in clinical lesions. As lesions developed from normal to diseased feet, an increase in several previously implicated bacterial families was noted, which included the Mycoplasmataceae, Porphyromonadaceae, and Campylobacteraceae families. In a closer look at the Spirochaetaceae family, there was found a change in the *Treponema* spp in preclinical lesions versus clinical lesions; 4 *Treponema* spp that were previously in very low numbers (<3%) in preclinical lesions (*T* PT8, *T denticola*, *T pedis*, and *T medium*) were found to comprise greater than 65% of the *Treponema* population in clinical lesions. Accompanying this increase in the population of these 4 species was a rapid decline in 4 of the 5 highly abundant *Treponema* spp identified in preclinical lesion, which then comprised less than 1% of the *Treponema* population in clinical lesions.

Although there is a consistent presence of multiple *Treponema* spp in DD lesions,[16,25–27,29,31–35,44–46] attempts to induce disease by skin inoculation with pure cultures of these microorganisms have largely failed to result in significant disease in a majority of the animals inoculated.[39] Additionally, the clinical use of vaccines focused against spirochetes provides limited protection against the disease process.[41] Although the consistent clinical response to antibiotic therapy suggests a bacterial agent involved in the etiology of the DD,[9,10,47–58] the fulfillment of Koch's postulates in identifying the key bacterial constituent necessary to produce disease has yet to be proved. The association of DD lesions with a variety of bacterial agents, the response of the lesions to antibiotics, and the failure to induce or protect from the disease using monovalent vaccines strongly suggest that DD is a polymicrobial disease process.[41,59,60]

Similarities to Other Polymicrobial Treponema-associated Diseases

Several research teams have recognized that the bacterial community composition of DD has notable similarities to that of human periodontal disease. Given that human periodontal disease has had significantly greater investments of research time and money, it is prudent to evaluate the similarities between it and DD to gain insights into these complex polymicrobial communities. The bacterial progression of periodontal disease has been extensively studied and develops with successive waves of bacterial colonization.[59,61–65] These waves are consistent in their bacterial composition and are largely driven by the ability of each stage to set up a favorable ecologic environment (in terms of available nutrient sources, oxygen tension, and so forth) for the colonization and growth of the following wave of bacterial agents. Several key themes emerge from this comparison that are helpful in better understanding DD.

First, the 2 disease processes share significant similarities in bacterial populations at the family and genus levels. Early colonizers of periodontal disease include the gram-positive cocci, followed by a wave of gram-positive and gram-negative rods and finally the anaerobic gram-negative rods. The early and midstage colonizers share notable overlap with organisms that are routinely isolated from DD lesions, including *Campylobacter* spp, *Bacteroiodes* spp, and *Fusobacterium* spp. As these organisms colonize they start to push the microenvironment away from a purely aerobic environment toward a more anaerobic niche at the microscopic scale. This process is critical to the development of disease given that the later bacterial colonizers are largely microaerophilic or anaerobic and do not readily grow in the initial aerobic environment of the oral cavity of humans or the skin of cattle. Additionally, as these organisms transition the microenvironment to an anaerobic one, they also transition the overall metabolic profiles of the bacterial community from largely saccharolytic (use glucose and sugars for energy) to one that relies more heavily on proteolytic metabolism of proteins.[66] This transition in local metabolism is believed critical in providing an environment for the colonization of the later colonizers of both disease processes that include the *Treponema* spp and *Porphyromonas* spp that exclusively utilize volatile fatty acids (VFAs) as an energy source as opposed to sugars. The transitions of microbial populations over disease progression described for DD[3] share remarkable similarities with the well-described changes in periodontal disease, which makes biological sense when considering the need for the final-stage organisms (namely the *Treponema* spp and *Porphyromonas* spp) to have an environment conducive to their growth.

Second, an improved understanding of the role that this sequential bacterial colonization process plays in the establishment of a conducive growth environment for the subsequent organism provides insights into explaining how an anaerobic organism, such as the *Treponema* spp, can colonize an aerobic environment like the surface of the skin. In summary, the early colonizers (largely aerobic saccharolytic organisms) set up a favorable microenvironment for the midstage colonizers (facultative anaerobes that shift metabolism sugars to produce VFAs) that then allow for the final colonization of the late-stage organisms that cannot colonize the initial aerobic environment with minimal concentrations of the VFAs that they require for growth.[66]

Finally, there is a significant body of literature on the periodontal communities to demonstrate that the late-stage colonizers, *T denticola* and *Porphyromonas gingivalis*, not only communicate with each other but also actually have direct contact between the cells.[62–64,67,68] This interaction has been demonstrated as critical to the virulence and pathogenicity of these organisms and is the focus of much of the ongoing research in this field. Based on the similarities of these 2 disease processes and that these organisms share significant genetic similarity to the specific species isolated from DD lesions, it seems prudent to consider that similar cross-species interactions are occurring and important in DD. As such, consideration of the *Treponema* spp as part of a larger bacterial community that plays a role in the progressive development and manifestation of DD lesions seems biologically prudent.

Epidemiology of Digital Dermatitis

DD has been found to have the greatest impact on welfare of all bovine lameness disorders due to high incidence and long duration.[69] With lame cows having proved difficult to identify and vastly underestimated by producers,[70] the use of lameness as an estimate for DD prevalence has also been shown unreliable, with only 39% of cows with severe DD lesions showing signs of lameness.[71] Estimates of prevalence have been published across multiple countries[7,11,24,72–78] and range from 1.4% in 14 Norwegian herds to 39% in 5 Danish herds. The large range of prevalence reported from these studies was highly variable based on location, management system, and prevention measures used. For herds in free-stall barns, most estimates suggest a prevalence of 20% to 25% of animals affected. These estimates are based on the prevalence of clinical DD lesions that have been described as having the typical characteristics of end-stage DD lesions.

Several longitudinal studies have attempted to report the rate at which DD lesions develop. Three unique studies in 3 different countries (United States, United Kingdom, and France) found the rate of DD lesion development approximately 4 cases per 100 cow foot–months in the absence of preventative measures,[79–81] with the average time for a lesion to develop from normal skin to a DD lesion between 133 days and 146 days.[79,81] Additionally, lameness is always associated with a macroscopically clinical DD lesion and not any of the preclinical DD morphologies. Krull and colleagues found that the average time from the development of a clinical DD lesion to the onset of lameness was 161 days. This is similar to a study by Frankena and colleagues[71] that found only 39% of cows with clinical lesions were considered lame.

Economic Impact of Digital Dermatitis

Bovine DD is a leading cause of lameness in dairy cattle in the United States[82] but has also been reported at various levels in beef cattle.[11,42,83] In the most recent National Animal Health Monitoring System survey of US dairy farms, DD accounted for 61.8% of the lameness in bred heifers and 49.1% of the lameness in cows.[82] DD was determined the most costly of all foot disorders ($95 per case) in a stochastic simulation model when an estimated prevalence of 20% for clinical DD was used.[84] When milk production losses associated with treatment, decreased reproductive performance, and treatment were incorporated, the losses were estimated at $126 to $133 for every clinical case of DD.[85,86] The total economic losses to the dairy industry has been calculated at $190 million per year in the United States.[87] The estimated economic impact in the United States was based on the 17% prevalence from 1996 National Animal Health Monitoring System (NAHMS) report. The 2007 NAHAMS report estimates the current prevalence at 28%,[82] which suggests the $190 million per year estimate vastly underestimates the economic impact in the United States.

CLINICAL CORRELATION
Dairy

In dairy cattle operations, lesions are most commonly identified in the plantar aspect of the interdigital cleft of the rear feet of lactating cows. Larger lesions may extend into the interdigital space in some cows. Rarely, lesions form on the dorsal aspect of the rear feet. Although less common, lesions occasionally occur on the front feet where they most commonly are located on the dorsal surface of the foot. The reason for the higher incidence on the palmar aspect of the rear feet is unclear; however, several hypotheses have been raised. Some investigators have speculated that the rear feet are at higher risk for exposure and lesion development due to those feet having more exposure to manure slurry, remaining more moist in many tie-stall and free-stall type situations, and their having shorter heels due to a lower hoof angle. Additionally, the plantar aspect of the rear feet has the potential to have more exposure and trauma to the stall mats when an animal is laying in a normal position, in contrast to the forelimbs, which have more exposure to the stall mats on the dorsal aspect of the claw. Lesions in younger animals and dry animals are reportedly less commonly observed by producers but are known to occur and may have a high prevalence in some herds. In many cases, the softer bedding (bedded pack vs free stall), lower body weight, and lower requirement for walking significant distances to be milked may result in a decreased ability to identify these lesions in younger animals or may delay recognition of lesions until the animal freshens and enters the lactating pen.

DD has been considered a leading cause of lameness in the dairy cattle industry for the past several decades; however, its role in beef cattle lameness has more recently emerged as a concern. Based on that fact, the first US clinical descriptions of lesions consistent with what is now called DD were identified in beef cattle.[88,89] Despite these early descriptions in beef cattle, disease identification and control efforts have been largely focused on dairy cattle management, where the lesions have historically caused the most problems. Given the high farm-level prevalence of the disease (finding a negative farm is rare), most dairy operations have been forced to development management protocols that control the animal-level incidence and severity of disease. These protocols typically revolve around a combination of approaches (discussed later) but often focus on the use of intermittent footbathing in combination with targeted treatment of lesions associated with lameness. Within-herd prevalence varies considerably, with some herds maintaining infection rates relatively low using control methods and good biosecurity and other herds having very high incidence of lesions.

Lesions develop over a series of stages that have morphologic differences that can be observed on physical examination (**Fig. 1**). This has led to the development of a variety of lesion staging systems that can be applied based on lesion appearance. The application of lesion staging in clinical medicine has potential benefits regarding treatment decision-making and monitoring treatment success. The decision of which scoring system provides the most information for a clinician should be driven by the needs and desired outcomes of the monitoring. In research settings, more complex systems with a higher number of stages might be useful for monitoring progress of therapy in higher resolution, whereas in many field situations a simpler staging system (for example a system based on description of the lesion — early or advanced) may provide the needed information while making it easier to train employees and get consistent observations. More advanced lesions are the ones associated with clinical lameness and likely shed massive numbers of infectious bacteria into the environment, so accurate diagnosis of those is potentially beneficial in terms of identifying lesions at high risk for causing lameness and treatment to lesson environmental pathogen load. Earlier lesions, although less likely to induce clinical disease, are key targets for management interventions to prevent their progression to more advanced lesions associated with clinical disease and potentially lameness. The period over which lesions develop from normal skin to advanced clinical lesions has also been studied by several groups. In a 3-year prospective observational study of cattle that received no blanket DD prevention measures, the authors showed that the average time from the first evidence of skin changes to the development of a classic clinical lesion (score = M2 or Iowa stage 3) averaged 133 days (range = 38–315 d, median = 105 d).[79] These results were similar to a multifarm study of 4000 cows in France, where the investigators found an average period of 146 days.[81] Both of these studies relied on observations of the feet while each individual was restrained in a trimming chute for detailed assessment of the skin. In many field situations, where observations are made simply by observing animals standing in stalls or in the milk parlor, it is likely that very early lesions may be missed, making the period of development seem shorter. It is also critical to realize that these progression periods are in the absence of

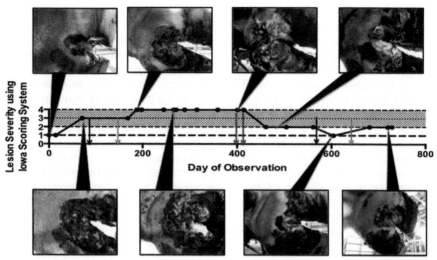

Fig. 1. A representative progression of a digital dermatitis lesion observed over a 2-year period. All pictures are of the same left rear foot of a Holstein dairy cow that was not exposed to any footbaths or management procedures other than routine hoof trimming. Blue arrows denote dry-off of the cow, green arrows denote freshening, and red arrows denote topical treatment with oxytetracycline due to significant lameness (locomotion score of >3 on 5-point scale). The lesion severity is recorded in the center timeline of the image using the linear Iowa DD scoring system.[3,79] The gray shaded area denotes lesions considered advanced lesions (stages 3–4) and the white area denotes preclinical lesions (stages 1–2). Several points are illustrated by these data. (1) In the absence of footbaths and treatment, the lesions are chronic in nature and progress very slowly. (2) This animal was regularly monitored during this 2-year period and treated with topical oxytetracycline when a locomotion score greater than 3/5 was observed (*red arrows*). Thus, despite having an obvious lesion for the entirety of this 2-year period, there were only a handful of days where this animal demonstrated significant lameness. (3) After 2 sequential topical treatments with oxytetracycline, the lesion decreases to a lower severity score but remains present as a lower severity for the full 200 days remaining in the observation period. (4) After both freshening dates (*green arrows*), the lesion on this foot increased severity score; however, this trend is not consistent across all cows observed and is likely influenced by a variety of other factors, including weather, genetics, and concurrent disease. (5) After treatment, lesions that do not heal develop a morphologic appearance similar to early lesions and contain a bacterial community identical to that of the early lesions. (*Adapted from* Krull AC, Shearer JK, Gorden PJ, et al. Deep sequencing analysis reveals temporal microbiota changes associated with development of bovine digital dermatitis. Infect Immun 2014;82:3359–73; and Krull AC, Shearer JK, Gorden PJ, et al. Digital dermatitis: Natural lesion progression and regression in Holstein dairy cattle over 3 years. J Dairy Sci 2016;99:3718–31, with permission.)

any prevention or treatment measures. Therefore, the dynamics of lesion changes are likely to occur differently in the face of routine management or therapeutic interventions.

Beef

Over the past decade, identification and interest in DD lesions in beef cattle have increased considerably. The most common clinical presentation in the feedlot situation involves development of lameness in heavy cattle that are close to marketing.

This timing of lameness development presents significant challenges for effected feedlots, because there are significant concerns associated with residues that may be incurred due to lesions treatment and due to concerns transporting lame cattle to slaughter. At present, it is unclear exactly when and how the lesions develop in feedlots, and more work is currently under way to investigate these issues. Based on anecdotal observations, a portion of cattle enter the feedlot with early lesions that have started development prior to arrival. The number of cattle that fall into this category is likely influenced by a variety of factors, including the number of sources of cattle (commingled vs single source), prevalence of DD on farms of origin, breed/ genetics, and age of the cattle. It seems likely that these cattle are more prone to developing lesions earlier during the feeding period than those that enter with no lesions. The authors also hypothesize that many cattle that enter the feedlot without lesions develop new lesions associated with exposure to either infected animals in the pen (discussed previously) or due to a contaminated pen environment. In feedlots that do not practice routine DD management strategies, lameness associated with heavy cattle is consistent with a similar timeline for lesion progression of dairy cattle in the absence of management interventions, at approximately 4 months.[79]

Nontypical Lesions (White Line, Sole Ulcer, and So Forth)

In recent years, there has been increasing reports of other claw horn lesions of cattle that seem to not be healing after routine therapy.[90] Specific examples include sole ulcers that fail to heal after therapeutic trimming and wooden block placement or white line lesions that fail to heal after appropriate trimming. There are some data to suggest that in some of these cases the corium that is exposed in these lesions has become infected with DD-associated organisms. Once infected, these lesions become significantly more difficult to heal and additional therapy focused on bacterial infections may be necessary in addition to routine trimming.

OTHER BOVINE LESIONS ASSOCIATED WITH DIGITAL DERMATITIS TREPONEMES

There is a growing body of evidence to demonstrate that a large variety of bovine skin lesions of the limbs and udder contain similar bacterial organisms to those of DD. Although full comparisons of the microbial compositions of many of these lesions are lacking, focus has been on identifying similar treponemal organisms to those observed in DD. These organisms have been identified in bovine ulcerative mammary dermatitis,[91,92] bovine teat ischemic necrosis,[93] toe necrosis,[94,95] and hock skin lesions.[96] The identification of these same organisms over a wide variety of bovine skin-related diseases suggest that these organisms have found a favorable niche for colonization in open wounds of cattle skin, although to date there is no evidence that this association has proved causation.

TREATMENT
Patient Evaluation Overview

Treatment or management interventions are likely to take 2 basic forms: individual focused therapeutic interventions of cattle with clinical lameness or obvious advanced lesions and herd-based prevention strategies designed to minimize the progression of lesions to advanced stages associated with clinical disease. Successful programs generally need to use a comprehensive variety to interventions to control the disease once it is endemic. Based on present-day clinical experience, eradication of DD from herds that are infected is not likely to be accomplished and management of the process to minimize clinical disease should be the goal. As with most herd health programs, monitoring of lesion prevalence and clinical disease assists clinicians in identifying gaps in the management program and allows for continual process improvement. A variety of helpful tools ranging from lesions scoring systems to record-keeping software packages have been developed and may be considered for application in management strategies[97] (Zinpro Corporation, Eden Prairie, Minnesota; Supervisor Systems, Dresser, Wisconsin).

Treatment of individual cows with DD lesions is usually based on 1 of 2 mechanisms. First, during routine foot trimming, cows with DD lesions should be identified and treated. Although there are few data regarding the cost benefit of this type of treatment, it is generally regarded as beneficial and important to DD management. In most cases, all identified lesions are treated regardless of the clinical stage of lesion development. Observation and recording of lesion prevalence and lesion severity are beneficial in monitoring disease status in the herd and modifying management strategies based on outcome. In addition, most individual animal treatment systems incorporate treatment of DD lesions that are identified in cattle exhibiting clinical lameness. Most DD lesions are painful to the touch, but a majority of DD lesions are not associated with lameness.[79] DD may also occur concurrent to other hoof lesions in cattle, so a complete physical examination and hoof evaluation should be conducted. Clinical lameness associated with DD is confined to animals with advanced lesions.[79] As such, identification of early lesions in cattle with significant lameness should warrant further investigation for another cause of the lameness. Treatment of DD in such cases, along with appropriate treatment of any additional cause of lameness, is warranted. Additionally, in cases of other claw horn lesions that result in exposure of corium, the possibility of a concurrent bacterial infection of the corium associated with DD organisms that could delay or prevent appropriate healing should be considered.

Pharmacologic Treatment Options

Pharamacologic treatment of DD generally focuses on a single application of a topical antimicrobial applied directly to the lesion. The most commonly used products include oxytetracycline soluble powder or tetracycline powder. Few data are available regarding appropriate dosing, and many clinicians and professional hoof trimmers empirically report a dose of between 2 g and 25 g of powder applied topically to the lesion. There is no evidence that the higher dose provides improved treatment outcomes over lower doses, whereas using lower doses decreases the use of antibiotics. Clinicians are directed to consult the Food Animal Residue Avoidance Databank for withdrawal recommendations; however, it has been suggested that there is likely minimal risk of milk residues with the lower doses when the number of cows treated at one time in the herd is limited.[98] Although the dose is commonly applied and held in place with a light bandage, there is no evidence that this practice leads to improved outcomes and it has been speculated to actually be counterproductive due to trapping debris, footbath solution, and manure against the lesion for a prolonged period of time.[99] Furthermore, topical treatment with a paste made from the oxytetracycline powder has been shown as effective as applying the dose with a wrap.[48,98] Dosing of 2 g of oxytetracycline paste applied in a paste made of 3:1 glycol to water has been recommended.[98] If a clinician does elect to use a wrap, it is recommended that the wrap be minimal in nature and designed to fall off or be removed after several days.

In cases of treatment applied to a cow with clinical lameness associated with the DD lesion, the lameness generally improves 1 to 2 locomotion scores within a couple-day period after treatment. The lesions typically turn blackish in color and develop a thick scab after oxytetracycline treatment. Although many people assume that these lesions are healing, the data suggest that in many cases infection remains below the scab and the lesions recrudesce once the scab falls off or is removed. Evaluation of 43 cows that were observed for a minimum of 50 days after therapy revealed that although a majority (93%) of them had an improvement in lesion score after treatment, only 9% of them returned to normal skin.[79] These data demonstrate that single-application therapy for topical oxytetracycline is likely to aid in improving acute lameness and reduce the severity of the lesion; however, it is unlikely to resolve the infection. In addition, approximately half of those animals that did not have the skin completely healed had lesion regression over the following year, and many of them required retreatment.[79] These findings suggest that clinicians need to be cautious when stating that animals that are repeatedly treated for DD are getting reinfected (as is commonly stated in the literature). It is more likely that these animals were never completely cured and are simply having a recrudescence of disease.

The application of systemic antibiotic therapy for the control of DD has been recently reviewed elsewhere in detail.[100] Although in vitro sensitivity testing has been described, there are no validated methods for this procedure that are approved by international laboratory testing authorities and there are no confirmed set points for Minimum Inhibitory Concentration (MIC) classification. As a consequence, results from these studies need to be interpreted with caution. With that in mind, in vitro sensitivity testing suggests that the DD-associated treponemes have only intermediate sensitivity to lincomycin, spectinomycin, oxytetracycline, ceftiofur, and gentamicin. In contrast, those treponemes had higher levels of sensitivity to penicillin, penicillin derivatives, and the macrolides.[49,54,101] Given the polymicrobial and polytreponemal nature of DD, clinicians should be cautious in making blanket assessments of drug susceptibility based on single-organism testing; however, these results suggest that many of the most commonly used antibiotics in dairy cattle of the United States (tetracyclines and cephalosporins) may have poor efficacy against the most prevalent bacteria in these lesions. This observation is supported by clinical data that demonstrate that concurrent therapy with these commonly used antibiotics had no significant impact on DD lesion severity.[79] In vitro sensitivities to penicillin were better for the treponemes, and there are data to suggest that systemic penicillin (aqueous procaine penicillin G; intramuscularly; 3 days; 18,000 U/kg; twice daily) does improve clinical lesions[1]; such a treatment regimen would not be clinically applied in most US dairy systems due to milk residues and the time associated with twice-daily application of antibiotics to the large number of animals commonly infected in US dairies.

Nonpharmacologic Treatment Options

In recent years there has been significant interest in the importance of macro and micro mineral nutrition in hoof health and lameness. At present, there is 1 commercial mineral mix that includes higher than typically recommended levels of organic trace minerals and iodine marketed for aid in maintaining appropriate hoof health. This mineral mix was specifically tested under research conditions for its ability to reduce the incidence of experimentally induced DD lesions.[102] Although the investigators were able to demonstrate a trend toward a decrease incidence of lesion formation and overall size of the lesion, neither result reached the level of statistical significance. Mineral nutrition, however, is beneficial in general hoof health and lameness; therefore, clinicians are encouraged to consider these issues and assure appropriate mineral nutrition in farms with significant lameness problems.

There is also a diverse range of commercially available therapies marketed for the control of DD. In almost all cases there are few to no evidence-based medicine trials to suggest improved therapeutic efficacy and control. Many products cite anecdotal reports or the results of poorly controlled studies; however, clinicians should consider these reports in light of the standard evidence-based medicine principles. There is a significant need for additional work comparing the efficacy of these products to the current gold standard–type therapies using strong unbiased research approaches that allow for direct comparison of treatment efficacy. Another commonly encountered problem in these types of trials is the use of inappropriate outcomes or comparisons. For instance, many companies try to use resolution of clinical lameness or lameness prevalence as a measure of treatment efficacy. Given that only a small percentage of animals with DD experiences clinical lameness, however, use of this measure as a proxy for lesion prevalence is risky and generally misleading.

Treatment Resistance/Complications

As discussed previously, there is a high rate of treatment failure after the single application of topical oxytetracycline when animals are monitored for periods of time sufficient for the initial scab formed by the treatment to fall off. Several shorter-term studies that followed animals for 14 days to 30 days post-treatment with a single dose of topical tetracycline have reported moderate to good cure rates, ranging from 68% to 87%, although 1 showed cure rates of only 14%.[2,55,103] Given that the scab that forms looks smooth, dry, and less painful, it is fairly easy to see why these lesions are considered healed. In contrast, when following these animals for longer periods of time that allow for the scab to fall off, a different picture emerges. When animals were followed a minimum of 50 days with an average of 289 days, only 9% returned to normal skin; 40 of the 43 animals had improvement of at least 1 score after treatment; however, only 4 went to normal skin and 17 of the others demonstrated an increased lesion severity during the follow-up period.[79]

An additional complication is the secondary invasion of these organisms in any other claw horn lesions that result in exposure of the corium. When cattle with sole ulcers, white line lesions, or toe necrosis fail to heal as expected, the potential for concurrent infection with DD-associated organisms in these lesions should be considered.

MANAGEMENT/PREVENTION

Management of DD in dairies or feedlots requires an integrated multifaceted approach that relies on a variety of tools and interventions. Key to this process is monitoring the disease prevalence and treatment success, and these measures should be emphasized at all levels of management. Record keeping of lameness, etiology of lameness, treatment success, eventual outcome, and footbath usage should be emphasized and required.

Most effective management approaches rely on a combination of individual animal treatment of advanced lesions and footbathing to assist in controlling the progression of early lesions to clinical disease. For a more detailed discussion of footbathing, see Nigel B. Cook's article, "A Review of the Design and Management of Footbaths for Dairy Cattle," in this issue. Footbaths require management and monitoring and, therefore, time, cost, and energy. In feedlots, use of footbaths is increasingly common. As opposed to the single-lane footbaths that are routinely used in dairies, these feedlots often install wider and longer baths that allow larger loads of animals to walk through as a group. Although there is no consensus at present on when and how often to footbath feedlot cattle, common times include entry into the feedlot and perhaps several times during the feeding period (ie, at reimplant and so forth). In terms of biosecurity, moving animals through the footbath on arrival may provide some additional benefit for control of animals entering with the disease, especially animals with early lesions.

Biosecurity of the farm is also a consideration. Care should be taken to not purchase and introduce animals into the housing facility from herds known to have DD. This is especially important for dairies and feedlots that currently have minimal issues with the disease. When possible, animals should be purchased from trusted sources in which the risk of DD can be adequately assessed prior to purchase. In addition, there is a documented increased risk of having significant DD problems in farms that use professional traveling foot trimmers. As such, training and implementation of in-house foot care teams provide significant benefits in limiting biosecurity risk. DD-associated organisms have been identified on foot-trimming equipment, and these instruments should be regularly disinfected after use on animals with DD lesions when feasible.[92,104]

REFERENCES

1. Read DH, Walker RL. Papillomatous digital dermatitis (footwarts) in California dairy cattle: clinical and gross pathologic findings. J Vet Diagn Invest 1998; 10:67–76.
2. Manske T, Hultgren J, Bergsten C. Topical treatment of digital dermatitis associated with severe heel-horn erosion in a Swedish dairy herd. Prev Vet Med 2002;53:215–31.
3. Krull AC, Shearer JK, Gorden PJ, et al. Deep sequencing analysis reveals temporal microbiota changes associated with development of bovine digital dermatitis. Infect Immun 2014;82:3359–73.
4. Dopfer D, ter Huurne AAHM, Cornelisse JL, et al. Histological and bacteriological evaluation of digital dermatitis in cattle, with special reference to spirochaetes and Campylobacter faecalis. Vet Rec 1997;140:620–3.
5. Nielsen BH, Thomsen PT, Green LE, et al. A study of the dynamics of digital dermatitis in 742 lactating dairy cows. Prev Vet Med 2012;104:44–52.
6. Dopfer D, Holzhauer M, Boven M. The dynamics of digital dermatitis in populations of dairy cattle: model-based estimates of transition rates and implications for control. Vet J 2012;193:648–53.
7. van Amstel SR, van Vuuren S, Tutt CL. Digital dermatitis: report of an outbreak. J S Afr Vet Assoc 1995;66:177–81.
8. Capion N, Boye M, Ekstrom CT, et al. Infection dynamics of digital dermatitis in first-lactation Holstein cows in an infected herd. J Dairy Sci 2012;95:6457–64.
9. Berry SL, Read DH, Famula TR, et al. Long-term observations on the dynamics of bovine digital dermatitis lesions on a California dairy after topical treatment with lincomycin HCl. Vet J 2012;193:654–8.
10. Berry SL, Read DH, Walker RL, et al. Clinical, histologic, and bacteriologic findings in dairy cows with digital dermatitis (footwarts) one month after topical treatment with lincomycin hydrochloride or oxytetracycline hydrochloride. J Am Vet Med Assoc 2010;237:555–60.
11. Brown CC, Kilgo PD, Jacobsen KL. Prevalence of papillomatous digital dermatitis among culled adult cattle in the southeastern United States. Am J Vet Res 2000;61:928–30.
12. Milinovich GJ, Turner SA, McLennan MW, et al. Survey for papillomatous digital dermatitis in Australian dairy cattle. Aust Vet J 2004;82:223–7.
13. Shibahara T, Ohya T, Ishii R, et al. Concurrent spirochaetal infections of the feet and colon of cattle in Japan. Aust Vet J 2002;80:497–502.

14. Rebhun WC, Payne RM, King JM, et al. Interdigital papillomatosis in dairy cattle. J Am Vet Med Assoc 1980;177:437–40.
15. Bassett HF, Monaghan ML, Lenhan P, et al. Bovine digital dermatitis. Vet Rec 1990;126:164–5.
16. Blowey RW, Sharp MW. Digital dermatitis in dairy cattle. Vet Rec 1988;122: 505–8.
17. Blowey RW, Done SH, Cooley W. Observation on the pathogenesis of digital dermatitis in cattle. Vet Rec 1994;135:115–7.
18. Cheli R, Mortellaro CM. Digital dermatitis in cattle. In: 8th International Meeting on Diseases of Cattle. Piacenza (Italy), 1974. p. 208–13.
19. Untersuchungen über Bakterien: V. Die Ätiologie der Milzbrand-Krankheit, begründet auf die Entwicklungsgeschichte des Bacillus anthracis. Investigations into bacteria: V. The etiology of anthrax, based on the ontogenesis of Bacillus anthracis. Cohns Beitrage zur Biologie der Pflanzen (in German) 1876;2(2): 277–310.
20. Walker RL, Read DH, Loretz KJ, et al. Spirochetes isolated from dairy cattle with papillomatous digital dermatitis and interdigital dermatitis. Vet Microbiol 1995; 47:343–55.
21. Demirkan I, Carter SD, Hart CA, et al. Isolation and cultivation of a spirochaete from bovine digital dermatitis. Vet Rec 1999;145:497–8.
22. Schrank K, Choi BK, Grund S, et al. Treponema brennaborense sp. nov., a novel spirochaete isolated from a dairy cow suffering from digital dermatitis. Int J Syst Bacteriol 1999;49(Pt 1):43–50.
23. Trott DJ, Moeller MR, Zuerner RL, et al. Characterization of Treponema phagedenis-like spirochetes isolated from papillomatous digital dermatitis lesions in dairy cattle. J Clin Microbiol 2003;41:2522–9.
24. Knappe-Poindecker M, Gilhuus M, Jensen TK, et al. Interdigital dermatitis, heel horn erosion, and digital dermatitis in 14 Norwegian dairy herds. J Dairy Sci 2013;96:7617–29.
25. Klitgaard K, Boye M, Capion N, et al. Evidence of multiple Treponema phylotypes involved in bovine digital dermatitis as shown by 16S rRNA gene analysis and fluorescence in situ hybridization. J Clin Microbiol 2008;46:3012–20.
26. Rasmussen M, Capion N, Klitgaard K, et al. Bovine digital dermatitis: possible pathogenic consortium consisting of Dichelobacter nodosus and multiple Treponema species. Vet Microbiol 2012;160:151–61.
27. Choi BK, Nattermann H, Grund S, et al. Spirochetes from digital dermatitis lesions in cattle are closely related to treponemes associated with human periodontitis. Int J Syst Bacteriol 1997;47:175–81.
28. Moter A, Leist G, Rudolph R, et al. Fluorescence in situ hybridization shows spatial distribution of as yet uncultured treponemes in biopsies from digital dermatitis lesions. Microbiology 1998;144(Pt 9):2459–67.
29. Nordhoff M, Moter A, Schrank K, et al. High prevalence of treponemes in bovine digital dermatitis-a molecular epidemiology. Vet Microbiol 2008;131:293–300.
30. Schlafer S, Nordhoff M, Wyss C, et al. Involvement of Guggenheimella bovis in digital dermatitis lesions of dairy cows. Vet Microbiol 2008;128:118–25.
31. Rijpkema SG, David GP, Hughes SL, et al. Partial identification of spirochaetes from two dairy cows with digital dermatitis by polymerase chain reaction analysis of the 16S ribosomal RNA gene. Vet Rec 1997;140:257–9.
32. Collighan RJ, Woodward MJ. Spirochaetes and other bacterial species associated with bovine digital dermatitis. FEMS Microbiol Lett 1997;156:37–41.

33. Brandt S, Apprich V, Hackl V, et al. Prevalence of bovine papillomavirus and Treponema DNA in bovine digital dermatitis lesions. Vet Microbiol 2011;148: 161–7.

34. Yano T, Moe KK, Yamazaki K, et al. Identification of candidate pathogens of papillomatous digital dermatitis in dairy cattle from quantitative 16S rRNA clonal analysis. Vet Microbiol 2010;143:352–62.

35. Klitgaard K, Foix Breto A, Boye M, et al. Targeting the treponemal microbiome of digital dermatitis infections by high-resolution phylogenetic analyses and comparison with fluorescent in situ hybridization. J Clin Microbiol 2013;51:2212–9.

36. Zuerner RL, Heidari M, Elliott MK, et al. Papillomatous digital dermatitis spirochetes suppress the bovine macrophage innate immune response. Vet Microbiol 2007;125:256–64.

37. Walker RL, Read DH, Loretz KJ, et al. Humoral response of dairy cattle to spirochetes isolated from papillomatous digital dermatitis lesions. Am J Vet Res 1997;58:744–8.

38. Demirkan I, Walker RL, Murray RD, et al. Serological evidence of spirochaetal infections associated with digital dermatitis in dairy cattle. Vet J 1999;157: 69–77.

39. Gomez A, Cook NB, Bernardoni ND, et al. An experimental infection model to induce digital dermatitis infection in cattle. J Dairy Sci 2012;95:1821–30.

40. Krull AC, Cooper VL, Coatney JW, et al. A Highly Effective Protocol for the Rapid and Consistent Induction of Digital Dermatitis in Holstein Calves. PLoS One 2016;11:e0154481.

41. Berry SL, Ertze RA, Read DH, et al. Field evaluation of Prophylactic And Therapeutic Effects of a Vaccine Against (Papillomatous) Digital Dermatitis of Dairy Cattle in Two California Dairies. In: 13th International Symposium on Ruminant Lameness. Slovenija (Maribor). February 11–15, 2004.

42. Sullivan LE, Evans NJ, Blowey RW, et al. A molecular epidemiology of treponemes in beef cattle digital dermatitis lesions and comparative analyses with sheep contagious ovine digital dermatitis and dairy cattle digital dermatitis lesions. Vet Microbiol 2015;178(1–2):77–87.

43. Moe KK, Yano T, Misumi K, et al. Detection of antibodies against Fusobacterium necrophorum and Porphyromonas levii-like species in dairy cattle with papillomatous digital dermatitis. Microbiol Immunol 2010;54:338–46.

44. Evans NJ, Brown JM, Demirkan I, et al. Three unique groups of spirochetes isolated from digital dermatitis lesions in UK cattle. Vet Microbiol 2008;130:141–50.

45. Evans NJ, Brown JM, Demirkan I, et al. Association of unique, isolated treponemes with bovine digital dermatitis lesions. J Clin Microbiol 2009;47:689–96.

46. Klitgaard K, Nielsen MW, Ingerslev HC, et al. Discovery of bovine digital dermatitis-associated Treponema spp. in the dairy herd environment by a targeted deep-sequencing approach. Appl Environ Microbiol 2014;80:4427–32.

47. Apley MD. Clinical evidence for individual animal therapy for papillomatous digital dermatitis (hairy heel wart) and infectious bovine pododermatitis (foot rot). Vet Clin North Am Food Anim Pract 2015;31:81–95, vi.

48. Cutler JH, Cramer G, Walter JJ, et al. Randomized clinical trial of tetracycline hydrochloride bandage and paste treatments for resolution of lesions and pain associated with digital dermatitis in dairy cattle. J Dairy Sci 2013;96:7550–7.

49. Evans NJ, Brown JM, Demirkan I, et al. In vitro susceptibility of bovine digital dermatitis associated spirochaetes to antimicrobial agents. Vet Microbiol 2009;136:115–20.

50. Hernandez J, Shearer JK. Efficacy of oxytetracycline for treatment of papillomatous digital dermatitis lesions on various anatomic locations in dairy cows. J Am Vet Med Assoc 2000;216:1288–90.

51. Laven RA, Hunt H. Comparison of valnemulin and lincomycin in the treatment of digital dermatitis by individually applied topical spray. Vet Rec 2001;149:302–3.

52. Loureiro MG, Rodrigues CA, Nascimento ES, et al. Efficacy of topical and systemic treatments with oxytetracycline for papillomatous digital dermatitis in cows. Arquivo Brasileiro de Medicina Veterinária e Zootecnia 2010;62:13–22.

53. Shearer JK, Hernandez J. Efficacy of two modified nonantibiotic formulations (Victory) for treatment of papillomatous digital dermatitis in dairy cows. J Dairy Sci 2000;83:741–5.

54. Yano T, Moe KK, Chuma T, et al. Antimicrobial susceptibility of Treponema phagedenis-like spirochetes isolated from dairy cattle with papillomatous digital dermatitis lesions in Japan. J Vet Med Sci 2010;72:379–82.

55. Nishikawa A, Taguchi K. Healing of digital dermatitis after a single treatment with topical oxytetracycline in 89 dairy cows. Vet Rec 2008;163:574–6.

56. Silva LA, Silva CA, Borges JR, et al. A clinical trial to assess the use of sodium hypochlorite and oxytetracycline on the healing of digital dermatitis lesions in cattle. Can Vet J 2005;46:345–8.

57. Ando T, Fujiwara H, Kohiruimaki M, et al. Peripheral blood leukocyte subpopulation of dairy cows with digital dermatitis and effect of hoof trimming with antibiotic treatment. J Vet Med Sci 2009;71:391–5.

58. Laven RA. Efficacy of systemic cefquinome and erythromycin against digital dermatitis in cattle. Vet Rec 2006;159:19–20.

59. Edwards AM, Dymock D, Jenkinson HF. From tooth to hoof: treponemes in tissue-destructive diseases. J Appl Microbiol 2003;94:767–80.

60. Logue DN, Offer JE, Laven RA, et al. Digital dermatitis–the aetiological soup. Vet J 2005;170:12–3.

61. Diaz PI, Hoare A, Hong BY. Subgingival microbiome shifts and community dynamics in periodontal diseases. J Calif Dent Assoc 2016;44:421–35.

62. Grenier D. Nutritional interactions between two suspected periodontopathogens, Treponema denticola and Porphyromonas gingivalis. Infect Immun 1992;60:5298–301.

63. Ito R, Ishihara K, Shoji M, et al. Hemagglutinin/Adhesin domains of Porphyromonas gingivalis play key roles in coaggregation with Treponema denticola. FEMS Immunol Med Microbiol 2010;60:251–60.

64. Nilius AM, Spencer SC, Simonson LG. Stimulation of in vitro growth of Treponema denticola by extracellular growth factors produced by Porphyromonas gingivalis. J Dental Res 1993;72:1027–31.

65. Socransky SS, Haffajee AD, Cugini MA, et al. Microbial complexes in subgingival plaque. J Clin Periodontol 1998;25:134–44.

66. Takahashi N. Oral microbiome metabolism: from "Who Are They?" to "What Are They Doing?". J Dent Res 2015;94:1628–37.

67. Simonson LG, McMahon KT, Childers DW, et al. Bacterial synergy of Treponema denticola and Porphyromonas gingivalis in a multinational population. Oral Microbiol Immunol 1992;7:111–2.

68. Yao ES, Lamont RJ, Leu SP, et al. Interbacterial binding among strains of pathogenic and commensal oral bacterial species. Oral Microbiol Immunol 1996;11:35–41.

69. Bruijnis MR, Beerda B, Hogeveen H, et al. Assessing the welfare impact of foot disorders in dairy cattle by a modeling approach. Anim Int J Anim Biosci 2012;6: 962–70.
70. Fabian J, Laven RA, Whay HR. The prevalence of lameness on New Zealand dairy farms: a comparison of farmer estimate and locomotion scoring. Vet J 2014;201:31–8.
71. Frankena K, Somers JG, Schouten WG, et al. The effect of digital lesions and floor type on locomotion score in Dutch dairy cows. Prev Vet Med 2009;88: 150–7.
72. Becker J, Steiner A, Kohler S, et al. Lameness and foot lesions in Swiss dairy cows: I. Prevalence. Schweiz Arch Tierheilkd 2014;156:71–8.
73. Capion N, Thamsborg SM, Enevoldsen C. Prevalence and severity of foot lesions in Danish Holstein heifers through first lactation. Vet J 2009;182:50–8.
74. Capion N, Thamsborg SM, Enevoldsen C. Prevalence of foot lesions in Danish Holstein cows. Vet Rec 2008;163:80–5.
75. Cramer G, Lissemore KD, Guard CL, et al. Herd- and cow-level prevalence of foot lesions in Ontario dairy cattle. J Dairy Sci 2008;91:3888–95.
76. Holzhauer M, Hardenberg C, Bartels CJ, et al. Herd- and cow-level prevalence of digital dermatitis in the Netherlands and associated risk factors. J Dairy Sci 2006;89:580–8.
77. Hulek M, Sommerfeld-Stur I, Kofler J. Prevalence of digital dermatitis in first lactation cows assessed at breeding cattle auctions. Vet J 2010;183:161–5.
78. van der Linde C, de Jong G, Koenen EP, et al. Claw health index for Dutch dairy cattle based on claw trimming and conformation data. J Dairy Sci 2010;93: 4883–91.
79. Krull AC, Shearer JK, Gorden PJ, et al. Digital dermatitis: natural lesion progression and regression in Holstein dairy cattle over 3 years. J Dairy Sci 2016;99: 3718–31.
80. Hedges J, Blowey RW, Packington AJ, et al. A longitudinal field trial of the effect of biotin on lameness in dairy cows. J Dairy Sci 2001;84:1969–75.
81. Relun A, Lehebel A, Bruggink M, et al. Estimation of the relative impact of treatment and herd management practices on prevention of digital dermatitis in French dairy herds. Prev Vet Med 2013;110:558–62.
82. USDA. Dairy 2007, part IV: reference of dairy cattle health and management practices in the United States. Fort Collins (CO): USDA: APHIS:VS, CEAH; 2009.
83. Sullivan LE, Carter SD, Blowey R, et al. Digital dermatitis in beef cattle. Vet Rec 2013;173:582.
84. Bruijnis MR, Hogeveen H, Stassen EN. Assessing economic consequences of foot disorders in dairy cattle using a dynamic stochastic simulation model. J Dairy Sci 2010;93:2419–32.
85. Cha E, Hertl JA, Bar D, et al. The cost of different types of lameness in dairy cows calculated by dynamic programming. Prev Vet Med 2010;97:1–8.
86. Wilshire JA, Bell NJ. An economic review of cattle lameness. Cattle Practice 2009;17:136–41.
87. Losinger WC. Economic impacts of reduced milk production associated with papillomatous digital dermatitis in dairy cows in the USA. J Dairy Res 2006; 73:244–56.
88. Lindley WH. Malignant verrucae of bulls. Vet Med Small Anim Clin 1974;69: 1547–50.
89. Barthold SW, Koller LD, Olson C, et al. Atypical warts in cattle. J Am Vet Med Assoc 1974;165:276–80.

90. Evans NJ, Blowey RW, Timofte D, et al. Association between bovine digital dermatitis treponemes and a range of 'non-healing' bovine hoof disorders. Vet Rec 2011;168(8):214.

91. Evans NJ, Timofte D, Carter SD, et al. Association of treponemes with bovine ulcerative mammary dermatitis. Vet Rec 2010;166:532–3.

92. Rock C, Krull A, Gorden P, et al. Metagenomic evaluation of the dairy farm environment and facilities for evidence of digital dermatitis associated bacteria. In: International Ruminant Lameness Conference, Valdivia (Chile). November 22–25, 2015.

93. Clegg SR, Carter SD, Stewart JP, et al. Bovine ischaemic teat necrosis: a further potential role for digital dermatitis treponemes. Vet Rec 2016;178:71.

94. Minini S, Crowhurst F, Nicolás J, et al. Toe necrosis and non-healing hoof lesions in commercial dairy herds in Argentina. In: 17th International Symposium and 9th International Conference on Lameness in Ruminants. Bristol (United Kingdom). August 11–14, 2013.

95. Acevedo J, Chesterton R, Hurtado C, et al. Bovine digital dermatitis and non-healing lesions and toe necrosis in grazing dairy herds in Chile. In: 17th International Symposium and 9th International Conference on Lameness in Ruminants. Bristol (United Kingdom). August 11–14, 2013.

96. Clegg SR, Bell J, Ainsworth S, et al. Isolation of digital dermatitis treponemes from cattle hock skin lesions. Vet Dermatol 2016;27:106–12.e29.

97. Tremblay M, Bennett T, Dopfer D. The DD check App for prevention and control of digital dermatitis in dairy herds. Prev Vet Med 2016;132:1–13.

98. Cramer G, Johnson R. Evaluation of risks of violative milk residues following extra-label topical administration of tetracycline for digital dermatitis in dairy cattle. In: American Association of Bovine Practitioners. Albuquerque (NM). September 18–20, 2014.

99. Shearer JK, Plummer PJ, Schleining J. Perspectives on the treatment of claw lesions in cattle. Vet Med Res Rep 2015;6:273–92.

100. Evans NJ, Murray RD, Carter SD. Bovine digital dermatitis: current concepts from laboratory to farm. Vet J 2016;211:3–13.

101. Evans NJ, Brown JM, Hartley C, et al. Antimicrobial susceptibility testing of bovine digital dermatitis treponemes identifies macrolides for in vivo efficacy testing. Vet Microbiol 2012;160:496–500.

102. Gomez A, Bernardoni N, Rieman J, et al. A randomized trial to evaluate the effect of a trace mineral premix on the incidence of active digital dermatitis lesions in cattle. J Dairy Sci 2014;97:6211–22.

103. Berry DB 2nd, Sullins KE. Effects of topical application of antimicrobials and bandaging on healing and granulation tissue formation in wounds of the distal aspect of the limbs in horses. Am J Vet Res 2003;64:88–92.

104. Sullivan LE, Blowey RW, Carter SD, et al. Presence of digital dermatitis treponemes on cattle and sheep hoof trimming equipment. Vet Rec 2014;175:201.

Pathogenesis and Treatment of Bovine Foot Rot

David C. Van Metre, DVM

KEYWORDS

- Cattle • Lameness • Foot rot • Interdigital necrobacillosis
- *Fusobacterium necrophorum* • Antimicrobial therapy

KEY POINTS

- Bovine foot rot is an infectious disease of the interdigital skin and subcutaneous tissues of cattle feet.
- The disease is characterized by progressive lameness; symmetric swelling of the affected foot; and the development of foul-smelling, necrotic cutaneous fissures.
- The gram-negative anaerobes *Fusobacterium necrophorum*, *Porphyromonas levii*, and *Prevotella intermedia* are common bacterial isolates from affected tissue.
- Treatment with systemic antimicrobial therapy early in the course of disease is expected to be curative, whereas delays in treatment may result in deep digital sepsis and a poor prognosis.

INTRODUCTION

Bovine foot rot (BFR) is an infectious bacterial disease of the interdigital skin and subcutaneous tissue of the feet of cattle. The geographic distribution of this disease is broad, with published reports of cases in North America[1,2] South America,[3] Australia,[4,5] New Zealand,[6] Europe,[7,8] Asia,[9,10] and Africa.[11] BFR is a common cause of lameness in dairy[1,4,5] and feedlot[12,13] cattle. BFR has been reported in housed and pastured cattle under a variety of climatic and management conditions. Equally diverse is the nomenclature that has been applied to BFR; it has also been referred to as interdigital necrobacillosis, interdigital pododermatitis, interdigital phlegmon, foul in the foot, and foot abscess. The anaerobic bacterium *Fusobacterium necrophorum*, formerly *Sphaerophorus necrophorum*, has long been considered to be centrally involved in the pathogenesis of BFR,[14–16] but additional bacteria such as *Porphyromonas levii* and *Prevotella*

Disclosure: The author has nothing to disclose.
Department of Clinical Sciences, College of Veterinary Medicine and Biomedical Sciences, Colorado State University, 300 W. Drake Road, Fort Collins, CO 80523-1678, USA
E-mail address: dcvanm@colostate.edu

Vet Clin Food Anim 33 (2017) 183–194
http://dx.doi.org/10.1016/j.cvfa.2017.02.003
0749-0720/17/© 2017 Elsevier Inc. All rights reserved.

vetfood.theclinics.com

intermedia may be involved in the pathogenesis.[2,14–16] This article focuses on the pathogenesis and treatment of this disease.

CLINICAL SIGNS

The clinical course of BFR begins with the acute onset of variable lameness, typically involving 1 foot in the affected animal.[4,5] The hind feet may be involved more often than the front feet.[4,5] Swelling and erythema are evident in the interdigital space and the coronary band. Progression of swelling causes separation of the digits. Swelling may extend to the fetlock or occasionally into the soft tissues covering the metacarpus or metatarsus.[14] When viewed from the rear of the animal, the dew claws of the affected foot may be seen to be spread further apart than those of the unaffected feet.[17] In the standing animal, careful inspection of the affected foot reveals that the swelling is symmetric relative to the axial midline of the foot (**Fig. 1**). Variable reduction of appetite and fever are common. Milk production in lactating animals is expected to decline precipitously. Left untreated, lameness may become severe.[14]

The clinical diagnosis of BFR is confirmed on careful examination of the well-restrained, affected foot. The characteristic lesion is 1 or more coalescing fissures of the interdigital skin that vary in size from 1 to 2 cm to spanning the entire length of the interdigital cleft.[14] The edges of the fissure are dark and necrotic. A fetid odor is characteristic.[14–16] The interdigital lesion matures over 2 to 4 days into moist, gaping, and markedly painful fissures. Necrosis and sloughing of the subcutaneous tissues and overlying interdigital skin are apparent. Exudate is variable in color and low in volume. Rarely, swelling, erythema, and pain develop in the absence of a visible lesion of the interdigital skin, a condition termed blind foot rot or blind foul. It is possible that blind foul represents BFR in an early stage.[18]

In the subacute to chronic phase, generalized weight loss and muscle atrophy of the affected limb are usually apparent. Granulation tissue may develop in the interdigital space (**Fig. 2**). Secondary invasion of the lesion by other bacterial pathogens, such as *Trueperella pyogenes*, may result in the development of abscesses in the subcutaneous tissue of the affected foot. Fistulous tracts may develop near the coronet or pastern.[14] At this stage, discharge typically becomes more voluminous than in the acute stage.

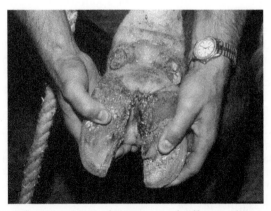

Fig. 1. Foot rot in a Holstein cow. Note the presence of diffuse swelling proximal to the coronary band. The swelling is symmetric relative to the axial midline of the foot.

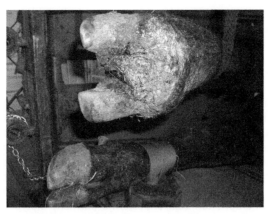

Fig. 2. Chronic foot rot in an Angus bull. There is extensive granulation tissue protruding from the interdigital skin and deep sepsis of the medial digit.

If BFR is left untreated or is treated unsuccessfully, extension of the infection from the interdigital subcutaneous space into adjacent bony, ligamentous, and synovial structures of 1 or both of the digits is possible. This condition has been termed deep sepsis of the digit.[4,19] When a single digit of a foot develops deep sepsis, swelling of the foot becomes asymmetric relative to the axial midline, with swelling more pronounced over the digit with the infected bone and/or synovial structures.[17] Septic arthritis of the distal interphalangeal joint seems to be a common complication to BFR, owing to the proximity of the synovial space to the interdigital subcutaneous tissue.[19] Septic tenosynovitis, navicular bursitis, retroarticular abscess, osteitis of the third phalangeal and navicular bone, and osteomyelitis of the second phalangeal bone are other possible sequelae to spread of infection from a BFR lesion. Radiographs may be necessary to fully ascertain the extent of bone and joint involvement. A rapidly progressive form of BFR has been reported in the United Kingdom.[20] In this form of so-called super foul, development of deep sepsis can occur within 2 days of the onset of disease. For most cases of deep sepsis secondary to BFR, surgical and medical treatment are necessary, and the prognosis is guarded to poor.[20]

The diagnosis of BFR is often made by clinical signs alone. Biopsy of interdigital skin or anaerobic culture of swabs of exudate may be used as confirmatory tests. Swabs for culture should be placed in transport medium suitable for support of anaerobic bacteria.[2] Bacteriologic examination typically reveals heavy growth of *F necrophorum*.[14–16] However, a variety of other species of anaerobic or facultative anaerobic bacteria may be isolated from naturally occurring and experimentally induced BFR, most notably *Bacteroides melaninogenicus*,[14–16] a bacterial species now taxonomically reclassified to 2 different genera and species: *Porphyromonas levii and P intermedia*.[21] Depending on environmental conditions, stage of disease, and sampling technique, it is possible that fecal or saprophytic bacteria may be isolated as well.

Differential diagnoses for BFR include laceration of the interdigital space, a foreign body introduced via a penetrating wound, and deep sepsis of the digit. In addition, cattle with interdigital fibroma (interdigital hyperplasia) may develop secondary bacterial dermatitis of the fibroma or of the deep skin clefts that often exist at the base of the fibroma. Digital dermatitis involving the interdigital skin (variably termed interdigital dermatitis) may result in a malodorous, erosive to ulcerative interdigital lesion, but there is no generalized swelling of the digit and the lesion is confined to the interdigital skin.[18] These conditions can be differentiated from BFR by careful examination of the lesion, including visualization of the distribution of swelling in the affected foot. Local anesthesia of the affected foot may be necessary to enable a thorough examination.

PATHOGENESIS

BFR is an infectious bacterial disease, the occurrence of which seems to be strongly influenced by environmental and management factors. Based on the preponderance of published data, BFR does not seem to be a highly contagious disease, primarily because occurrence seems to be sporadic[14] and outbreaks seem to occur uncommonly.[20] *F necrophorum*, a gram-negative, pleomorphic rod–shaped, anaerobic bacterium, is the agent most consistently incriminated as a primary pathogen in BFR.[14–16] Two subspecies of this agent exist: *F necrophorum* ssp *necrophorum* (formerly biotype A) and *F necrophorum* ssp *funduliforme* (formerly biotype B).[22] The former is considered more virulent and more commonly found in infections than the latter.[22] *F necrophorum* can be isolated from the gastrointestinal tract of healthy cattle.[22–25] Fecal contamination of the digital skin seems to be the primary route of infection,[14,22] although exudate from BFR lesions may contaminate the environment and serve as a source of infection for other cattle.[18,26]

The role of other bacterial agents in the pathogenesis of BFR remains unclear at present. This lack of clarity stems primarily from differences in the design of experimental challenge studies (including methodology of bacterial culture), disparities in the virulence of bacteria used among different studies, and taxonomic reclassification of putative pathogens.[2,14–16,21,27] A brief review of the history of BFR research may help to clarify these issues.

In 1975, Berg and Loan[14] isolated *F necrophorum*, *B melaninogenicus*, and various other anaerobic bacteria from 8 of 8 acute, naturally occurring cases of BFR in Missouri. Culture of biopsy specimens taken from affected interdigital skin yielded *F necrophorum* and *B melaninogenicus* in high numbers (10^6–10^9 colonies per gram); other anaerobic bacteria were isolated less frequently or in lesser numbers. Using these isolates of *F necrophorum* and *B melaninogenicus*, these investigators successfully induced BFR in healthy cattle. These two bacterial species could be reisolated from BFR lesions, thereby fulfilling the Koch postulates. Importantly, topical inoculation of healthy interdigital skin with these agents did not induce disease; scarification of the interdigital skin with a rasp at the time of topical inoculation was necessary for BFR to develop.[14] Poor pen sanitation increased the proportion of affected feet with severe lesion scores. These findings lent support to the contention that injury of interdigital skin by abrasion, maceration, chapping, or heavy bacterial contamination is an important factor in pathogenesis of this disease.[28]

Berg and Loan[14] also found that intradermal injection of cultures of *F necrophorum* and *B melaninogenicus* in the interdigital space resulted in successful recreation of BFR, as did intradermal injection of *F necrophorum* alone. *B melaninogenicus* could be isolated from BFR lesions that had been inoculated solely with *F necrophorum*, suggesting that the former organism could be carried in cattle feces and could colonize or infect BFR lesions after *F necrophorum*. When used as the sole bacterium in the intradermal injection, *B melaninogenicus* failed to induce BFR.

In 1976, Berg and colleagues[15] were also able to experimentally induce BFR in Missouri feedlot cattle by intradermal inoculation of a mixture of *F necrophorum* and *B melaninogenicus*. These isolates were obtained from naturally occurring and experimentally induced BFR. Feet inoculated with *B melaninogenicus* alone either developed no lesions or developed superficial dermatitis that was uncharacteristic of

BFR. When added to the ration, the chemicals ethylenediamine dihydriodide (a source of organic iodine) and urea did not influence the occurrence of BFR.

Roughly a decade later, Clark and colleagues[16] conducted a similar study on healthy pastured cattle in Australia, inducing BFR through intradermal and subcutaneous inoculation of field strains of *F necrophorum* and *B melaninogenicus*. Mixed inocula containing both bacteria produced characteristic BFR lesions, as did inocula containing *F necrophorum* alone. No difference in lesion severity was detected between feet inoculated with the 2 bacteria and those receiving inocula of *F necrophorum* alone. Injection of *B melaninogenicus* alone failed to induce lesions.[15] Therefore, by the mid-1980s, based on published data to date, *F necrophorum* seemed to play a primary role in the pathogenesis of BFR, owing to its capacity to induce characteristic disease when inoculated as the sole agent. A secondary role seemed to be most plausible for *B melaninogenicus*, given the failure of multiple investigators to induce BFR with this bacterium alone.

In 1994, Jang and Hirsch[29] described the anaerobic microorganisms that had been coisolated with the genus *Fusobacterium* in clinical specimens from ruminants and other animals in California. For ruminants, specimens that yielded this genus were most commonly obtained from abscesses and the respiratory tract. Out of 491 ruminant samples, *F necrophorum* was the predominant species isolated, (468 samples, 95%). A broad variety of other obligate anaerobic bacteria were coisolated with *Fusobacterium* spp in ruminants. These bacteria included a preponderance of *Bacteroides* spp, as well as *Porphyromonas* spp, *Prevotella* spp, and *Peptostreptococcus* spp. Facultative anaerobes coisolated from ruminant specimens included *Trueperella* (then *Actinomyces*) *pyogenes*, *Escherichia coli*, and *Pasteurella multocida*. Thus, polymicrobial infections seemed to be common in specimens that yielded *Fusobacterium* spp, suggesting potential synergy among these organisms in causing infections, as well as the potential for necrotic lesions to harbor a variety of isolates.

In 1995, through advances in genetic sequencing and biochemical characterization, organisms previously classified as *B melaninogenicus* were reclassified into 3 distinct genera and 17 species.[21] The novel genus *Prevotella* was established for saccharolytic species, and *Porphyromonas* for asaccharolytic species, with retention of *Bacteroides* as the genus designation for species closely related to *Bacteroides fragilis*. This change in taxonomy fostered concerns that isolates of *B melaninogenicus* used in previous studies of BFR may have been more diverse than originally appreciated.[27] Notably, in their seminal experiment, Berg and Loan[14] identified 2 morphologically and biochemically distinct isolates of *B melaninogenicus* from field cases of BFR, a finding that lent credence to these subsequent concerns.

In 1998, in a study of BFR in western Canadian feedlot steers, Morck and colleagues[2] isolated multiple anaerobic bacteria, including *B fragilis*, *Porphyromonas levii*, *Peptostreptococcus indolicus*, *Bifidobacterium* spp, and *P intermedia* in biopsy specimens of naturally occurring cases. The numbers of these different bacterial isolates were not measured in this study, so it is not clear whether there was a preponderance of any given isolate. Of particular interest was the absence of *F necrophorum* in the diverse array of isolates obtained from these BFR cases.

Dichelobacter (formerly *Bacteroides*) *nodosus* is a gram-negative anaerobe that is considered to be the primary causal agent of contagious ovine foot rot.[30,31] This agent can be found on the feet of healthy cattle.[32] The potential role of *D nodosus* in the pathogenesis of BFR was first established in 1981, when this agent was identified by culture and immunofluorescent staining in BFR lesions from live and slaughtered cattle in Sweden.[33] Owing to the fastidious nature of this organism, conventional culture may be less sensitive than polymerase chain reaction (PCR)[34]; ostensibly, this problem could have limited its detection by culture in earlier studies of BFR. Bennet and colleagues[35] detected *F necrophorum*, and, far less frequently, *D nodosus*, by PCR in hoof scrapings obtained from lame dairy cattle in New Zealand. Importantly, in a more recent experiment, topical inoculation of *D nodosus* onto the macerated interdigital skin of heifers resulted in interdigital dermatitis, not BFR.[36] The role, if any, of *D nodosus* in the pathogenesis of BFR remains to be elucidated.

When compiled, the results of these studies bring to light the difficulty in finding absolute clarity in the role of various bacteria in the pathogenesis of BFR. *F necrophorum*, *P levii*, and *P intermedia* seem to be the most consistent isolates across different studies. As has recently been accomplished for other infectious digital diseases of ruminants, novel application of PCR test methodologies is likely to better define the roles of these and other bacteria in the pathogenesis of BFR.

BACTERIAL FACTORS

A variety of bacterial virulence factors have been implicated in the pathogenesis of BFR. For *F necrophorum*, these virulence factors include endotoxin (lipopolysaccharide), hemolysin (phospholipase), hemagglutinin, adhesins (pili), proteases, and leukotoxin.[22,37] Of these, leukotoxin is the most extensively studied. The leukotoxin of *F necrophorum* is a large (336 kDa), water-soluble exotoxin that is cytotoxic for ruminant neutrophils, macrophages, hepatocytes, and ruminal epithelial cells.[37] At low concentrations, this exotoxin induces apoptosis of these cells; at higher concentrations, cell lysis occurs. Destruction of these host defense cells (with release of lysosomal enzymes and reactive oxygen species) is hypothesized to cause tissue necrosis and induce local anaerobiosis. In an Australian study, strains of *F necrophorum* that produced negligible levels of leukotoxin failed to induce BFR when inoculated into the interdigital skin of calves, whereas inoculation of leukotoxin-producing strains produced characteristic disease.[38] Notably, the leukotoxin of *F necrophorum* shares no sequence homology with the RTX (repeats in toxin) family of exotoxins produced by other gram-negative bacteria, including the leukotoxin of *Mannheimia hemolytica*.[37]

P levii is a pleomorphic, gram-negative, anaerobic, rod-shaped bacterium that has been cultured or detected by PCR in cases of bovine metritis,[39] bovine necrotic vulvovaginitis,[40] bovine digital dermatitis,[41] and BFR.[2] In vitro, *P levii* does not induce strong chemotactic or oxidative burst responses in bovine macrophages.[42] Further, this organism produces an enzyme that cleaves bovine immunoglobulin (Ig) G_2, thereby potentially reducing the host's capacity to opsonize the organism for neutrophil-mediated phagocytosis.[43] Together, the virulence factors of *P levii* have been hypothesized to impair or delay the host's response to infection, facilitating establishment of BFR by this and other bacteria.[42]

P intermedia is a gram-negative, anaerobic rod that has been isolated from humans[44] and dogs[45] with various oral infections, as well as from cases of BFR.[2] Virulence factors identified for this organism include a potentially robust antimicrobial resistance profile.[44] Specifically, β-lactamase production seems to be common among members of this genus.[21] *P intermedia* also can form biofilms during infection, which limit access of antimicrobials to the bacterium.[44] The role of these virulence factors in the pathogenesis of BFR remains undefined.

HOST FACTORS

Recent calving (early lactation) seems to be a risk factor for BFR. In a large, 2-year study of dairy cows in Denmark, Alban and colleagues[46] found that nearly 40% of BFR cases occurred in the first 30 days after calving; the incidence during the first month postpartum was 6-fold higher than in any other month postpartum as well as the month preceding calving. This finding is consistent with studies of BFR in dairy cattle in the United Kingdom[47,48] and the United States.[1,49] The metabolic, immunologic, nutritional, and environmental changes experienced by freshening dairy cows are speculated to be involved in this spike in incidence of BFR during the postpartum period.[1,46] In contrast, associations between parity and BFR risk were not consistent between studies in dairy cattle in Denmark,[46] the United Kingdom,[47,48] and the United States.[1]

Differences in risk of BFR by breed were also identified in the Danish study, but the investigators hypothesized that these differences could have been confounded by breed disparities in milk production.[46] However, when measured in Holstein cows, milk production did not influence the risk for BFR.[49] Estimates of the heritability of BFR susceptibility are variable (0.09–0.38).[49]

The immune response to natural cases of BFR remains poorly characterized. In Berg and Loan's[14] experiments, 2 cattle that had recovered after treatment from experimentally induced BFR were reinoculated; both developed recurrent BFR. This finding suggested that protective immunity had not been induced by the previous infection. In a study of large dairy herds in California, Oberbauer and colleagues[49] found that estimates of repeatability for BFR were high, suggesting that naturally occurring cases can recur. Dairy cattle with BFR were shown to have higher plasma IgG concentrations than healthy herd mates, but the specificity of the immunoglobulins was not determined.[9] In contrast, immune compromise from bovine viral diarrhea infection may render cattle more susceptible to BFR.[50]

ENVIRONMENTAL AND MANAGEMENT FACTORS

Warm, moist environmental conditions are commonly considered to be conducive to BFR. This association may reflect enhanced survival of causative bacteria in the environment or a tendency for cattle to congregate and defecate in shaded or wet areas. In temperate climates, BFR has been documented to occur more frequently in warmer months of the year,[46–48] although this trend is not consistent across all studies.[1,49,51] Similarly, periods of rainfall have been shown to increase the incidence of lameness in pastured cattle; this association has been attributed to muddy conditions, maceration of the digital skin, and carriage of stones from cattle paths (tracks) into concrete-floored areas of the dairy.[4,5] However, monthly rainfall was not associated with the total monthly number of treatments for BFR in Denmark.[46] It is important to consider that seasonal rainfall may coincide with calving season in certain operations, and the increased risk of BFR brought about by parturition may be attributed erroneously to precipitation.[46]

Cattle maintained in tie stall barns may be at lower risk than loosely housed cattle, which may reflect a lesser risk of interdigital trauma, drier conditions, and reduced fecal contamination of feet in the former setting.[46,52] Mineral supplementation,[52] footbath use,[52] and supplementation of the diet with biotin[53] may be variably protective against BFR. Poor pen hygiene, dried mud, rocks, crop stubble, twigs, frozen rough ground, and ice in the environment have been incriminated in the pathogenesis, because these may incite traumatic injury to the interdigital skin.[20,54,55] In the author's practice, low-lying cacti are problematic for pastured cattle. Careful scrutiny of the ground near feed bunks, waterers, sources of shade, and salt or mineral feeders is warranted.[55]

Dairy cows treated for other causes of lameness were found to be at greater risk of BFR, which alludes to the presence of common risk factors for both conditions.[46]

Table 1
Antimicrobials currently approved in the United States for treatment of bovine foot rot

Generic Name and Formulation	Dosage (mg/kg)	Approved Routes	Treatment Interval	Use Restrictions for Cattle
Ceftiofur sodium	1.1–2.2	IM, SC	Every 24 h for 3–5 d	None
Ceftiofur hydrochloride	1.1–2.2	IM, SC	Every 24 h for 3–5 d	None
Ceftiofur crystalline free acid	6.6	SC[a]	Once	Specific route of injection[a]
Florfenicol	20	IM	Second dose in 48 h	Not for use in female dairy cattle 20 mo of age or older or in calves to be processed for veal
	40	SC	Once	As above
Oxytetracycline	6.6–11	SC, IV IM (some products)	Every 24 h not to exceed 4 consecutive days As above	None None
Sulfadimethoxine				
Bolus	25 (day 1), then 12.5	PO	Every 24 h not to exceed 5 consecutive days	Not for use in calves to be processed for veal
40% solution	55 (day 1), then 27.5	IV	Every 24 h for 3–5 d	As above
Sulfamethazine				
Bolus	As directed on product label	PO	Second dose in 72 h if signs persist	Not for use in female dairy cattle 20 mo of age or older. Not for use in calves <1 mo of age or calves being fed an all-milk diet
Soluble powder	237.6 (day 1), then 118.8	PO in drinking water[b] or as a drench	Every 24 h not to exceed 5 consecutive days	As above
Tulathromycin	2.5	SC	Once	Not for use in female dairy cattle 20 mo of age or older
Tylosin	17.6	IM	Every 24 h not to exceed 5 consecutive days	Not for use in female dairy cattle 20 mo of age or older, (including dry dairy cows) or in calves intended to be processed for veal

Abbreviations: IM, intramuscular; IV, intravenous; PO, per os (oral); SC, subcutaneous.

[a] For subcutaneous injection in the posterior aspect of the ear where it attaches to the head (base of the ear) in lactating dairy cattle. For subcutaneous injection in the middle third of the posterior aspect of the ear or in the posterior aspect of the ear where it attaches to the head (base of the ear) in beef and nonlactating dairy cattle.

[b] As of January 1, 2017, antimicrobials used in water in the United States require a prescription from a licensed veterinarian.

Data from Compendium of Veterinary Products. Available at: https://bayerall.naccvp.com/?u=bayer&p=dvm. Accessed December 1, 2016. Search terms used on this Web site: Species filter = Cattle; Product Use Category = "Footrot [*Fusobacterium necrophorum* and/or *Porphyromonas levii* (*Bacteroides* spp)], control and/or treatment."

TREATMENT

Early intervention with systemic antimicrobial therapy is considered essential for effective treatment of BFR.[14,20,54,55] The currently approved antimicrobials for treatment of this condition in the United States are shown in **Table 1**. Ceftiofur (1 mg/kg intramuscular [IM] every 24 h × 3 days) was shown to be as effective as oxytetracycline (6.6 mg/kg IM every 24 h × 3 days) in treating affected feedlot steers.[2] The shorter withholding time of ceftiofur may make it a more suitable choice for animals that are near market weight. Procaine penicillin (22,000 IU/kg IM) has been recommended,[54] but this constitutes extralabel use in the United States. Outside of this country, tilmicosin (5 mg/kg subcutaneously) may be used successfully for treatment of BFR,[56] as may regional perfusion with ceftiofur sodium.[57] Published treatment success rates with parenteral antimicrobial therapy include 68% (oxytetracycline),[2] 73% to 99% (ceftiofur sodium),[2,10,58] 74% (tilmicosin),[56] and 99.5% (ceftiofur crystalline free acid).[58] Cook and Cutler[20] reported successful parenteral and topical antimicrobial therapy in 16 of 22 (73%) British cattle affected by severe, rapidly progressive BFR; notably, 5 of 9 (56%) cases that had deep sepsis at the time of initial diagnosis did not recover.[20] Spontaneous resolution of infection is expected in approximately 15% of affected cattle.[56]

Resistance to penicillin and potentiated sulfonamides was detected in _F necrophorum_ isolates obtained from rapidly progressive BFR in the United Kingdom.[20] Morck and colleagues[2] detected susceptibility to oxytetracycline and ceftiofur in isolates of _P levii_, _P intermedia_, and _T pyogenes_ obtained from BFR in feedlot cattle. Across other studies, the antimicrobial susceptibility of bacterial isolates from BFR is not well described. This problem may reflect limited capacity for antimicrobial susceptibility testing of anaerobic bacteria in some veterinary diagnostic laboratories. Further, the expectation for reasonable success with early antimicrobial therapy may prompt few practitioners to submit samples for culture and sensitivity. The imminent development of rapid DNA sequencing technology is likely to facilitate more rapid pathogen identification and detection of antimicrobial resistance than conventional culture and antimicrobial sensitivity methods.

In conjunction with systemic antimicrobial therapy, debridement of necrotic tissue and bandaging are optional adjunct treatments.[54] Although there are various compounds (eg, zinc sulfate, benzalkonium chloride) labeled for topical application for foot rot and related conditions of livestock, these have not been proved to augment or replace systemic therapy.

REFERENCES

1. DeFrain JM, Socha MT, Tomlinson DJ. Analysis of foot health records from 17 confinement dairies. J Dairy Sci 2013;96:7329–39.
2. Morck DW, Olson ME, Louie TJ, et al. Comparison of ceftiofur sodium and oxytetracycline for treatment of acute interdigital phlegmon (foot rot) in feedlot cattle. J Am Vet Med Assoc 1998;212:254–7.
3. Silva LAF, Cunha PHJ, Fioravanti MCS, et al. The prevalence of locomotor system diseases in cattle raised in extensive and semi-intensive production system[s] from different regions of Goiás state. Vet Noticias 2001;7:93–101.
4. McLennan MW. Incidence of lameness requiring veterinary treatment in dairy cattle in Queensland. Aust Vet J 1988;65:144–7.
5. Jubb TF, Malmo J. Lesions causing lameness requiring veterinary treatment in pasture-fed dairy cows in East Gippsland. Aust Vet J 1991;68:21–4.

6. Zhou H, Bennett G, Hickford JGH. Variation in *Fusobacterium necrophorum* strains present on the hooves of footrot infected sheep, goats, and cattle. Vet Microbiol 2009;135:363–7.

7. Haggman J, Junni R, Simojoki H, et al. The costs of interdigital phlegmon in four loose-housed Finnish dairy herds. Acta Vet Scand 2015;57:90.

8. Russell AM, Rowlands GJ, Shaw SR, et al. Survey of lameness in British dairy cattle. Vet Rec 1982;111:155–60.

9. Sun D, Zhang H, Guo D, et al. Shotgun proteomic analysis of plasma from dairy cattle suffering from footrot: Characterization of potential disease-associated factors. PLoS One 2013;8:e55973.

10. Sano K, Taguchi K, Maruyama N, et al. Efficacy of ceftiofur given intramuscularly at 1 or 2 mg/kg for 3 days in the treatment of bovine foot rot in Japan. J Vet Med Japan 2007;60:203–8.

11. Mgasa MN. Footrot in cattle in Morogoro, Tanzania. Bull Anim Health Prod Afr 1987;35:332–5.

12. Frank GR, Salman MD, MacVean DW. Use of a disease reporting system in a large beef feedlot. J Am Vet Med Assoc 1988;192:1063–7.

13. Terrell SP, Thompson DU, Reinhardt CD, et al. Perception of lameness management, education, and effects on animal welfare of feedlot cattle by consulting nutritionists, veterinarians, and feedlot managers. Bov Pract 2014;48:53–60.

14. Berg JN, Loan RW. *Fusobacterium necrophorum* and *Bacteroides melaninogenicus* as etiologic agents of foot rot in cattle. Am J Vet Res 1975;36:1115–22.

15. Berg JN, Brown LN, Ennis PG, et al. Experimentally induced foot rot in feedlot cattle fed rations containing organic iodide (ethylenediamine dihydriodide) and urea. Am J Vet Res 1976;37:509–12.

16. Clark BL, Stewart DJ, Emery DL. The role of *Fusobacterium necrophorum* and *Bacteroides melaninogenicus* in the aetiology of interdigital necrobacillosis in cattle. Aust Vet J 1985;62:47–9.

17. Van Metre DC, Wenz JR, Garry FB. Lameness in cattle: rules of thumb. Proceedings, 38th Annual Convention, American Association of Bovine Practitioners. Utah, September 25, 2005.

18. Shearer JK. Infectious disorders of the foot skin. In: Anderson DE, Rings DM, editors. Current veterinary therapy: food animal practice. 5th edition. St Louis (MO): Saunders Elsevier; 2009. p. 234–42.

19. Baxter GM, Broome TA, Lakritz J, et al. Alternatives to digit amputation in cattle. Compend Cont Ed Pract Vet 1991;13:1022–35.

20. Cook NB, Cutler NK. Treatment and outcome of a severe form of foul-in-the-foot. Vet Rec 1995;136:19–20.

21. Jousimies-Somer HR. Update on the taxonomy and the clinical and laboratory characteristics of pigmented anaerobic gram-negative rods. Clin Infect Dis 1995;20(Suppl 2):S187–91.

22. Nagaraja TG, Narayanan SK, Stewart GC, et al. *Fusobacterium necrophorum* infections in animals: pathogenesis and pathogenic mechanisms. Anaerobe 2005; 11:239–46.

23. Smith GR, Thornton EA. The prevalence of *Fusobacterium necrophorum* biovar A in animal faeces. Epidemiol Infect 1993;110:327–31.

24. Amachawadi RG, Nagaraja TG. Liver abscesses in cattle: A review of incidence in Holsteins and of bacteriology and vaccine approaches to control in feedlot cattle. J Anim Sci 2016;94:1620–32.

25. Berg JN, Scanlon CM. Studies of *Fusobacterium necrophorum* from bovine hepatic abscesses: biotypes, quantitation, virulence, and antimicrobial susceptibility. Am J Vet Res 1982;43:1580–6.

26. Radostits OM, Gay CG, Hinchcliff KW, et al. Diseases associated with bacteria – V. Veterinary medicine. 10th edition. St Louis (MO): Saunders Elsevier; 2007. p. 1061–156.

27. Walter MRV, Morck DW. In vitro expression of tumor necrosis factor α, interleukin 1β, and interleukin 8 mRNA by bovine macrophages following exposure to *Porphyromonas levii*. Can J Vet Res 2002;66:93–8.

28. Adams OR. Foot rot in cattle. J Am Vet Med Assoc 1960;136:589–99.

29. Jang SS, Hirsch DC. Characterization, distribution, and microbiological associations of *Fusobacterium* spp. in clinical specimens of animal origin. J Clin Microbiol 1994;32:384–7.

30. Raadsma HW, Egerton JR. A review of footrot in sheep: aetiology, risk factors, and control methods. Livest Sci 2013;156:106–14.

31. Witcomb LA, Green LE, Kaler J, et al. A longitudinal study of the role of *Dichelobacter nodosus* and *Fusobacterium necrophorum* load in initiation and severity of footrot in sheep. Prev Vet Med 2014;115:48–55.

32. Laing EA, Egerton JR. The occurrence, prevalence, and transmission of *Bacteroides nodosus* infection in cattle. Res Vet Sci 1978;24:300–4.

33. Forshell LP, Andersson L. *Bacteroides nodosus* infection in bovine interdigital necrobacillosis. Svensk Veterinart 1981;33:551–3.

34. Moore LJ, Woodward MJ, Grogono-Thomas R. The occurrence of treponemes in contagious ovine digital dermatitis and the characterization of associated *Dichelobacter nodosus*. Vet Microbiol 2005;111:199–209.

35. Bennett G, Hickford J, Zhou H, et al. Detection of *Fusobacterium necrophorum* and *Dichelobacter nodosus* in lame cattle on dairy farms in New Zealand. Res Vet Sci 2009;87:413–5.

36. Knappe-Poindecker M, Jorgensen HJ, Jensen TK, et al. Experimental infection of cattle with ovine *Dichelobacter nodosus* isolates. Acta Vet Scand 2015;57:55.

37. Narayanan SK, Nagaraja TG, Chengappa MM, et al. Leukotoxins of Gram-negative bacteria. Vet Microbiol 2002;84:337–56.

38. Emery DL, Vaughan JA, Clark BL, et al. Cultural characteristics and virulence of strains of *Fusobacterium necrophorum* isolated from the feet of cattle and sheep. Aust Vet J 1985;62:43–6.

39. Santos TMA, Gilbert RO, Bicalho RC. Metagenomic analysis of the uterine bacterial microbiota in healthy and metritic postpartum dairy cows. J Dairy Sci 2011;94: 291–302.

40. Elad D, Friedgut O, Alpert N, et al. Bovine necrotic vulvovaginitis associated with *Porphyromonas levii*. Emerg Infect Dis 2004;10:505–7.

41. Nielsen MW, Strube ML, Isbrand A, et al. Potential bacterial core species associated with digital dermatitis in cattle herds identified by molecular profiling of interdigital skin samples. Vet Microbiol 2016;186:139–49.

42. Walter MRV, Morck DW. Chemotaxis, phagocytosis, and oxidative metabolism in bovine macrophages exposed to a novel interdigital phlegmon (foot rot) lesion isolate, *Porphyromonas levii*. Am J Vet Res 2002;63:757–62.

43. Lobb DA, Loeman HJ, Sparrow DG, et al. Bovine polymorphonuclear neutrophil-mediated phagocytosis and an immunoglobulin G_2 protease produced by *Porphyromonas levii*. Can J Vet Res 1999;63:113–8.

44. Jang E, Kim M, Noh MH, et al. *In vitro* effects of polyphosphate against *Prevotella intermedia* in planktonic phase and biofilm. Antimicrob Agents Chemother 2016; 60:818–26.

45. Jeusette IC, Roman AM, Torre C, et al. 24-hour evaluation of dental plaque bacteria and halitosis after consumption of a single placebo or dental treat by dogs. Am J Vet Res 2016;77:613–9.

46. Alban L, Lawson LG, Agger JF. Foul in the foot (interdigital necrobacillosis) in Danish dairy cows – frequency and possible risk factors. Prev Vet Med 1995; 24:73–82.

47. Eddy RG, Scott CP. Some observations on the incidence of lameness in dairy cattle in Somerset. Vet Rec 1980;106:140–4.

48. Rowlands GJ, Russell AM, Williams LA. Effects of stage of lactation, month, age, origin and heart girth on lameness in dairy cattle. Vet Rec 1985;117:576–80.

49. Oberbauer AM, Berry SL, Belanger JM, et al. Determining the heritable component of dairy cattle foot lesions. J Dairy Sci 2012;96:605–13.

50. Daniel R, Davies H, Davies A, et al. Severe foul-in-the-foot and BVD infection [letter]. Vet Rec 1995;137:647.

51. Murray RD, Downham DY, Clarkson MJ, et al. Epidemiology of lameness in dairy cattle: description and analysis of foot lesions. Vet Rec 1996;138:586–91.

52. Faye B, Lescourret F. Environmental factors associated with lameness in dairy cattle. Prev Vet Med 1989;7:267–87.

53. Hedges J, Blowey RW, Packington AJ, et al. A longitudinal field trial of the effect of biotin on lameness in dairy cows. J Dairy Sci 2001;84:1969–75.

54. Rebhun WC, Pearson EG. Clinical management of bovine foot problems. J Am Vet Med Assoc 1982;181:572–7.

55. Stokka GL, Lechtenberg K, Edwards T, et al. Lameness in feedlot cattle. Vet Clin North Am Food Anim Pract 2001;17:189–207.

56. Merril JK, Moark DW, Olson ME, et al. Evaluation of the dosage of tilmicosin for the treatment of acute bovine footrot (interdigital phlegmon). Bov Pract 1999; 33:60–2.

57. Kamiloglu A, Baran V, Klc E, et al. The use of local and systemic ceftiofur sodium application in cattle with acute interdigital phlegmon. Veteriner Cerrahi Dergisi 2002;8:13–8.

58. Van Donkersgoed J, Dussalt M, Knight P, et al. Clinical efficacy of a single injection of ceftiofur crystalline free acid sterile suspension versus three daily injections of ceftiofur sodium sterile powder for the treatment of footrot in cattle. Vet Ther 2008;9:157–62.

A Review of the Design and Management of Footbaths for Dairy Cattle

Nigel B. Cook, BSc, BVSc Cert, CHP, DBR, MRCVS

KEYWORDS

- Dairy cattle • Footbaths • Infectious hoof disease

KEY POINTS

- Footbaths may play a significant role in the prevention of infectious hoof disease in confinement housed dairy herds.
- Copper sulfate appears to be the most effective antibacterial agent, but there are legitimate concerns regarding disposal and lifetime accumulation of copper in the soil.
- Alternatives to copper sulfate exist, but relatively few have been subjected to scientific testing in the field.
- Scientific testing of footbaths requires greater standardization of footbath design and management and assessment of outcomes.
- Design and management of the footbath are critical to the success of the program.

INTRODUCTION

Use of a footbath in the dairy industry for the control of infectious hoof disease is widespread in North America and elsewhere around the world. Most confinement housed dairy herd owners use a regular footbath protocol, and frequent use was a feature of the well-managed freestall housed dairy herds maintaining high levels of milk production with low levels of lameness in a recent Wisconsin survey.[1] However, the benefits of footbaths are not universally accepted, because some authors have associated footbath use with increased risk for lameness problems.[2]

The cost of using a footbath is considerable. For a 1000-cow dairy using a 5% copper sulfate footbath once a day for 4 days per week through a typical 200-L (~50 US gallons) bath, changing the bath solution every 200 cow passes, with a 23-kg (50 lb) bag of copper sulfate costing ~$80 US, the annual cost would be ~$41,600 or ~$42 US per cow per year. This cost would rival what many farms would spend on

Disclosure Statement: The author has nothing to disclose.
Department of Medical Sciences, University of Wisconsin-Madison, School of Veterinary Medicine, 2015 Linden Drive, Madison, WI 53706, USA
E-mail address: nigel.cook@wisc.edu

Vet Clin Food Anim 33 (2017) 195–225
http://dx.doi.org/10.1016/j.cvfa.2017.02.004
0749-0720/17/© 2017 Elsevier Inc. All rights reserved.

vetfood.theclinics.com

animal medications and treatments in a typical dairy herd, yet there are no national guidelines for prudent footbath use or requirements for control or oversight as there would be for other antimicrobial use in the United States.

In some countries, there are stricter controls on footbath use however, and these are likely to be embraced globally in the future. Since 2006, copper sulfate has been illegal for footbath use in the European Union as a result of the EU biocide directive,[3] put in place largely due to environmental concerns. Formaldehyde, also commonly used in footbaths, is a carcinogen in humans[4] and is considered a hazard in the workplace. As such, it is likely that the use of this chemical on the farm will come under increasing scrutiny and control.

Clearly, if one is to continue to use a footbath as an aid in lameness prevention programs, one must look to the scientific literature and other available evidence to develop best practice recommendations for their use, and be mindful of the human health and environmental risks associated with them.

In this review, the author summarizes the current peer-reviewed literature on footbath use and management to date and attempts to create a best-practice protocol for use on the dairy farm based on the available evidence.

CURRENT FOOTBATH MANAGEMENT PRACTICES
Antibacterial Choice

There are few reports of footbath practices in North America and elsewhere. Cook and colleagues[5] reported on a survey of 65 freestall housed dairy herds averaging 1023 milking cows in size with a range from 100 to 4100 cows. The herds originated from United States, Spain, Japan, United Kingdom, and New Zealand. Forty-two percent of herds used more than one antibacterial agent in rotation. Copper sulfate was the most commonly used antibacterial, with 63% of herds using it at concentrations of between 1% and 10%. Formaldehyde was used by 34% of herds at between 2% and 5% formalin solution. Of note in this survey was that antibiotics, including lincomycin and oxytetracycline, were used by only 5% of herds, and then only as a second-choice agent. Although antibiotics have been recommended for use in footbaths by some,[6] such use cannot be justified from the perspective of prudent drug use. However, there are distinct regional and herd level differences. For example, in a sample of larger high-producing upper Midwest herds, where mean lameness prevalence was 13%, copper sulfate was used by 100% of the herds, only 8% used formaldehyde, but 17% used an antibiotic in their footbath.[1] Similarly, Solano and colleagues[7] reported on footbath management on 141 farms in Quebec, Ontario, and Alberta. Again, a high proportion of herds used more than one product (62%): 41% used both copper sulfate and formaldehyde; 37% only used copper sulfate; 15% relied solely upon formaldehyde; and 7% used other products.

There are a myriad of alternative footbath agents marketed to the dairy industry in North America. These products are largely untested and unregulated and appear not to have been embraced by the industry given the perceived efficacy of copper sulfate and formaldehyde. However, if use of these agents is more tightly controlled, there is scope for increased use of other products if they can be shown to be efficacious.

Footbath Design

Given that there has been no standardized footbath design recommended in the dairy industry, there are substantial differences in bath designs in use in the field. The median footbath measured 0.81 m wide, was 2.03 m long, and was filled to a depth of

0.11 m in the survey by Cook and colleagues,[5] but there was considerable variation. For example, bath length ranged from 1.57 to 4.55 m. Median capacity was 189 L, but the range was from 80 to 1417 L, an 18-fold variation. Similar dimensions were found in the survey of Canadian herds by Solano and colleagues,[7] with median footbath length 2.2 m, width 0.74 m, and depth 0.15 m. Footbath length averaged 2.3 m with a range from 1.5 m to 4.1 m in the 66 herds examined by Cook and colleagues.[1]

It is known that footbath design influences the delivery of antibacterial to the cow's feet, which impacts the efficacy of whatever antibacterial agent is in use. Cook and colleagues[5] showed that to achieve at least 2 immersions per rear foot with a probability of greater than 95%, the footbath needed to be at least 3.0 m in length, with approximately half of rear feet receiving 3 immersions when the bath was extended further to 3.7 m. In order to minimize bath volume, this study also demonstrated that cows tolerated a narrow bath width (0.6 m) and a relatively high step-in height (0.28 m), reducing the cost of maintaining the bath. An "ideal footbath" design is shown in **Fig. 1**.

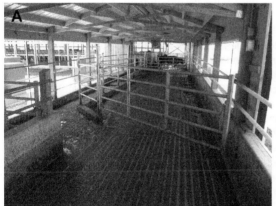
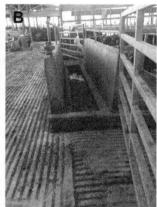
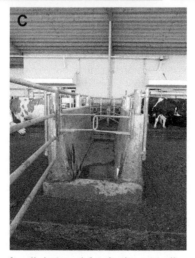

Fig. 1. Some examples of well-designed footbaths, typically measuring 3.7 m long, 0.6 m wide at the base with a 25-cm step in height.

Logue and colleagues[8] were able to show a significant beneficial impact on digital dermatitis lesion severity of a longer footbath (4.4 m compared with 2.2 m) with 2 different test antibacterial agents, and most recently, Solano and colleagues[9] showed that standardizing the footbath program and switching to a footbath 3.0 m in length improved the control of digital dermatitis in herds that were using the same antibacterial (copper sulfate) before the study. The success of this standardized protocol, particularly in herds with a high prevalence of digital dermatitis at the start of the study, could have been related to changes to bath design, but also preparation of the chemical (fixed 5% solution), a fixed upper limit on cow passes before chemical refreshment (200 cow passes), and a constant footbath frequency (4 milkings per week).

Wash baths positioned before the cows entering the treatment bath have long been recommended by some.[10,11] They may benefit the footbath program by removing manure contamination from the foot before the cow entering the treatment bath and by reducing manure contamination of the treatment bath, thereby enhancing the duration of effect of the antibacterial used. Manning and colleagues[12] demonstrated that use of a wash bath did indeed reduce the organic matter transferred to the treatment bath on one farm. However, this is not always the case; Cook and colleagues[13] documented an increased rate of defecation in the treatment bath (8.5% cows) compared with the preceding wash bath (5.8% cows) on 3 farms, and these herds had larger group sizes, with a greater number of cow passes before the chemical was changed than the study by Manning and colleagues.[12] Use of a wash bath also adds a considerable amount of water to the manure management system. For example, a 1000-cow dairy, a 200-L (50 gallon) wash bath used 4 days per week, refreshed every 200 cow passes, would add approximately 200,000 L (52,000 gallons) of water per year to the manure management system.

Those producers wishing to use a wash bath may use water or a salt solution in the existing treatment bath as an adjunct to use of another antibacterial agent. Speijers and colleagues[14] examined the use of a water or 10% salt bath when alternated weekly with a 5% copper sulfate bath. Compared with a control group receiving only the copper sulfate baths every 2 weeks, the groups receiving the additional wash baths demonstrated some minor improvements, although the results were somewhat equivocal overall.

Frequency of Use

Despite the general advice that footbaths should be used regularly to be effective,[15] there is a wide range of times per day and days per week of use employed by farms. The median frequency of footbath use on the farms surveyed by Cook and colleagues[5] was once a day, with a range from 1 to 4 times daily, and 3 days per week with a range from 1 to 7 days. The Midwest herds surveyed by Cook and colleagues[1] used the footbath on average 4.5 milkings per week, with 18% of the herds bathing for 6 to 7 milkings per week, whereas in the Canadian herd survey by Solano and colleagues,[7] 52% of herds used a footbath 2 or more days per week, with the others using the bath less frequently. Clearly, the industry is seeking better guidelines on frequency of use, given the significant variation observed from farm to farm. In some herds, overuse of chemicals is clearly an economic problem, and it could be an environmental issue.

Duration of Efficacy

The number of cow passes between solution changes varied widely between 80 and 3000 cows, with a median of 250 cows in the herds studied by Cook and colleagues.[5] Empirical advice for changing footbath solutions every 100 to 300 cows appears to be followed by most farms, but is challenged on larger dairies, where this recommendation would require chemical changes for every pen of cows milked: some herds are obviously reluctant to do this, and there is very little in the scientific literature to help producers with their decision making.

Dr Dörte Döpfer has suggested performing sequential sampling of footbaths during their use and measuring the bacterial load, suggesting that the solution be changed when either the aerobic or the anaerobic bacterial load exceeds 100,000 CFU/mL or the growth between samples becomes exponential (personal communication, Dörte Döpfer, personal communication 2016). Such an approach is somewhat time consuming and intensive, but between herds under a variety of different circumstances, solution changes have been recommended typically after 100 to 300 cow passes. Predictably, degree of soiling, pH, bath volume, and perhaps water quality influence the duration of activity.

Ideally, in the future, there would be a bath side test to tell when the solution needs to be changed. However, until then, the empirical recommendation of ~200 cow passes appears to have merit and in large herds matches typical pen sizes, so that solutions can be changed between pens as they are milked. In order to facilitate this rapid change, a large vat, such as an old bulk milk tank, fitted with an agitator paddle should be used to mix the required amount of chemical before it is needed (**Fig. 2**). The solution can then be directly pumped into the bath. Several milking machine manufacturers have already invested in automated equipment to facilitate footbath mixing in large herds.

HOW DO FOOTBATHS WORK?

Given that use of a footbath is common and of significant cost, financially and in terms of potential environmental contamination, one should consider the potential positive actions of a footbath. Related to the improvement of hoof health and prevention of lameness, there are 3 potential modes of action:

1. They may serve to harden the hoof.
2. They may improve hoof hygiene.
3. They may control the microbial population present on and around the hoof.

Do Footbaths Harden the Hoof?

Use of a footbath to harden the hoof is a statement commonly made by dairy producers, and there is some scientific evidence to support this claim. Fjeldaas and

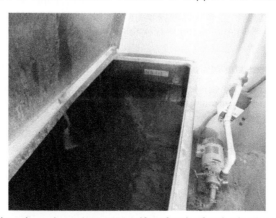

Fig. 2. A bulk milk tank used to mix copper sulfate for the footbath. The pump delivers the solution to the bath rapidly and safely.

colleagues[16] measured hoof hardness using a Shore durometer in 4 locations of the right lateral rear claw of cows under a variety of treatments. Although flushing hooves in a bath with water significantly softened the hoof wall after 12 weeks, use of a 7% copper sulfate footbath significantly hardened the hoof wall compared with unbathed control cows, likely a result of the astringent effect of copper sulfate.[17] No other footbath study has measured hoof hardness as an outcome, so the evidence is limited. Also unknown is the potential impact of a harder hoof wall on lameness prevention. It would have little impact on infectious hoof diseases, such as digital and interdigital dermatitis, which affects the epidermal skin layer usually proximal to the interdigital space, but there may be some as yet unquantifiable effect on heel horn erosion and white line disease incidence.

In summary, copper sulfate footbaths do indeed harden the hoof wall; however, the significance of this is questionable and likely does not justify use of this type of footbath for this purpose alone.

Do Footbaths Improve Hoof Hygiene?

Because hoof hygiene has been recognized as a risk factor for infectious hoof diseases, digital dermatitis in particular,[18–20] it is possible that footbaths may function to improve hoof hygiene and thereby reduce the risk for new infection through this mode of action. The ultimate test for this hypothesis is to test the use of a wash bath using only water to improve hoof hygiene, in the absence of the use of an antibacterial agent.

Given the stricter controls on the use of formaldehyde and copper sulfate in the European Union, there has been increased interest in the use of wash baths in the control of infectious hoof disease. Several commercial automated wash baths have become available, and some have been put to the test under experimental conditions. Thomsen and colleagues[20] showed that when hooves were washed with water through an automated flush bath compared with hooves that remained unwashed and untreated, the washed hooves were cleaner, but importantly, not at reduced risk for new digital dermatitis infection. Fjeldaas and colleagues[16] similarly found no benefit in the control of interdigital dermatitis or heel horn erosion with the use of a water flush bath compared with untreated controls, and no difference in claw hygiene. These authors pointed out that return to the contaminated environment of the stall housing likely made any impact on hoof hygiene relatively brief.

In summary, the available evidence does not support the use of a footbath in improving hoof hygiene as a major factor in the control of infectious hoof disease. The use of a wash bath containing only water appears to have minimal impact on infectious hoof disease.

Do Footbaths Control the Microbial Population on and Around the Hoof?

Infectious hoof lesions have a strong bacterial component, and manipulation of the hoof microbiota through regular footbathing is a reasonable mode of action for their role in lameness control and the prevention and cure of infectious hoof diseases. Digital dermatitis is by far the most common and important infectious hoof disease to control on dairy farms, and control of this disease through the use of footbaths has received the most interest in the scientific literature. However, foot rot (interdigital necrobacillosis or phlegmon) and heel horn erosion (slurry heel) are also very common and should not be forgotten in assessment of footbath efficacy.

Various *Treponema* spp have been identified as the bacteria most commonly associated with the development of active digital dermatitis lesions: *Treponema denticola*, *Treponema maltophilum*, *Treponema medium*, *Treponema putidum*, *Treponema phagedenis*, and *Treponema paraluiscuniculi* being the most commonly found in the United States.[21] Although other bacteria may be involved in the disease, such as *Candidatus Amoebophilus asiaticus*[21] and other species belonging to several other phyla,[22] Treponemes are consistently found and were major contributors to the development of experimental lesions.[23]

It would be reasonable to expect that a footbath should contain an antibacterial with some efficacy against *Treponema* spp, and one method to examine their usefulness in this regard would be to test their efficacy against these bacterial populations in vitro. Hartshorn and colleagues[24] described such an approach to establish the in vitro minimum bactericidal concentration (MBC) and minimum inhibitory concentration (MIC) against a *T phagedenis*-like organism isolated from the field. The approach also examined the impact of the presence of manure and different exposure times. The study confirmed the relative efficacy of copper sulfate compared with formaldehyde, glutaraldehyde, and the other agents tested. Zinc sulfate performed very poorly under all the conditions of the test. Duration of exposure (30 seconds vs 10 minutes) impacted most chemicals in a relatively small way, whereas the significance of manure contamination was of greater importance, especially in relation to copper sulfate and formaldehyde use, where the MBC and MIC increased markedly in the presence of 20% manure. Manure and organic matter may bind Cu^{2+} ions, preventing their action, or it may inhibit the ability of the salt to dissociate.[25] It should however be noted that field use of copper sulfate, even at 2.5%, was far greater than the recorded MBC in the presence of manure (0.31%), but the study does highlight the importance of footbath management and hygienic practices.

In vivo testing of footbaths for the control of infectious hoof disease has received relatively scant attention in the scientific literature, but the available peer-reviewed published field studies since 2000 are summarized in **Tables 1** and **2**. The 15 reports represent 38 different footbath regimens tested in a variety of different ways. Overall, most of these studies demonstrate efficacy of copper sulfate, formaldehyde, and some other antibacterial agents in footbaths in the field in the control of infectious hoof disease, presumably due to some antibacterial action on the microbiota of the hoof. However, the methodologies used in these studies raise significant questions regarding the optimal approach that needs to be taken in the field, worthy of examination.

FOOTBATH TESTING
Study Design and Outcomes

Of note, across the studies documented in **Tables 1** and **2** is a definitive lack of standardized testing criteria related to methodology and analysis, which reflects the wide range of footbathing practices in the field previously discussed. Footbath design and management parameters with significant variation between studies include footbath design (for example, footbath length varied from 1.5 to 4.0 m), use of a wash bath or washing of the feet before the treatment bath (19/38 tests did not use a wash bath), frequency of changing the footbath chemical (ranged from 31 to 300 cow passes), number of times per day the footbath was used (15 regimens used once a day bathing and 23 regimens used twice daily), and frequency of use (ranging from once daily for 7 days to just 4 days in every 28 days).

The vast majority of studies were primarily focused on control of digital dermatitis, although a few studies included heel horn erosion,[16,26] interdigital dermatitis,[16] and lameness[31] as additional outcomes of interest. Across the 38 regimen tests, the number of cows included in the sample ranged from 14 to 960 cows housed in 1 to 12

Table 1
Summary of the peer-reviewed scientific literature testing footbaths in the field with a description of the duration of the study, its design, the outcomes measured, and the criteria used for measuring success

Citation, Date	No. of Cows	No. of Herds	Antibacterial Agent	Concentration	Treatment Duration (wk)	Treatment and Follow-Up Period (wk)	Study Design	Outcomes Measured	Success Criteria
Manske et al,[26] 2002	44	1	Acidic ionized copper (Hoofpro+)	0.60%	5 × ~10 d periods	24	Split bath, negative water control, natural exposure study monitoring digital dermatitis (DD) and heel horn erosion (HHE)	DD 6-point (pt) score, 1–3 active, 0, 4, or 5 inactive, HHE 2-pt score	Cure of existing lesions and reduction in new cases
Holzhauer et al,[27] 2012	110	1	Acidified ionized copper sulfate (Digiderm+)	—	16	16	Split bath positive control treatment comparison with test product	5-pt M-stage classification for DD lesions,[28] interdigital dermatitis (ID), and HHE	New active M2 vs cured M2 adjusted for presence of ID and HHE
Relun et al,[29] 2012	805	10	Copper and zinc chelates (Hoof-Fit)	5%	24	24	Footbath regimen comparison with negative control herds using only individual cow treatment	DD 5-pt M-stage classification scored in parlor, leg hygiene	Hazard for cure from active (M1 M2) to cured (M0 M4) lesion scores
Relun et al,[29] 2012	960	12	Copper and zinc chelates (Hoof-Fit)	5%	24	24	Footbath regimen comparison with negative control herds using only individual cow treatment	DD 5-pt M-stage classification scored in parlor, leg hygiene	Hazard for cure from active (M1 M2) to cured (M0 M4) lesion scores

Study			Product	Concentration			Study design	Outcome measures	Objective
Laven & Hunt,[30] 2002	31	1	Copper sulfate	2%	1	3	Cows with DD lesions only, treatment effect comparison, no negative control	DD lesion 4-pt score for depth and color, lesion size	Improvement in lesion score and lesion size and presence
Teixeira et al,[31] 2010	356	1	Copper sulfate	10%	4	4	Treatment group comparison with test product, crossover design	Active painful DD lesion vs healed inactive DD lesion and locomotion score	Resolve active painful lesions, prevent new lesions, reduce lameness
Logue et al,[8] 2012	165	6	Copper sulfate	5%	16	16	Split bath positive control treatment comparison with test product	DD lesion size, 4-pt lesion score; healing, chronic, raw	Conversion to binary score for healing or no lesion vs acute and chronic lesions
Smith et al,[32] 2014	120–200	3	Copper sulfate	5%	9	9	Split bath, positive control comparison with copper sulfate as the control	5-pt M-stage classification for DD lesions[28]	Prevalence of M1-2 active and M0, 3, 4 inactive lesions compared between treatments
Fjeldaas et al,[16] 2014	45	1	Copper sulfate	7%	12	12	Group comparison with negative untreated control	ID, DD, and HHE scored 1–3, lameness, hoof hardness, hygiene	Risk for becoming diseases and risk for cure
Solano et al,[9] 2017	152 cows per herd	9	Copper sulfate	5%	12	22	Response to intervention within herds before and after change in program	DD 6-pt M-stage classification including M4.1 stage[38]	Prevalence of active M2 and 4.1 lesions

(continued on next page)

Table 1
(continued)

Citation, Date	No. of Cows	No. of Herds	Antibacterial Agent	Concentration	Treatment Duration (wk)	Treatment and Follow-Up Period (wk)	Study Design	Outcomes Measured	Success Criteria
Speijers et al,[14] 2010	40	1	Copper sulfate	5%	5	5	Treatment group comparison with a negative control group	5-pt M-stage classification for DD lesions[28]	Prevalence of active M1 and M2 lesions and rate of "healed" lesions (improved transition)
Speijers et al,[14] 2010	19	1	Copper sulfate	5%	8	8	Treatment group comparison	5-pt M-stage classification for DD lesions[28]	Prevalence of active M1 and M2 lesions and rate of "healed" lesions (improved transition)
Speijers et al,[14] 2010	20	1	Copper sulfate	2%	8	8	Treatment group comparison	5-pt M-stage classification for DD lesions[28]	Prevalence of active M1 and M2 lesions and rate of "healed" lesions (improved transition)
Speijers et al,[14] 2010	39	1	Copper sulfate	5%	8	8	Treatment group comparison	5-pt M-stage classification for DD lesions[28]	Prevalence of active M1 and M2 lesions and rate of "healed" lesions (improved transition)

Speijers et al,[14] 2010	39	1	Copper sulfate	2%	8	8	Treatment group comparison	5-pt M-stage classification for DD lesions[28]	Prevalence of active M1 and M2 lesions and rate of "healed" lesions (improved transition)
Speijers et al,[33] 2012	29	1	Copper sulfate	5%	13	13	Treatment group comparison	5-pt M-stage classification for DD lesions[28]	Prevalence of active M1 and M2 lesions and rate of "healed" lesions (improved transition)
Speijers et al,[14] 2012	32	1	Copper sulfate	5%	13	13	Treatment group comparison	5-pt M-stage classification for DD lesions[28]	Prevalence of active M1 and M2 lesions and rate of "healed" lesions (improved transition)
Speijers et al,[14] 2012	26	1	Copper sulfate	5%	13	13	Treatment group comparison	5-pt M-stage classification for DD lesions[28]	Prevalence of active M1 and M2 lesions and rate of "healed" lesions (improved transition)
Speijers et al,[33] 2012	27	1	Copper sulfate	5%	13	13	Treatment group comparison	5-pt M-stage classification for DD lesions[28]	Prevalence of active M1 and M2 lesions and rate of "healed" lesions (improved transition)

(continued on next page)

Table 1
(continued)

Citation, Date	No. of Cows	No. of Herds	Antibacterial Agent	Concentration	Treatment Duration (wk)	Treatment and Follow-Up Period (wk)	Study Design	Outcomes Measured	Success Criteria
Laven & Hunt,[30] 2002	52	1	Erythromycin	2.1 g/L	1	3	Cows with DD lesions only, treatment effect comparison, no negative control	DD lesion 4-pt score for depth and color, lesion size	Improvement in lesion score and lesion size and presence
Laven & Proven,[6] 2000	111	6	Erythromycin	35 mg/L	1	1.5	Cows with DD lesions only, treatment effect, no negative control	DD lesion type (exudation, reddening, creaminess, scabbing), lesion size, pain and lameness	Change in lesion score and size, pain and lameness
Laven & Hunt,[30] 2002	42	1	Formalin	6%	1	3	Cows with DD lesions only, treatment effect comparison, no negative control	DD lesion 4-pt score for depth and color, lesion size	Improvement in lesion score and lesion size and presence
Holzhauer et al,[34] 2008	15	1	Formalin	4%	24	24	Treatment group comparison, no negative control	5-pt M-stage classification for DD lesions[28]	Prevalence of active M2, type I unaffected cows, type II new infection, type III chronic infection

Reference									
Holzhauer et al,[34] 2008	62	1	Formalin	4%	24	24	Treatment group comparison, no negative control	5-pt M-stage classification for DD lesions[28]	Prevalence of active M2, type I unaffected cows, type II new infection, type III chronic infection
Teixeira et al,[31] 2010	406	1	Formalin	5%	4	4	Treatment group comparison with test product, crossover design	Active painful DD lesion vs healed inactive DD lesion and locomotion score	Resolve active painful lesions, prevent new lesions, reduce lameness
Holzhauer et al,[27] 2012	110	1	Formalin	4%	16	16	Split bath positive control treatment comparison with test product	5-pt M-stage classification for DD lesions,[28] ID, and HHE	New active M2 vs cured M2 adjusted for presence of ID and HHE
Thomsen et al,[35] 2008	82	4	Glutaraldehyde (Virocid)	1.50%	8	8	Split bath, negative control natural exposure study monitoring DD	DD 6-pt score, 1–4 active (including healing dry lesions), 5 chronic inactive	Prevention of new active DD lesions and cure of existing active DD lesions
Thomsen et al,[35] 2008	82	4	Hydrogen peroxide, peracetic and acetic acids (Kick Start 2)	1%	8	8	Split bath, negative control natural exposure study monitoring DD	DD 6-pt score, 1–4 active (including healing dry lesions), 5 chronic inactive	Prevention of new active DD lesions and cure of existing active DD lesions
Holzhauer et al,[34] 2008	16	1	Multicompound (Feetcare) for 20 min	2%	24	24	Treatment group comparison, no negative control	5-pt M-stage classification for DD lesions[28]	Prevalence of active M2, type I unaffected cows, type II new infection, type III chronic infection

(continued on next page)

Table 1
(continued)

Citation, Date	No. of Cows	No. of Herds	Antibacterial Agent	Concentration	Treatment Duration (wk)	Treatment and Follow-Up Period (wk)	Study Design	Outcomes Measured	Success Criteria
Holzhauer et al,[34] 2008	15	1	Multicompound (Feetcare) walkthrough	2%	24	24	Treatment group comparison, no negative control	5-pt M-stage classification for DD lesions[28]	Prevalence of active M2, type I unaffected cows, type II new infection, type III chronic infection
Laven & Hunt,[30] 2002	44	1	Peracetic acid	1%	1	3	Cows with DD lesions only, treatment effect comparison, no negative control	DD lesion 4-pt score for depth and color, lesion size	Improvement in lesion score and lesion size and presence
Teixeira et al,[31] 2010	356	1	Phenoxyethanol (Dragonhyde)	5%	4	4	Treatment comparison with copper sulfate, crossover design	Active painful DD lesion vs healed inactive DD lesion and locomotion score	Resolve active painful lesions, prevent new lesions, reduce lameness
Teixeira et al,[31] 2010	406	1	Phenoxyethanol (Dragonhyde)	5%	4	4	Treatment group comparison with formalin, crossover design	Active painful DD lesion vs healed inactive DD lesion and locomotion score	Resolve active painful lesions, prevent new lesions, reduce lameness

Thomsen et al,[35] 2008	82	4	2%	Quaternary ammonium (Hoofcare DA)	8	8	Split bath, negative control natural exposure study monitoring DD	DD 6-pt score, 1–4 active (including healing dry lesions), 5 chronic inactive	Prevention of new active DD lesions and cure of existing active DD lesions
Holzhauer et al,[34] 2008	14	1	3%	Sodium carbonate	24	24	Treatment group comparison, no negative control	5-pt M-stage classification for DD lesions[28]	Prevalence of active M2, type I unaffected cows, type II new infection, type III chronic infection
Silva et al,[36] 2005	30	1	1%	Sodium hypochlorite	4.3	6.4	Cows with DD lesions only after surgical removal, treatment effect compared with non-footbath groups	DD presence or absence	Absence of DD lesion, pain and inflammation
Speijers et al,[14] 2010	39	1	2%	Sodium hypochlorite	5	5	Treatment group comparison with a negative control group	5-pt M-stage classification for DD lesions[28]	Prevalence of active M1 and M2 lesions and rate of "healed" lesions (improved transition)
Smith et al,[32] 2014	120–201	3	3%	Tea tree oil and organic acid (Provita Hoofsure Endurance)	9	9	Split bath, positive control comparison with copper sulfate	5-pt M-stage classification for DD lesions[28]	Prevalence of M1-2 active and M0, 3, 4 inactive lesions compared between treatments

Table 2
Summary of the peer-reviewed scientific literature testing footbaths in the field with a description of the footbath design, program used, and the outcome of the regimen tested

Citation, Date	No. of Cows	No. of Herds	Antibacterial Agent	Concentration	Footbath Description	Wash Bath Use (Y or N)	No. of Cow Passes Before Footbath Solution Changed	Times per Day	Days per Week	Summary Findings
Manske et al,[26] 2002	44	1	Acidic ionized copper (Hoofpro+)	0.60%	NA	N	300	2	3–16 d	Improved cure of DD vs water alone in rear feet, no significant preventive effect identified
Holzhauer et al,[27] 2012	110	1	Acidified ionized copper sulfate (Digiderm+)	—	2.33 m long, 0.32 m wide, 0.18 m deep	N	231	2	5	Reduction in risk for developing a new M2 lesion lower than formalin use every 14 d
Relun et al,[29] 2012	805	10	Copper and zinc chelates (Hoof-Fit)	5%	2.33 m long, 0.32 m wide, 0.19 m deep, 160-L capacity	N	151	2	2 every 28	Footbathing every month was insufficient to enhance cure from individual topical treatment
Relun et al,[29] 2012	960	12	Copper and zinc chelates (Hoof-Fit)	5%	2.33 m long, 0.32 m wide, 0.19 m deep, 160-L capacity	N	150	2	2 every 14	Footbathing every 2 wk enhanced cure over individual topical treatment alone, with healing improved by cleanliness of the feet, and early detection and smaller lesion size

Study									
Laven & Hunt,[30] 2002	31	1	Copper sulfate	2%	3.0 m long, 0.13 m deep	N	31	1	7	Greatest improvement in DD lesion score and presence after 21 d compared with other treatments (erythromycin, formalin, peracetic acid)
Teixeira et al,[31] 2010	356	1	Copper sulfate	10%	1.5 m long, 1.0 m wide, 0.1 m deep bath, 150-L capacity	Y	45	1	2	18% new lesion rate, no difference with Dragonhyde for prevalence of DD or lameness
Logue et al,[8] 2012	165	6	Copper sulfate	5%	2.2 m long, 0.95 m wide, 0.36 m deep	Y	165	2	3	Copper sulfate resulted in a greater reduction in severity score than a test product. Effect was enhanced by use of a longer footbath
Smith et al,[32] 2014	120–200	3	Copper sulfate	5%	2.33 m long, 0.325 m wide, 80-L capacity × 2	N	NA	1	.5	Significant reduction in prevalence of active lesions between start and end of study
Fjeldaas et al,[16] 2014	45	1	Copper sulfate	7%	2.33 m long, 0.74 m wide, 0.17–0.22 m deep	N	90	2	2 every 14	Beneficial effect of 7% copper sulfate on prevention of HHE compared with negative control

(continued on next page)

Table 2
(continued)

Citation, Date	No. of Cows	No. of Herds	Antibacterial Agent	Concentration	Footbath Description	Wash Bath Use (Y or N)	No. of Cow Passes Before Footbath Solution Changed	Times per Day	Days per Week	Summary Findings
Solano et al,[9] 2017	152 cows per herd	9	Copper sulfate	5%	3.0 m long, 0.25 m wide × 2, 0.15 m deep, 225-L capacity	Y	200	2	2	Intervention with a standardized footbath protocol reduced proportion of active lesions over time, especially in high DD prevalence herds at start of study
Speijers et al,[14] 2010	40	1	Copper sulfate	5%	2.07 m long, 0.79 m wide, 0.17 m deep, 270-L capacity	Y	200	2	2	Prevalence of active lesions decreased over time relative to negative control group (~56% to 21%) and healing rate higher for copper sulfate than hypochlorite or control
Speijers et al,[14] 2010	19	1	Copper sulfate	5%	2.07 m long, 0.79 m wide, 0.17 m deep, 270-L capacity	Y	200	2	2 every 14	Less frequent use at 5% resulted in more cows without DD at end of study with fewer M1 and M4 cows compared with 2% group, but overall less effective than more frequent use

Study										Findings
Speijers et al,[14] 2010	20	1	Copper sulfate	2%	2.07 m long, 0.79 m wide, 0.17 m deep, 270-L capacity	Y	200	2	2 every 14	Less frequent use at 2% was the least effective program compared with 5% copper sulfate and more frequent use programs, but prevalence of active lesions still declined
Speijers et al,[14] 2010	39	1	Copper sulfate	5%	2.07 m long, 0.79 m wide, 0.17 m deep, 270-L capacity	Y	200	2	2	More frequent use at 5% resulted in more cows without DD at the end of the study compared with 2% group and higher rate of healing of active lesions and the most rapid decrease in prevalence of active lesions
Speijers et al,[14] 2010	39	1	Copper sulfate	2%	2.07 m long, 0.79 m wide, 0.17 m deep, 270-L capacity	Y	200	2	2	More frequent use at 2% was effective, but less so than 5% concentration, with less healing effect on active lesions
Speijers et al,[33] 2012	29	1	Copper sulfate	5%	2.07 m long, 0.79 m wide, 0.17 m deep, 270-L capacity	Y	200	1	4	Weekly copper sulfate use resulted in no active DD lesions, more cows with no DD lesions and fewer cows in the healing stage than use every 2 wk

(continued on next page)

Table 2
(continued)

Citation, Date	No. of Cows	No. of Herds	Antibacterial Agent	Concentration	Footbath Description	Wash Bath Use (Y or N)	No. of Cow Passes Before Footbath Solution Changed	Times per Day	Days per Week	Summary Findings
Speijers et al,[33] 2012	32	1	Copper sulfate	5%	2.07 m long, 0.79 m wide, 0.17 m deep, 270-L capacity	Y	200	1	4 every 14	Copper sulfate use every 2 wk resulted in no active DD lesions, but fewer cows with no DD lesions and more cows in the healing stage compared with weekly use
Speijers et al,[33] 2012	26	1	Copper sulfate	5%	2.07 m long, 0.79 m wide, 0.17 m deep, 270-L capacity	Y	200	1	4 every 14	Copper sulfate use every 2 wk resulted in more cows without DD and fewer cows in the healing stage compared with monthly use
Speijers et al,[33] 2012	27	1	Copper sulfate	5%	2.07 m long, 0.79 m wide, 0.17 m deep, 270-L capacity	Y	200	1	4 every 28	Monthly copper sulfate use was the least effective program compared with more frequent use weekly or every 2 wk
Laven & Hunt,[30] 2002	52	1	Erythromycin	2.1 g/L	3.0 m long, 0.13 m deep	N	52	1	2	Improvement in DD lesion score, but performed worse than copper sulfate and formalin

Reference										
Laven & Proven,[6] 2000	111	6	Erythromycin	35 mg/L	NA	N	111	2	2	Erythromycin in a footbath improved clinical signs of DD and reduced lameness
Laven & Hunt,[30] 2002	42	1	Formalin	6%	3.0 m long, 0.13 m deep	N	42	1	7	Second best improvement in DD lesion score and presence after 21 d, slightly poorer than copper sulfate
Holzhauer et al,[34] 2008	15	1	Formalin	4%	3.0 m long, 0.8 m wide, 0.15 m deep, 288-L capacity	N	NA	2	1 every 14	Higher proportion of type III chronic cows than group bathed once a week
Holzhauer et al,[34] 2008	62	1	Formalin	4%	3.0 m long, 0.8 m wide, 0.15 m deep, 288-L capacity	N	128	2	1	Reference group; lowest prevalence of active lesions compared with other treatments tested
Teixeira et al,[31] 2010	406	1	Formalin	5%	1.5 m long, 1.0 m wide, 0.1 m deep bath, 150L capacity	Y	45	1	2	15% new lesion rate but higher prevalence of DD than Dragonhyde and higher lameness prevalence
Holzhauer et al,[27] 2012	110	1	Formalin	4%	2.33 m long, 0.32 m wide, 0.18 m deep	N	230	2	1 every 14	Preventive effect less than for test product containing ionized copper, but cure rate similar
Thomsen et al,[35] 2008	82	4	Glutaraldehyde (Virocid)	1.50%	2.3 m long, 0.2 m deep	N	100	2	2	No difference in cure of DD and prevention of new DD lesions compared with negative control

(continued on next page)

Table 2
(continued)

Citation, Date	No. of Cows	No. of Herds	Antibacterial Agent	Concentration	Footbath Description	Wash Bath Use (Y or N)	No. of Cow Passes Before Footbath Solution Changed	Times per Day	Days per Week	Summary Findings
Thomsen et al,[35] 2008	82	4	Hydrogen peroxide, peracetic and acetic acids (Kick Start 2)	1%	2.3 m long, 0.2 m deep	N	100	2	2	No difference in cure of DD and prevention of new DD lesions compared with negative control
Holzhauer et al,[34] 2008	16	1	Multicompound (Feetcare) for 20 min	2%	4.0 m long, 3.0 m wide, 0.15 m deep, 1800-L capacity	N	NA	1	1	Less effective than reference group using formalin once weekly
Holzhauer et al,[34] 2008	15	1	Multicompound (Feetcare) walkthrough	2%	3.0 m long, 0.8 m wide, 0.15 m deep, 288-L capacity	N	NA	2	1	Outbreak (>30% limbs affected) of M2 lesions, lower % type I and more type II and type III cows
Laven & Hunt,[30] 2002	44	1	Peracetic Acid	1%	3.0 m long, 0.13 m deep	N	44	1	7	Improvement in DD lesion score, but performed worse than copper sulfate and formalin
Teixeira et al,[31] 2010	356	1	Phenoxyethanol (Dragonhyde)	5%	1.5 m long, 1.0 m wide, 0.1 m deep bath, 150-L capacity	Y	45	1	2	20% new lesion rate similar to copper sulfate, no difference in prevalence of DD or lameness

Study			Product	Concentration	Dimensions	Footbath				Outcome
Teixeira et al,[31] 2010	1	406	Phenoxyethanol (Dragonhyde)	5%	1.5 m long, 1.0 m wide, 0.1 m deep bath, 150-L capacity	Y	45	1	2	15% new lesion rate, lower prevalence of DD, and fewer lame cows than formalin
Thomsen et al,[35] 2008	4	82	Quaternary Ammonium (Hoofcare DA)	2%	2.3 m long, 0.2 m deep	N	100	2	2	No difference in cure of DD and prevention of new DD lesions compared with negative control
Holzhauer et al,[34] 2008	1	14	Sodium carbonate	3%	3.0 m long, 0.8 m wide, 0.15 m deep, 288-L capacity	N	NA	2	1	Outbreak (>30% limbs affected) of M2 lesions
Silva et al,[36] 2005	1	30	Sodium hypochlorite	1%	NA	Y	120	2	7	73% animals cured after surgical removal and footbath program compared with 50%—57% cure in non-footbathed groups
Speijers et al,[14] 2010	1	39	Sodium hypochlorite	2%	2.07 m long, 0.79 m wide, 0.17 m deep, 270-L capacity	Y	200	2	2	Prevalence of active lesions increased over time with no difference with negative control group
Smith et al,[32] 2014	3	120–201	Tea tree oil and organic acid (Provita Hoofsure Endurance)	3%	2.33 m long, 0.325 m wide, 80-L capacity × 2	N	NA	1	5	Significant reduction in prevalence of active lesions between start and end of study equivalent to copper sulfate control

herds, suggesting significant variance in power across studies, and a variety of testing approaches.

Essential to any assessment of the preventive or curative effects of a footbath is an understanding of the various stages of digital dermatitis infection and how they relate to each other dynamically. Most footbath studies use the M-stage scoring system developed by Döpfer and colleagues[37] and refined by Berry and colleagues.[38] M1 lesions are small, less than 20 mm in diameter, and may spontaneously resolve or expand into acute M2 lesions: the typical painful strawberry-type lesion, greater than 20 mm in diameter, on the plantar aspect of the interdigital space. If left untreated, M2 lesions expand and may become proliferative with long projections or pili developing due to uncontrolled skin proliferation, eventually becoming chronic M4 lesions. However, if treated effectively, M2 lesions will pass through an M3 scab stage before resolving. M4 lesions may recrudesce, developing small M1 lesions within the chronic lesion itself, referred to as M4.1 lesions. These lesions may transition back to M2 stages, causing pain and lameness. M0 represents a normal unaffected foot. Other scoring systems attempt to differentiate an active painful lesion from an inactive chronic or healing lesion (for example, see Refs.[8,26,31]), and in general, the M-stage system is collapsed into an active versus inactive lesion differentiation for analysis. In some studies, the M1 lesion is classified as active (for example, see Refs.[14,33]), whereas in others only M2 lesions are classified as active.[27,34] Given the difficulties viewing large numbers of lesions rapidly, as cows either pass through a chute, or are assessed in the parlor, it would seem necessary to attempt differentiation between active M2 lesions and inactive M3 and M4 lesions. A successful footbath program may be measured by enhancing the transition of active to inactive lesions, that is, cure, and by reducing the prevalence of new active lesions; that is, prevention. **Tables 1** and **2** documents the outcomes measured, the criteria for success, and the findings related to cure and prevention for each study regimen.

Study designs are quite variable, but appear to fit into 1 of 3 main approaches:

1. The first approach uses only diseased cows already affected by digital dermatitis, where the outcome of the study is solely focused on cure of the lesion.[6,30,36] Obviously, this study design precludes any assessment of the preventive effects of footbathing, thereby restricting the scope of the assessment. This study approach would also need to be careful in lesion type selection, making sure that the treatment cows consisted of cows with active lesions, rather than chronic M4 type lesions.
2. The second study design uses a split footbath where a treatment may be applied to one-half of the cow and compared with either a negative control with an empty bath,[35] a negative control with only water in the bath,[26] or a positive control with a standard agent, typically copper sulfate[8,32] or formalin.[27] The type of negative or positive control selected would affect sample size requirement. This study design has significant merit because it controls for cow level biases such as hygiene and parity, but because digital dermatitis infections tend to cluster within cow, the effect of any product may be underestimated and biased toward not finding an effect.[27]
3. The third design is a treatment group comparison where one group of cows is exposed to one treatment and compared with another group exposed to a second treatment. The approach may be done in a single herd or across multiple herds, and success is dependent on selection and balancing cows by parity, days in milk, and lesion type across groups. The design can be improved by incorporating a treatment crossover (eg, see Ref.[31]), but even then, pen and herd (if several herds are used) effects can influence the outcome and need to be taken into account.

Two further aspects of study design may impact the results of a footbath study. First, in most, but not all studies, cows affected by acute painful M2 lesions are treated individually with topical therapy. Studies will vary in the ability of the workers to find and treat these cows, and Relun and colleagues[29] showed that early detection of a digital dermatitis lesion tended to ensure a higher cure rate, which would obviously influence the perceived efficacy of the footbath being tested. Second, the duration of the study is thought to be important. Study duration varied from 1 week to 24 weeks in **Table 1**. Döpfer and colleagues[39] recommended that footbath trials last at least 12 weeks based on a study where an outbreak of active digital dermatitis occurred after 9 weeks, before which the test product group appeared to be performing well compared with a positive control group. Only 17/38 regimens reviewed met this criterion.

From the discussion thus far, the conclusion reached is that footbath studies are hard to do well, which is likely one of the reasons for the relative dearth of peer-reviewed studies. However, it is encouraging to see an increase in interest in more recent years and improvements in methodology and analysis that will likely add to the knowledge in the future. The studies reviewed here all passed through peer review and all garner merit, so much can still be learned from their findings.

Peer-Review Study Findings and Recommendations

The significance of footbath design and use of a wash bath has already been discussed, but of further interest when best management practices are to be considered is the range in frequency of use and the observed results. For example, Speijers and colleagues[14,33] tested copper sulfate across a range of frequencies applied weekly, every 2 weeks, and monthly. They showed clearly that more frequent use resulted in fewer cows affected by digital dermatitis at the end of each study, more rapid reduction in the prevalence of infection, and improved healing rates. Similarly, Holzhauer and colleagues[34] demonstrated that formaldehyde use weekly produced the lowest prevalence of active digital dermatitis lesions compared with use every 2 weeks, which resulted in a higher proportion of cows with chronic digital dermatitis lesions. Using a copper and zinc chelate solution, Relun and colleagues[29] also determined that use every month was not as efficacious in enhancing digital dermatitis cure from individual topical treatment compared with footbathing every 2 weeks. Together, it can be concluded that an optimal footbath program should be applied weekly rather than less frequently. The number of times per week the bath should be used is still open for debate based on variation from 2 to 4 milkings per week across these studies. Four milkings per week is close to the mean approach being taken in the field, reported by Cook and colleagues,[1] and was the frequency chosen by Solano and colleagues[9] in their standardized approach. Less frequent use may still work well enough in some herds, and the results of these studies do not preclude the finding that more frequent use may be even more successful, but bathing for 4 milkings each week appears to be a good starting recommendation, from which adjustments can be made based on results.

In regard to antibacterial agent and concentration of products used across studies, some common findings also emerge. Some agents simply do not appear to work or require more evidence for them to be recommended in a footbath program, among this group would be glutaraldehyde, quaternary ammonium, hydrogen peroxide,[35] sodium carbonate,[34] and sodium hypochlorite.[14]

Although antibiotics such as erythromycin have been shown to be effective in a footbath,[6,30] they should not be routinely used in this manner on farm.

Other antibacterial agents have been shown to work well in footbaths for the control of infectious hoof disease. Copper sulfate has been shown to outperform several other antibacterial agents it has been tested against. Copper sulfate was superior to a negative control,[16] erythromycin, formalin, peracetic acid,[30] and sodium hypochlorite,[14] and comparable to phenoxyethanol[31] and tea tree oil.[32] In addition, products containing acidified ionized copper were superior to water[26] and had a greater preventive effect against digital dermatitis infection than formaldehyde used every 14 days.[27] Concentrations of copper sulfate between 2% and 10% have been used across studies.[14,16,30–32] Although lower concentrations retain some efficacy, Speijers and colleagues[14] demonstrated improved digital dermatitis control at 5% compared with 2%, with less healing effect on active lesions at the lower concentration, thus making 5% copper sulfate a reasonable choice where it can be used. Even when use is permissible, there is considerable interest in using cooper sulfate at lower concentrations. The ionic form of copper, Cu^{2+}, is the bioactive form, reacting with thiol groups in target organisms, which requires acid pH typically in the range 3.5 to 4.0 for optimal results. There are now many commercial acidifiers being used to acidify solutions to improve solvency and activity. However, there exists some concern for overacidification, to a point where the skin may be damaged. One report examined the effect of pH in a single herd over a 4-year period, where pH use of a copper sulfate bath changed from pH less than 1.4 to greater than 3.0. The change was associated with a reduction in the prevalence of digital dermatitis and corns, heel horn erosion, and foot rot, and a reduction in treatment wraps. The higher pH also decreased active (M1, 2, and 4.1) lesions, while increasing chronic lesions (M4 stage). There was also a reduction in proliferative lesions, especially in chronic M4 lesions.[40] Thus, although acidifiers may be used to reduce the concentration of copper sulfate being used to ~2% to 3%, and thereby reduce the environmental risk associated with its use, pH should be moderated greater than 3.0 in order to avoid skin damage. The presence of proliferative lesions in affected cattle can be used as a marker for this damage.

Formaldehyde is commonly used in footbaths as a 2% to 6% solution of formalin at a pH of 3 to 5, which is itself a 37% to 39% solution of formaldehyde. Efficacy has been reported across multiple studies when used at a concentration of 4% to 6%.[27,30,31,34] However, in several of these studies, it was outperformed by copper-based products as previously mentioned, and it resulted in a higher prevalence of digital dermatitis and more lame cows compared with a product containing phenoxyethanol.[31] Under temperatures of 15°C, polymerization may occur, which may impact the effectiveness of formalin products, but the addition of methanol to commercially available solutions should offset this problem to some degree. That said, directions for the use of formalin footbaths would generally recommend use above temperatures of 18°C, precluding winter use in much of North America. A commercial trend toward using lower concentration solutions at less than 4% is untested in the peer-reviewed literature.

There are many other footbath products marketed, but it is surprising how few have been subjected to a peer-reviewed report of their use in the field in a controlled manner. Left untested, it is difficult to recommend any of these products, and the user should be wary of poor results or adverse effects. Some commercially available products containing acidified ionized copper,[26,27] copper and zinc chelates,[29] and tea tree oil[32] have been tested, with evidence of efficacy, and they should be considered as potential alternatives.

ENVIRONMENTAL AND HUMAN HEALTH CONCERNS

Use of large quantities of chemicals in footbaths on farms is a source of some concern, from a human health perspective and when disposal of the spent footbath solution is considered.

There are obvious concerns related to the use of formaldehyde, given that it is a carcinogen to humans,[4] but it is noncorrosive, biodegradable, and rapidly degraded in the presence of manure.

Although no such human health risk exists for copper sulfate, there has been growing concern regarding its disposal.[41] Soil copper concentration is of interest because high levels can become toxic to plants and the animals ingesting them, and obviously, the copper impacts the microorganism composition of the soil.[42] That said, these concerns do not preclude use of this chemical in footbaths, because soil and plant levels of copper are affected by several factors. These include the following:

1. The frequency of footbath use: clearly the less frequently the product is used to control infectious hoof disease, the less the environmental concern.
2. The concentration of copper sulfate used: a typical footbath of 5% copper sulfate will use ~11.4 kg copper sulfate per bath. Because copper sulfate pentahydrate crystals have 25% available copper, this would yield 2.8 kg copper for each bath. Use of a 10% bath would double this amount, and using 2.5% instead would halve this amount.
3. The overall concentration of copper in the manure being spread needs to be measured.
4. The availability of the copper in the manure system: ~90% to 95% of the copper is rendered unavailable, held in organic phases in the waste lagoon, but the remainder remains soluble when it is applied to the land.[42]
5. The application rate of manure to the land: typically manure application rate is limited by nitrogen rates, but application rates of 5.2 to 11.8 kg copper per hectare (4.6–10.4 lb per acre) annually have been recorded from 4 Wisconsin herds.[43]
6. The availability of the copper in the soil: 60% to 75% of the remaining copper in the soil is available to the plant once applied to the soil.
7. The uptake of copper from the soil: this is limited to ~0.1 kg per hectare (0.1 lb per acre) for most crops, meaning that soil copper loading rates can easily exceed plant uptake, leading to lifetime accumulation problems that are irredeemable once plant toxicity is identified.

Given these variables, small herds with a reasonable land base for spreading manure are unlikely to suffer problems using a copper sulfate footbath once or twice per week as long as application rates are less than 6 kg copper per hectare (5 lb copper per acre). However, larger herds using the product more frequently at higher concentrations, with a limited land base, may see issues arise related to lifetime accumulation of copper in the soils. Indeed, 75% of Oregon herds were identified with high levels of copper (>2 ppm) in one study.[41] Routine soil copper measurement is considered essential in order to gauge the risk on any given farmstead and determine whether current use levels can be sustained.

Because copper sulfate appears very effective in a footbath program, it likely needs to be retained in the arsenal of antibacterial agents to be used in footbaths. However, best practice demands that as little of it as is necessary be used to control infectious hoof disease.

RECOMMENDATIONS FOR PRUDENT FOOTBATH USE

Based on the review of the literature and field observations of current practices, the following best practice can be proposed for footbath management. Footbaths should be used strategically as a tool to assist in the prevention of infectious hoof disease in all ages of cattle, from breeding heifers to lactating and dry cows. They are not a crutch for poor leg hygiene caused by poor pen design, infrequent manure removal, overstocking, or poor lame cow surveillance and treatment. Footbaths should also not be relied on to cure active digital dermatitis lesions. There should be a program in place to survey cows' feet for early signs of active M2 lesions, and these cows should be topically treated independent of the footbath program. Footbaths will be viewed as most successful when their potential to prevent new active lesions is relied on, rather than relying on them to cure existing lesions. The approach should therefore be to footbath as little as possible to control infectious hoof disease.

In herds endemically infected with digital dermatitis, the goal should be to keep active lesions to less than 5% of cows, and the following approach is suggested:

1. A well-designed treatment bath should be used, correctly located to ensure smooth passage by cows and heifers.

The footbath should be 3.0 to 3.7 m long, 0.6 m wide at the base with a 0.25-m high step-in height, with sloped sidewalls to 0.9 m wide at a height of 0.9 m above the floor of the bath. Ideally, the bath should be located on a level surface. One side should allow access to the bath; the other can be plastic, stainless steel, or concrete with solid side walls to prevent cows seeing over the top. At this time, a separate wash bath cannot be justified, but the treatment bath may be used as a wash bath if the producer wishes to use water, salt, or a surfactant to help clean the feet. Ensure that there is easy access to the bath, with a straight walk through so that cows can follow each other easily. In larger herds, multiple baths can be positioned side by side to improve cow flow.

2. A mixing tank should be located immediately adjacent to the footbath with a pump to transfer the agitated chemical into the bath.

Mixing should occur outside the footbath in a clean area where chemicals can be transferred safely by workers wearing appropriate protective clothing. The bath should be filled to a depth of 10 cm to ensure that the solution washes the interdigital space of cows passing through the bath. Empirically, refresh the solution each day, or after between 100 and 300 cow passes, whichever best fits with pen size and management on the farm. Bacterial count testing can be used to determine whether the bath requires refreshing more or less frequently. Solution pH should be checked. Where acidifiers are in use, pH of the bath should be verified so that it lies between 3.0 and 4.5 throughout the use period. Evidence of proliferation of digital dermatitis lesions may alert the farm to skin damage caused by solutions that are too acidic.

3. Start using the footbath for 4 milking per week and adjust frequency based on outcome.

After 4 to 6 weeks, if infectious hoof disease goals are being reached, the frequency of footbathing can be reduced by one milking per week and performance can be reassessed. The adjustment may be repeated in order to find the minimum frequency where control is maintained. If goals are not being met, frequency can be increased, or antibacterial choice and concentration can be changed.

4. Choose an antibacterial with evidence of efficacy for the prevention of new digital dermatitis lesions and foot rot.

Where copper sulfate can be used, it is clearly the first choice antibacterial to be considered. Concentration of copper sulfate should not be higher than 5%, and with use of an acidifier, concentrations of 2% to 3% may be used as long as pH is not lowered less than 3.0. Farms should monitor manure and soil copper levels routinely to limit lifetime loading. If soils or regulations preclude the use of copper sulfate, formaldehyde or another alternative product can be used in its place in a similar manner. Other products likely will not match copper sulfate for their curative potential, so it is essential to ensure that cows are being surveyed for new active lesions, and they should be treated individually. Evidence for skin damage, such as proliferation of digital dermatitis lesions, should be monitored as a warning sign that footbath chemicals are too caustic.

SUMMARY

In this article, the author has attempted to review current footbath practices used in dairy herds, questioned the mechanism by which footbaths function, and reviewed the available scientific literature for guidelines to assist in the creation of best practices for their use. Footbaths have a significant role to play in the control of infectious hoof disease in confinement housed dairy facilities, but they are not a replacement for good hygienic practices and lame cow surveillance and treatment. Copper sulfate appears the most efficacious agent to include in a footbath program, but disposal concerns should limit the frequency of its use. Other agents, such as formaldehyde, have some merit when used with care but also carry human health concerns. Whatever antibacterial is used, the footbath should be designed to allow for easy flow of cows through the bath and ensure adequate delivery of the solution to the cows' feet. Footbaths should be used as infrequently as possible to achieve lameness prevention goals for the herd.

ACKNOWLEDGMENTS

The author thanks Dr Arturo Gomez and Dr Dörte Döpfer, 2 exceptional colleagues that have helped advance our understanding of the control of digital dermatitis in the field.

REFERENCES

1. Cook NB, Hess JP, Foy MR, et al. Management characteristics, lameness and body injuries of dairy cattle housed in high performance dairy herds in Wisconsin. J Dairy Sci 2016;99:5879–91.
2. Amory JR, Kloosterman P, Barker ZE, et al. Risk factors for reduced locomotion in dairy cattle on nineteen farms in The Netherlands. J Dairy Sci 2006;89:1509–15.
3. Anonymous, 2006.
4. Collins JJ, Lineker GA. A review and meta-analysis of formaldehyde exposure and leukemia. Regul Toxicol Pharmacol 2004;40:81–91.
5. Cook NB, Rieman J, Gomez A, et al. Observations on the design and use of footbaths for the control of infectious hoof disease in dairy cattle. Vet J 2012;193:669–73.
6. Laven RA, Proven MJ. Use of an antibiotic footbath in the treatment of bovine digital dermatitis. Vet Rec 2000;147:503–6.
7. Solano L, Barkema HW, Pajor EA, et al. Prevalence of lameness and associated risk factors in Canadian Holstein-Friesian cows housed in freestall barns. J Dairy Sci 2015;98:6978–91.
8. Logue DN, Gibert T, Parkin T, et al. A field evaluation of a footbathing solution for the control of digital dermatitis in cattle. Vet J 2012;193:664–8.

9. Solano L, Barkema HW, Pickel C, et al. Effectiveness of a standardized footbath protocol for prevention of digital dermatitis. J Dairy Sci 2017;100(2):1295–307.

10. van Amstel SR, Shearer JK. Manual for treatment and control of lameness in cattle. 1st edition. Oxford (United Kingdom): Blackwell Publishing; 2006.

11. Blowey R. Factors associated with lameness in dairy cattle. In Pract 2005;27: 154–62.

12. Manning AD, Mahendran SA, Hurst BS, et al. Effect of a prewash on footbath contamination: a randomized control trial. Vet Rec 2016;180(5):121.

13. Cook NB, Rieman J, Burgi K, et al. Behavioral observations on hoofbath design. In: Proceedings of 16th Symposium and 8th Conference Lameness in Ruminants: Lameness – A Global Perspective. Rotorua (New Zealand), 2011. p. 22.

14. Speijers MHM, Baird LG, Finney GA, et al. Effectiveness of different footbath solutions in the treatment of digital dermatitis in dairy cows. J Dairy Sci 2010;93: 5782–91.

15. Blowey R. Factors associated with lameness in dairy cattle. In Pract 2005;27: 154–62.

16. Fjeldaas T, Knappe-Poindecker M, Bøe KE, et al. Water footbath, automatic flushing, and disinfection to improve the health of bovine feet. J Dairy Sci 2014;97: 2835–46.

17. Trent AM, Redic-Kill KA. Clinical pharmacology. In: Greenough PR, Weaver AD, editors. Lameness in cattle. London: WB Saunders; 1997. p. 57–70.

18. Relun A, Lehebel A, Bareille N, et al. Effectiveness of different regimens of a collective topical treatment using a solution of copper and zinc chelates in the cure of digital dermatitis in dairy farms under field conditions. J Dairy Sci 2013;95: 3722–35.

19. Rodriguez-Lainz A, Melendez-Retamal P, Hird DW, et al. Farm- and host-level risk factors for papillomatous digital dermatitis in Chilean dairy cattle. Prev Vet Med 1999;42:87–97.

20. Thomsen PT, Ersbøll AK, Sørensen JT, et al. Short communication: Automatic washing of hooves can help control digital dermatitis in dairy cows. J Dairy Sci 2012;95:7195–9.

21. Zinicola M, Lima F, Lima S, et al. Altered microbiomes in bovine digital dermatitis lesions, and the gut as a pathogen reservoir. PLoS One 2015;10:e0120504.

22. Krull AC, Shearer JK, Gorden PJ, et al. Deep sequencing analysis reveals the temporal microbiota changes associated with the development of bovine digital dermatitis. Infect Immun 2014;82:3359–73.

23. Gomez A, Cook NB, Bernardoni ND, et al. An experimental infection model to induce digital dermatitis infection in cattle. J Dairy Sci 2012;95(4):1821–30.

24. Hartshorn RE, Thomas EC, Anklam K, et al. Short communication: minimum bactericidal concentration of disinfectants for bovine digital dermatitis-associated Treponema phagedenis-like spirochetes. J Dairy Sci 2013;96:3034–8.

25. Ippolito JA, Barbarick KA. Fate of biosolids trace metals in a dryland wheat agroecosystem. J Environ Qual 2008;37:2135–44.

26. Manske T, Hultgren J, Bergsten C. Topical treatment of digital dermatitis associated with severe heel horn erosion in a Swedish dairy herd. Prev Vet Med 2002; 53:215–31.

27. Holzhauer M, Bartels CJ, Bergsten C, et al. The effect of an acidified ionized copper sulfate solution on digital dermatitis in dairy cows. Vet J 2012;193:659–63.

28. Döpfer D, Koopmans A, Meijer FA, et al. Histological and bacteriological evaluation of digital dermatitis in cattle, with special reference to spirochaetes and Campylobacter faecalis. Vet Rec 1997;140:620–3.

29. Relun A, Lehebel A, Bareille N, et al. Effectiveness of different regimens of a collective topical treatment using a solution of copper and zinc chelates in the cure of digital dermatitis in dairy farms under field conditions. J Dairy Sci 2012;95: 3722–35.

30. Laven RA, Hunt H. Evaluation of copper sulfate, formalin and peracetic acid in footbaths for the treatment of digital dermatitis in cattle. Vet Rec 2002;151:144–6.

31. Teixeira AGV, Machado VS, Caixeta LS, et al. Efficacy of formalin, copper sulfate, and a commercial footbath product in the control of digital dermatitis. J Dairy Sci 2010;93:3628–34.

32. Smith AC, Wood CL, McQuerry KJ, et al. Effect of a tea tree oil and organic acid footbath solution on digital dermatitis in dairy cows. J Dairy Sci 2014;97: 2498–501.

33. Speijers MHM, Finney GA, McBride J, et al. Effectiveness of different footbathing frequencies using copper sulfate in the control of digital dermatitis in dairy cows. J Dairy Sci 2012;95:2955–64.

34. Holzhauer M, Döpfer D, de Boer J, et al. Effects of different intervention strategies on the incidence of papillomatous digital dermatitis in dairy cows. Vet Rec 2008; 162:41–6.

35. Thomsen PT, Sorensen JT, Ersboll AK. Evaluation of three commercial hoof-care products used in footbaths in Danish dairy herds. J Dairy Sci 2008;91(4):1361–5.

36. Silva LAF, Silva CA, Borges JRJ, et al. A clinical trial to assess the use of sodium hypochlorite and oxytetracycline on the healing of digital dermatitis lesions in cattle. Can Vet J 2005;46:345–8.

37. Döpfer D, Koopmans A, Meijer FA, et al. Histological and bacteriological evaluation of digital dermatitis in cattle, with special reference to spirochaetes and Campylobacter faecalis. Vet Rec 1997;140(24):620–3.

38. Berry SL, Read DH, Famula TR, et al. Long-term observations on the dynamics of bovine digital dermatitis lesions on a California dairy after topical treatment with lincomycin HCl. Vet J 2012;193:654–8.

39. Döpfer D, Gomez A, Burgi K, et al. 2011. Long-term evaluation of footbath agents for the prevention of infectious claw disease in dairy cattle. In: Proceedings of 16th Symposium and 8th Conference Lameness in Ruminants: Lameness – A Global Perspective. Rotorua (New Zealand), 2011. p. 2.

40. Burgi K, Dopfer D. The association between acid pH in CuSO4 footbaths with prevalence severity and chronicity of infectious claw diseases in a Wisconsin dairy herd. In: Proceedings of 18th International Symposium, 10th International Conference on Lameness in Ruminants. Valdivia (Chile), 2015. p. 157.

41. Downing TW, Stiglbauer K, Gamroth M, et al. Case study: Use of copper sulfate and zinc sulfate in footbaths on Oregon dairies. Professional Animal Scientist 2010;26:332–4.

42. Ippolito JA, Ducey T, Tarkalson D. Copper impacts on corn, soil extractability and the soil bacterial community. Soil Sci 2010;175:586–92.

43. Rankin M. Agronomic and environmental issues with footbath solution land spreading. In: Proceedings of the 4-state dairy conference. 2009.

The Relationship of Cow Comfort and Flooring to Lameness Disorders in Dairy Cattle

Marcia I. Endres, DVM, MS, PhD

KEYWORDS

• Cow comfort • Stall surface • Flooring • Management

KEY POINTS

- Cow comfort contributes to lameness incidence by increasing the risk for development of new cases and the time it takes for a cow to recover.
- Confinement housing can result in reduced cow comfort and greater incidence of lameness from increased exposure to hard flooring surfaces.
- Exposure of feet and legs to moisture and manure in confinement or pasture transfer lanes may contribute to development of infectious disorders of the foot, such as digital dermatitis and foot rot.
- The trigger factors for lameness, such as nutrition, hormonal changes at calving, infection, and trauma, can all be exacerbated by poor cow comfort.

INTRODUCTION

Ideally, cows would be housed on a comfortable, soft, and dry area at all times. This is not practically possible on dairy farms. That cattle evolved to walk on grass or dirt should be taken into consideration when building confinement facilities for dairy cattle to provide opportunity for the cow to rest comfortably and away from hard surfaces. For cattle on pasture, it is important to also pay attention to the flooring on transfer lanes and other areas they walk on a daily basis.

The trigger factors for lameness, such as nutrition, hormonal changes at calving, infection, and trauma, can all be exacerbated by poor cow comfort. Cow comfort can affect herd lameness incidence by increasing the risk for development of new cases of lameness and the time it takes for a cow to recover from a lameness event.

Disclosure Statement: The author has nothing to disclose.
Department of Animal Science, University of Minnesota, 1364 Eckles Avenue, St Paul, MN 55108, USA
E-mail address: miendres@umn.edu

There is a large variation in the prevalence of lameness across herds with similar housing types. A field study conducted by the research team in Minnesota[1] that included 53 randomly selected freestall dairy sites illustrates this variation (**Fig. 1**). Factors related to facility design and management on dairy farms most likely explain a good portion of this variability. Daily standing time, cow handling, management factors, and the flooring surface the cow is exposed to while standing can all contribute to lameness. In this article, the association of lameness with aspects of cow comfort and flooring surface are discussed based on research conducted primarily in North America, along with some work conducted in other parts of the world as applicable. The emphasis is on overall lameness prevalence or incidence with less discussion on specific types of foot lesions.

COW COMFORT
Stall Design and Surface

Most cows in North America are housed in confinement facilities with freestalls or tie stalls (78.6% of cows in the United States[2]). Stalls should be adequately designed (with appropriate dimensions) and have appropriate surface and bedding material to provide a comfortable resting space. Comfortable stalls will most likely result in longer resting times and a reduction of standing time on hard concrete; this reduction in standing time can potentially reduce herd lameness incidence.

Stall designs that impede the natural rising behavior of cows, especially with less cushioned stall surfaces, will reduce use of stalls and/or affect the number of daily lying bouts. Cows become more fearful of slipping when rising especially if they are already lame. A cow needs to transfer weight over the front knees and create a point of balance to rise on her rear legs safely and naturally. This requires her head to almost touch the ground in front of her, in an area referred to as the bob zone, when she lunges forward.[3] Dippel and colleagues[4] found a significant association between lameness prevalence and the presence of head lunge impediments or neck rail-to-

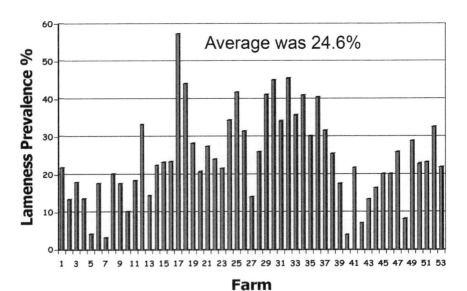

Fig. 1. Distribution of lameness prevalence in Minnesota from 2006 field study of randomly selected freestall herds.

curb diagonals that were too short. Espejo and Endres[5] reported that the height of the brisket board (if >10 cm or 4 in) was a risk factor for lameness independent of stall surface. In a recent study with automated milking system freestall barns,[6] average stall width and obstructed lunge space were significantly associated with lameness prevalence. An inability to fit the average stall width increased the odds of being lame 3.7 times in heifers and 1.3 times in mature cows.

Stall surface and bedding material are important factors associated with lameness prevalence in dairy herds. Various epidemiologic studies[1,7–9] have shown a significantly higher prevalence of lameness in herds using mattress-based freestalls compared with deep-bedded stalls (mostly sand). There has been approximately a 10% unit difference in overall prevalence (scores 3, 4, and 5; with 1 = normal gait; 5 = extremely lame) between the 2 surfaces. Herds with deep-bedded recycled manure solids also had a lower prevalence of lameness than herds with solids on top of mattresses. However, the percentage unit difference was about 5% instead of 10%, which might have been because farms were using large amounts of bedding on top of the mattresses.[10] Similarly, high-producing herds with mats or mattresses averaged 17.4% clinical lameness, whereas deep, loose-bedded herds were at 11.4%.[9] In a study with automated milking system farms in Minnesota and Wisconsin (J. Salfer and M. Endres, University of Minnesota, unpublished results, 2013), a lower prevalence of lameness was found in herds with deep-bedded sand stalls (22.5%), bedded packs (19.0%), or access to pasture (21.5%) than in herds with mattress-based stalls (40.9%). Within these datasets, there were mattress-based stall herds with a low prevalence of lameness, indicating that factors such as amount of bedding placed on top of the mattresses, early detection of lameness, and quick intervention could help reduce lameness incidence in herds with mattress-based stalls. Another option would be to move lame cows to a more comfortable facility, such as a bedded pack, until they recover.

When mattresses covered with 0, 1, or 7.5 kg (0, 2.2, or 16.5 lb) of kiln-dried sawdust were compared, longer daily lying times and increased number of daily lying bouts were reported with more bedding (from 12.3 hours lying and 8.5 bouts on bare mattresses to 13.8 hours lying and 10.0 bouts on mattresses with 7.5 kg of sawdust).[11] In addition, there was a reduction in daily perching time (standing with only the front feet in the stalls) when more sawdust was used. These results indicate that more bedding improved cow comfort in stalls with mattresses, which could result in lower lameness prevalence.

Time budgets of cows in freestall barns with mattress versus deep-sand stalls were compared using continuous video surveillance.[12] Locomotion score influenced time budgets. Lame cows spent less time feeding, less time in the alleys, and more time standing in the stalls in mattress herds but not in sand herds. In mattress herds, cows had a larger number of lying bouts of shorter duration than in sand herds (14.4 vs 10.2; and 1.0 vs 1.3 hours duration, respectively). Lameness was associated with an increase in time standing in the stall and a reduction in the number of lying bouts per day from 13.2 bouts per day for nonlame cows to 10.9 bouts per day for moderately lame cows, and an overall reduction in lying time in mattress herds compared with sand herds (11.5 vs 12.7 hours per day, respectively). The investigators concluded that stall-base type and lameness significantly affect time budgets of cows housed in freestall facilities.

Another study found that lame cows housed on deep-sand stalls had lying and stall standing times similar to nonlame cows.[3] However, lame cows on mattresses had increased time standing in the stall and reduced lying time by about 2 hours per day (moderately lame cows) compared with nonlame cows. These differences in behavior can influence how long it would take for a cow to recover from a lameness event because she is not resting as much as a cow on deep sand. Prevalence of lameness is measured at a point in time and, if it takes longer for cows to recover from a lameness event, the prevalence of lameness in mattress herds would be higher than deep-bedded sand herds (studies show that, on average, it is). It is suggested that cows stand longer in mattress-based stalls because mattresses do not offer the cushion and traction provided by deep-bedded stalls. There is pain associated with lameness in the rear feet (where most lesions occur) and a less cushioned surface makes it harder for a lame cow to get up and lie down. Therefore, early lameness detection and intervention is especially important for herds with mattress-based stalls.

Heat Abatement

Cows prefer to stand rather than lie down during periods of high ambient air temperature. An increase of 3 hours per day in standing time for cows housed at a temperature humidity index (THI) of 73.8 compared with a thermoneutral THI of 56.2 was observed in a study with freestall herds.[13] Longer standing time during the summer can be a contributing factor for increased lameness; therefore, dairy farms should implement effective heat abatement strategies.

Management Factors

Time away from the home pen

Cows prefer to rest 10 to 14 hours a day, so they should be allowed enough time to rest between milking times. Time away from the home pen for milking greater than 4 hours per day was found to be a risk factor for lameness in high-producing cows.[5] When comparing time budgets of cows in mattress-based freestall herds with cows in deep-sand herds, time spent milking varied between cows from 0.5 to 6.0 hours per day and averaged 2.7 plus or minus 1.1 hours per day and it was not influenced by type of stall surface.[12] Time spent milking was influenced by pen stocking density, and time spent milking negatively affected time cows spent feeding, lying down, and in the alley but not time spent standing in the stall. The investigators concluded that time away from the pen can significantly affect time budgets of cows housed in freestall facilities.

It is recommended that the total milking time per day be less than 4 hours for 3 times milking. For each trip to the parlor, calculate the time interval from the point at which the first cow leaves the pen to the point in time at which the last cow has returned to the pen and the gate is closed. If cows are on pasture, the negative consequences of long standing time might be less obvious. Attention should be given to how long cows are locked up for health checks or breeding at feed lanes or palpation rails; this time should ideally be limited to 60 minutes a day or less.

Cow handling

Low-stress cow handling is another important aspect of dairy cattle management that can benefit feet and leg health. Personnel should be trained on calmly and consistently moving cows from their pen to the milking parlor, adequately managing holding pens and crowd gates, and other human-animal interactions that could cause cows to slip, fall, run, or stand for long periods of time. These cow responses could potentially cause damage to the feet and legs, and result in increased incidence of lameness.

Overstocking

Stocking densities greater than 113% (cows per stalls) resulted in greater percentage of cows standing idle in the alleys.[14] Increased standing time in the alleys rather than resting in the stalls could potentially lead to stress on the feet and greater incidence of lameness. A small study with 35 heifers in Ireland housed in a 2:1 animal to stall ratio found a reduction in lying time and worse foot lesion scores for heifers that were over-crowded.[15] A direct relationship between overstocking and lameness has not been extensively reported in the literature. However, overstocking combined with pro-longed time away from the home pen, inadequate cow handling, or uncomfortable stalls should still be considered a risk factor for lameness. Overcrowding should espe-cially be avoided during the transition period when cows are more susceptible to lame-ness due to hormonal and body condition changes.

Flooring

Cows prefer soft surfaces for standing and walking. Flooring can affect lameness inci-dence by duration of standing on a hard surface, the roughness of the surface, how slippery and wet it is, and the distance cows have to walk, especially on an uncomfort-able surface. Concrete is the most practical flooring surface to be used in confinement systems but it is not an ideal surface for cows to walk and stand on for long periods of time. Concrete should be properly grooved or stamped to provide confident footing for cows.[16] The reader is referred to a review on flooring consideration for dairy cows[16] for details on concrete floor installation. Transfer lanes can have rocks, unevenness, or be very muddy during certain seasons of the year. Puncture of the sole, leading to sole lesions and abscess, can be caused by sharp rocks, wires, nails, and other traumatic elements on transfer lanes or alleys.

Lame cows with sole ulcers had better gait scores on soft, high-friction rubber than concrete alleys.[17] Cows with more severe lameness had the greatest improvement in gait scores. Rubber flooring decreased slipping, number of strides, and time for cows to traverse the experimental walkway when compared with concrete.[18] These re-sponses were most obvious at difficult sections of the walkway, such as at the start, at a right-angle turn, and across a gutter. These results indicate that soft flooring could help alleviate the pain and reduce the wear on feet, contributing to improvements in herd lameness incidence. There has been a trend in the United States to install rubber surfaces, especially in milking parlors, and holding pens, as well as sometimes in transfer lanes and barn alleys. Installing rubber flooring in freestall barn alleys is not recommended if the barn has uncomfortable stalls. This might cause cows to stand in the alley, therefore reducing their resting time or lead them to lie down in the alley. These would have negative effects on foot health and cow welfare.

Slippery or traumatic flooring surfaces are a major risk factor for white line disease, which is a common foot lesion in freestall dairy herds.[19] The white line is the softest area of the claw and its strength is influenced by the degree of keratinization of the claw. Laminitis influences the keratinization process but the white line is also affected by mechanical trauma because it is located between the hard horn of the wall and the softer horn of the sole.

The increase in thin soles and toe ulcers due to excessive wear of the feet has been recognized as another issue in freestall herds. The toe becomes short (less than 3 inches on the dorsal surface) and the sole at the toe becomes thin (less than 0.25 inches) when there is excessive wear of the feet.[19] Observational data indicate that thin soles can be more prevalent during summer months.[19] Thin soles can also be more vulnerable to punctures. Another area of concern in freestall herds is the expo-sure to greater amounts of manure slurry and moisture, which can lead to softer feet due to moisture absorption by the claw horn. Heel horn erosion is found almost exclu-sively in confinement-housed cattle and can be considered an example of what can happen with greater exposure to moisture.[19] Foot lesions of 2665 cows housed either in tie stalls or freestalls were recorded and 48% percent of cows housed in tie stalls had 1 or more claw lesions compared with 72% in freestalls, with white line hemorrhages, white line fissures in front feet, sole hemorrhages, and heel horn erosions being significantly higher.[20] Cows housed in tie stalls are less likely to spend as much time standing on concrete. However, there are other welfare concerns with housing cows in tie stalls that are related to issues other than lameness.

A study in Canada showed an improvement in locomotion scores over a 4-week period by moving cows from concrete to pasture,[21] despite that cows on pasture actually spent less time lying down than cows kept indoors (10.9 vs 12.3 hours per day). A study in Ireland[22] compared cows housed on pasture or a freestall housing system from day 85 after calving to the end of lactation. Pasture-housed cows had less severe foot disorders, better locomotion scores, and less clinical lameness than cows in the barn system. The pasture system also resulted in longer lying times that might have beneficial effects on lameness incidence. In a study with compost-bedded pack barns,[23] cows spent only 9.3 hours per day lying down during the summer but lameness prevalence in these herds was only 7.8%. Those cows spent most of their standing time on a soft, sawdust-bedded surface rather than on hard concrete. These studies show that time spent standing is especially a concern in confinement facilities with concrete floors. However, pasture systems can expose feet to a variety of pathogens and muddy conditions. Incidence of lameness in New Zealand, a pasture-based dairy industry, has been shown to vary from 5% to 50%[24] but, in general, most of the research indicates that confinement herds have greater lameness incidence or prevalence than pasture-based herds.

SUMMARY

Cow comfort and flooring contribute to lameness incidence in dairy herds. The trigger factors for lameness, such as nutrition, hormonal changes at calving, infection, and trauma, can all be exacerbated by poor cow comfort. Housing and management factors should be optimized to reduce lameness incidence on dairy farms.

REFERENCES

1. Espejo LA, Endres MI, Salfer JA. Prevalence of lameness in high-producing Holstein cows housed in freestall barns in Minnesota. J Dairy Sci 2006;89:3052–8.
2. NAHMS. US Department of Agriculture. National Animal Health Monitoring Services. Dairy 2014. Dairy cattle management practices in the United States. 2014. Available at: https://www.aphis.usda.gov/animal_health/nahms/dairy/downloads/dairy14/Dairy14_dr_PartI.pdf. Accessed December 11, 2016.
3. Cook NB, Bennett TB, Nordlund KV. Effect of free stall surface on daily activity patterns in dairy cows with relevance to lameness prevalence. J Dairy Sci 2004;87:2912–22.
4. Dippel S, Dolezal M, Brenninkmeyer C, et al. Risk factors for lameness in freestall-housed dairy cows across two breeds, farming systems, and countries. J Dairy Sci 2009;92:5476–86.
5. Espejo LA, Endres MI. Herd-level risk factors for lameness in high-producing Holstein cows housed in free stall barns. J Dairy Sci 2007;90:306–14.
6. Westin R, Vaughan A, de Passille AM, et al. Cow- and farm-level risk factors for lameness on dairy farms with automated milking systems. J Dairy Sci 2016;99:3732–43.
7. Cook NB. Prevalence of lameness among dairy cattle in Wisconsin as a function of housing type and stall surface. J Am Vet Med Assoc 2003;223:1324–8.

8. Chapinal NA, Barrientos K, von Keyserlingk MAG, et al. Herd-level risk factors for lameness in freestall farms in the northeastern United States and California. J Dairy Sci 2013;98:318–28.

9. Cook NB, Hess JP, Foy MR, et al. Management characteristics, lameness, and body injuries of dairy cattle housed in high-performance dairy herds in Wisconsin. J Dairy Sci 2016;99:5879–91.

10. Husfeldt AW, Endres MI. Association between stall surface and some animal welfare measurements in freestall dairy herds using recycled manure solids for bedding. J Dairy Sci 2012;96:5626–34.

11. Tucker CB, Weary DM. Bedding on geotextile mattresses: How much is needed to improve cow comfort? J Dairy Sci 2004;87:2889–95.

12. Gomez A, Cook NB. Time budgets of lactating dairy cattle in commercial freestall herds. J Dairy Sci 2010;93:5772–81.

13. Cook NB, Mentink RL, Bennett TB, et al. The effect of heat stress and lameness on time budgets of lactating dairy cows. J Dairy Sci 2007;90:1674–82.

14. Krawczel PD, Hill CT, Dann HM, et al. Effect of stocking density on indices of cow comfort. J Dairy Sci 2008;91:1903–7.

15. Leonard FC, O'Connell JM, O'Farrell KJ. Effect of overcrowding on claw health in first-calved Friesian heifers. Br Vet J 1996;152:459–72.

16. Gooch C. Flooring considerations for dairy cows. 2012. Available at: http://articles.extension.org/pages/65155/flooring-considerations-for-dairy-cows. Accessed December 11, 2016.

17. Flower FC, de Passille AM, Weary DM, et al. Softer, higher-friction flooring improves gait of cows with and without sole ulcers. J Dairy Sci 2007;90:1235–42.

18. Rushen J, de Passille AM. Effects of roughness and compressibility of flooring on cow locomotion. J Dairy Sci 2006;89:2965–72.

19. Shearer JK. Effect of flooring and/or flooring surfaces on lameness disorders in dairy cattle. In Proc. Western Dairy Herd Management Conf. Reno (NV), 2007. p. 1–12. Available at: http://wdmc.org/2007/shearer.pdf. Accessed December 11, 2016.

20. Sogstada ÅM, Fjeldaasa T, Østeråsa O, et al. Prevalence of claw lesions in Norwegian dairy cattle housed in tie stalls and free stalls. Prev Vet Med 2006;70: 191–209.

21. Hernandez-Mendo O, von Keyserlingk MAG, Veira DM, et al. Effects of pasture on lameness in dairy cows. J Dairy Sci 2007;90:1209–14.

22. Olmos G, Boyle L, Hanlon A, et al. Hoof disorders, locomotion ability and lying times of cubicle-housed compared to pasture-based dairy cows. Livest Sci 2009;125:199–207.

23. Endres MI, Barberg AE. Behavior of dairy cows in an alternative bedded pack housing system. J Dairy Sci 2007;90:4192–200.

24. Bennett G, Hickford J, Zhou H, et al. Detection of *Fusobacterium necrophorum* and *Dichelobacter nodosus* in lame cattle on dairy farms in New Zealand. Res Vet Sci 2009;87:413–5.

Mobility Scoring of Finished Cattle

Lily N. Edwards-Callaway, PhD[a],*, Michelle S. Calvo-Lorenzo, PhD[b],
John A. Scanga, PhD[c], Temple Grandin, PhD[d]

KEYWORDS

- Cattle • Fatigued cattle syndrome • Lameness • Mobility • Scoring system

KEY POINTS

- Lameness in cattle is detrimental to animal welfare and can negatively affect a variety of production parameters, leading to significant economic loss.
- Multiple locomotion scoring systems are available to assess lameness in dairy cattle, which vary in the number and type of gait attributes assessed.
- There has been little research conducted to understand, measure, and monitor mobility in finished cattle.
- The North American Meat Institute Mobility Scoring System is a useful tool to measure mobility in finished cattle.
- Recent events within the beef industry have led to increased industry efforts to monitor finished cattle mobility.

INTRODUCTION

Mobility and, more specifically, lameness, in all food animal species has been a long-term focus within the livestock industry because it has a significant impact on animal well-being and production parameters. Lameness has been identified by stakeholders in the dairy industry as the most important welfare and production issue affecting dairy cattle.[1,2] Lameness is an abnormal gait or stance. It is normally caused by pain that can result from a myriad of pathologic conditions.[3] Rather than being a disease itself, lameness is a description of abnormal behavior that is a symptom resulting from an underlying health condition.[4] Regardless of the reasons that cattle express conditions of lameness, lameness causes pain to the animal[5] and can negatively affect a variety

The authors have nothing to disclose.
[a] Animal Welfare Specialist, Callalily Consulting LLC, 716 E Ridgecrest Road, Fort Collins, CO 80524, USA; [b] Elanco Animal Health, Division of Eli Lilly Company, 2500 Innovation Way, Greenfield, IN 46140, USA; [c] Protein Product Analytics, Elanco Knowledge Solutions, Elanco Animal Health, Division of Eli Lilly Company, 2500 Innovation Way, Greenfield, IN 46140, USA; [d] Department of Animal Sciences, Colorado State University, Campus Delivery 1171, Fort Collins, CO 80521, USA
* Corresponding author.
E-mail address: lilynedwards@gmail.com

Vet Clin Food Anim 33 (2017) 235–250
http://dx.doi.org/10.1016/j.cvfa.2017.02.006
0749-0720/17/© 2017 Elsevier Inc. All rights reserved.

of production parameters, such as milk yield,[6,7] and is often associated with reduced reproductive efficiency[8,9] in dairy cattle that can ultimately lead to significant economic loss.[10,11]

The occurrence of lameness in dairy cattle varies between herds because it is affected by multiple environmental and management factors. A benchmarking study on cow comfort in North American freestall dairies published by von Keyserlingk and colleagues[12] reported that the prevalence of lameness averaged from 30% to 55%, varying by geographic region. Although finished cattle can certainly suffer from lameness and it can have significant economic impacts on feedyards,[13] impaired mobility has been relatively unstudied in finished cattle compared with dairy cattle. A recent survey of feedlot managers, consulting veterinarians, and nutritionists was conducted to assess the perception of lameness within the feedlot segment of the beef cattle industry.[14] On average, survey respondents estimated that lameness incidence in the feedyard was 3.8% and contributed to less than 10% of total feedyard mortality. Prior research indicates that dairy producers usually underestimate the percentage of lame cows existent in their operations.[15,16] A more accurate estimate of the degree of lameness or its prevalence in a herd may be achieved through the use of locomotion scoring by experienced or trained observers. Although perhaps not as prevalent In finished cattle, mobility issues in feedlot cattle can affect animal welfare and have a significant economic impact via increased costs from treatment, salvage loss, and potential performance losses.[13,17]

GROWING AWARENESS OF FINISHED CATTLE MOBILITY ISSUES

Observation of cattle arriving at packing plants during the summer of 2013 rapidly heightened the focus on mobility issues. At that time, there were anecdotal reports within the meat processing community of increased numbers of market-ready cattle delivered to packing plants that, although ambulatory on arrival, were unable or unwilling to walk at some time during their lairage at the plant. This ranged from a few animals in a lot (usually a lot is defined as a group or pen from a specific origin) exhibiting what appeared to be stiffness and/or sore feet, to most of a lot exhibiting this type of impairment. In addition, some individual animals exhibited such extreme mobility impairment that they were described as statue-like. Cattle displaying this type of altered gait behavior were often unable to keep up with contemporaries in their respective groups; the separation of which caused additional stress to the animal but also negatively affected operational efficiencies at the packing plant. In 2006, Dr Grandin[18,19] made similar observations in 3 different groups of cattle arriving at packing plants when temperatures were elevated above 90°F (32°C). Grandin reported that approximately 5% to 10% of cattle were panting from each truckload observed, some lying down and open-mouth breathing (ie, panting hard with their tongues extended), and some acting stiff and arthritic.

During the summer of 2013, the National Cattlemen's Beef Association (NCBA) held several industry discussions on the topic of cattle welfare, specifically highlighting perceived issues with beta-adrenergic agonist (BAA) growth promotants because this was an underlying concern with some of the impaired mobility observations. At the final NCBA meeting, video evidence of cattle with impaired mobility at packing plants was presented. This led to a cascade of events, resulting in the packing industry's voluntary refusal to purchase cattle fed with zilpaterol hydrochloride (Zilmax; Merck Animal Health; Desoto, KS, USA). This reaction was due to a perception that zilpaterol was the causative or common factor responsible for the reduced mobility of cattle observed. Unfortunately, at that time, neither the cattle nor pharmaceutical industries had sufficient data to quantify what was happening at packing plants, or data to support that the actions taken were justified or effective in improving the mobility of cattle arriving at and being held in lairage at packing plants.

MOBILITY AND LOCOMOTION SCORING SYSTEMS
Scoring Systems Used Primarily in Dairy Cattle

In the wake of the heightened interest in understanding the prevalence and impact of mobility issues in finished cattle, it became evident that a standard tool for measuring mobility of finished cattle was needed to capture aspects of cattle lameness and the inability of the animals to keep up with the pace of their contemporary group. There are multiple locomotion scoring systems used to assess lameness in dairy cattle. Practical uses for locomotion scoring might include the assessment of lameness severity in lame animals or as a tool for the estimation of herd lameness prevalence. Locomotion scoring is also used in lameness research and is an important criterion in welfare assessment and audit programs. Selected scoring systems are listed in **Table 1**. Established locomotion and mobility scoring systems were developed for use primarily in dairy cattle but vary in the number of categories within the scale, numerical assignment (ie, beginning with 0 vs beginning with 1), language used to describe each category, parameters used to assess locomotion, and the application of the measurement tool. Thus, a standard tool does not exist. Many of the locomotion scoring systems used in dairy cattle research assign a discrete score to an animal using a 5-point scale (eg, 1–5; 1, normal; 2, mildly lame; 3, moderately lame; 4, lame; 5, severely lame; see **Table 1**).[20–24] Much of the variation in the 5-point locomotion scoring systems is in the number and combinations of attributes used to determine the locomotion score, such as gait asymmetry, reluctance to bear weight, back arch, joint flexion, tracking up, and head bobbing. Several studies have demonstrated poor repeatability and lack of agreement between scorers when using these scales to score locomotion.[22,24] In addition, several reports indicate substantial variation in the ability of farm managers or farm owners to identify altered locomotion in dairy cattle compared with trained observers. Lameness detected by trained observers was 2.5 to 4 times higher than estimates by farm owners or managers.[16,25,26] Training and the use of more specific terms and detailed descriptions can help reduce observer variability.[24] The National Milk Producers Federation Farmers Assuring Responsible Management (FARM) Program (version 3.0) requires locomotion scoring as part of their dairy farm assessment and uses a 3-point locomotion scoring system (see **Table 1**).[27] This simplified system is intended to reduce interobserver variability among farm evaluators. Similarly, the researchers for the National Animal Health Monitoring System (NAHMS) Dairy Cattle benchmarking survey created a 3-point locomotion scoring system, rather than using a 5-point scale, to reduce complexity in scoring method when using such a large number of evaluators.[28]

Locomotion Scoring Systems Used Primarily in Finished Cattle

There does not exist an extensive body of literature on locomotion scoring in finished cattle. Terrell and colleagues,[29] at the Beef Cattle Institute at Kansas State University, developed a 4-point locomotion scoring system for use in finished cattle (see **Table 1**). Their system assesses clinical lameness using the animal's stride length, head movement, adduction or abduction of affected limb or limbs, willingness to move, and willingness to place weight on the limb. The Step-Up Locomotion Scoring program is part of the Zinpro Corporation Step-Up Management Program for Beef Cattle and was

Table 1
Selection of locomotion scoring systems used in dairy and finished cattle

	Locomotion and Mobility Numerical Score Category					
	0	1	2	3	4	5
Finished Cattle Locomotion Scoring Systems						
NAMI Mobility Scoring System[32]	—	Normal: Walks easily with no apparent lameness or change in gait.	Exhibits minor stiffness, shortness of stride or a slight limp but keeps up with normal cattle in the group.	Exhibits obvious stiffness, difficulty taking steps, an obvious limp or obvious discomfort, and lags behind normal cattle walking as a group.	Extremely reluctant to move even when encouraged by a handler. Described as statue-like.	—
Terrell,[29] 2016	Normal: Animal walks normally. No apparent lameness or change in gait.	Mild lameness: Animal exhibits shortened stride, may move head slightly side to side but no head bob.	Moderate lameness: Animal exhibits a limp, with an obviously identifiable limb or limbs affected and/or head bob present when walking. Limbs still bears weight.	Severe lameness: Animal applies little or no weight to affected limb while standing or walking. Animal reluctant or unable to move. While walking, animal's head dropped, back arched, with head bob and limp detected.	—	—

	1	2	3	4	5
Step-Up Locomotion Scoring System[30]	Normal: Animal walks normally with no apparent lameness or change in gait. Hind feet land in a similar location to front feet.	Mild lameness: Animal exhibits short stride when walking, dropping its head slightly. Animal does not exhibit a limp when walking.	Moderate lameness: Animal exhibits obvious limp, favoring affected limbs, which still bear weight. A slight head bob is present when the animal is walking.	Severe lameness: Animal applies little or no weight to affected limb and is reluctant or unable to move. While walking, animal's head is dropped and back arched, with head bob and limp detected.	—

Dairy Locomotion Scoring Systems

	1	2	3	4	5
Sprecher et al,[21] 1997	Normal: The cow stands and walks with a level-back posture. Her gait is normal.	Mildly lame: The cow stands and walks with a level-back posture but develops an arched-back posture while walking. Her gait remains normal.	Moderately lame: An arched-back posture is evident both while standing and walking. Her gait is affected and is best described as short-striding with 1 or more limbs.	Lame: An arched-back posture is always evident and gait is best described as 1 deliberate step at a time. The cow favors 1 or more limbs or feet.	Severely lame: The cow additionally demonstrates an inability or extreme reluctance to bear weight on 1 or more of her limbs or feet.
Zinpro Locomotion Scoring of Dairy Cattle	Normal: Stands and walks normally with a level back. Makes long confident strides.	Mildly lame: Stands with flat back but arches when walks. Gait is slightly abnormal.	Moderately lame: Stands and walks with an arched back and short strides with 1 or more legs. Slight sinking of dew-claws in limb opposite to the affected limb may be evident.	Lame: Arched back standing and walking. Favoring 1 or more limbs but can still bear some weight on them. Sinking of the dew-claws is evident in the limb opposite to the affected limb.	Severely lame: Pronounced arching of back. Reluctant to move, with almost complete weight transfer off the affected limb.

(continued on next page)

Table 1
(continued)

	Locomotion and Mobility Numerical Score Category			
FARM[27] Program Scoring System	—	Sound: Animal has normal posture and a normal gait.	Moderate lameness: Stands well but is noted to favor a limb when walking.	Severe lameness: Animal either unable to move or able to move but barely able to bear weight on the affected limb. Signs may also include back arch, poor body condition, head bob, and an inability to flex the lower leg joints. This cow is sore on her left rear leg, favoring it both standing and walking.	—

Category descriptions are listed under the corresponding numerical category. Descriptions signifying similar levels of locomotion across scoring systems are shaded similarly. If a numerical locomotion category within a system has an em dash, it was not shared by other scoring systems.

Data from Refs.[21,27,29,30,32]; and Zinpro Corporation Dairy Locomotion Scoring. Zinpro Corporation. 2016. Available at: http://www.zinpro.com/lameness/dairy/locomotion-scoring. Accessed January 2017.

created in conjunction with the aforementioned work of Terrell and colleagues.[29,30] A recent study by Simon and colleagues[31] assessing welfare parameters on cow-calf operations included a 3-point system to capture locomotion scores in cows (1, acceptable; 2, moderately lame; 3, severely lame). Similar to some of the other large-scale benchmarking studies or audit programs, this study assessed in part the feasibility of cow-calf on-farm animal welfare audits and, therefore, the scoring system would need to be easily trained and repeatable across multiple observers in the long-term.

As mentioned previously, the feedlot cattle industry recognized the need for a mobility scoring system to capture and measure cattle mobility at packing plants. To address this need, industry experts met to establish a locomotion scoring system for finished cattle with the packing plant application in mind. The parameter not included in the multiple dairy cattle and the limited number of fed beef cattle locomotion scoring systems is the consideration and identification of individual animals that cannot keep pace with their contemporaries. In the groups of cattle at packing plants reported to have impaired mobility, it was evident there was a clear difference between individuals in their ability to maintain the speed of their overall group (personal observations, Edwards-Callaway, 2013). Some animals exhibiting signs of stiffness or soreness were still able to maintain a normal walking speed, whereas others were so impaired they lagged behind most cattle in their group. This was an important distinction to be able to capture in a scoring system. The North American Meat Institute (NAMI) Animal Welfare Committee in collaboration with industry experts helped facilitate and guide the process of establishing what is now referred to as the NAMI Mobility Scoring System used in the packing industry.[32] This system has 4 categories of locomotion:

- Mobility score 1, normal, walks easily with no apparent lameness or change in gait
- Mobility score 2, exhibits minor stiffness, shortness of stride, or a slight limp but keeps up with normal cattle in the group
- Mobility score 3, exhibits obvious stiffness, difficulty taking steps, an obvious limp or obvious discomfort, and lags behind normal cattle walking as a group
- Mobility score 4, extremely reluctant to move even when encouraged by a handler; described as statue-like.

To enhance the use of this scoring system, NAMI developed a training video[32] that provides imagery for each score and guidance on the application of the scoring system at commercial operations. Thus far, this scoring system has been effective in capturing mobility issues in finished cattle arriving at packing facilities.

CURRENT RESEARCH ON MOBILITY IN FINISHED CATTLE

Cattle mobility concerns in the beef industry that were recently reported in the summer of 2013 involved cattle that were nonambulatory; slow and difficult to move; and, in some cases, experiencing sloughed hoof walls.[33,34] Discussions about these anecdotal reports between industry stakeholders and animal health experts revealed there was insufficient scientific evidence to determine specific causes at the time but initiated the development of industry mobility programs and scientific studies to better understand this disease-state in finished cattle. Likewise, finished cattle lameness in the United States has remained a welfare and economic loss issue for many years, with improvements needed in lameness identification, diagnosis, and treatment.[35] A recent survey indicated that there is still a knowledge gap on improving lameness-related issues in the feedlot industry and there continues to be increased concerns on the impact of lameness on cattle comfort and welfare.[14] Several research studies have indicated the benefits of using objective and subjective methods to improve evaluation of both mobility and lameness conditions in cattle. Objective methods include technologies used to measure the velocity of animal movement, stride length, posture, number of steps over time, and pressure or weight distribution by individual limbs when animals move across a platform (comprehensive reviews are available[35,36]). As mentioned, subjective scoring systems are available for routine use by farm or slaughter facility employees. Some of these have application in research, whereas others are used in welfare programs to monitor and improve beef cattle mobility conditions. However, there is little research published on impaired mobility of finished beef cattle and, therefore, there is much to be learned and applied from the dairy cattle lameness literature. Altogether, objective and subjective methods are needed to monitor the prevalence of mobility issues, understand the behavioral and physiologic changes associated with poor mobility, determine and mitigate factors related to impaired mobility conditions, and help establish effective treatment outcomes.

Locomotion scoring systems that have been used extensively in dairy cattle lameness research include subjective scoring systems that are typically based on the absence, presence, and/or alteration of the following behaviors: arching of the spine, limb favoring, altered stride lengths, tenderness, reduced speed, head bobbing, changes in placement of the claw, abduction or adduction in rotation of the feet, and reluctance to move.[20,21,23,24,37–39] Although many locomotion scoring systems are used in research to noninvasively quantify lameness and grade severity, the behaviors evaluated across these scoring systems will vary across investigators, may be prone to poor reliability and reproducibility, are influenced by the scorer's skill and perception, and little work has validated such systems in relation to pain and other welfare outcomes.[22,35,40,41] To overcome some of these limitations, several research groups have investigated quantitative measures of posture and gait in dairy cattle to detect painful lameness. These measures include assessing image analyses of back posture,[42] force per weighing platforms,[43–49] pressure mats,[50] kinematic gait variables,[39,51,52] electromyography,[53] accelerometers or pedometers,[23,54] nociceptive thresholds,[55,56] heart rate,[50] and cortisol concentrations.[50] Collectively, these exploratory studies emphasize that, although quantitative gait measures can be collected with a high degree of consistency, they do not necessarily provide a better measure of pain than the subjective scoring systems. This is because either approach, subjective or objective, will depend on the degree of pain experienced by the animal, the sensitivity and specificity of the measures, the efficacy and practicality of real-time measures on farms and slaughter facilities, and the training of the observer.[40] With regard to monitoring and studying finished cattle mobility, these aspects will need to be considered and emphasized as research progresses in understanding the disease-state of finished cattle experiencing mobility issues.

Many factors are hypothesized to be associated with poor mobility and research has been progressing over the last few years to investigate more of these factors. One factor that has been studied in relationship to cattle mobility is BAAs, which are fed to improve feed efficiency and increase lean muscle mass in finishing cattle.[57] BAAs have been challenged by welfare experts[19] and questioned when impaired mobility of BAA-fed cattle at slaughter facilities were coupled with clinical symptoms and serum biochemical abnormalities, now known as the fatigued cattle syndrome (FCS).[58] Therefore, mobility scoring systems have been used to help determine the impacts of BAA on mobility and other welfare concerns in cattle. For instance, a mobility scoring system (Tyson Foods mobility scoring system: 0, normal, through 4, nonambulatory or severe distress) was used to determine if zilpaterol hydrochloride (Zilmax;

Merck Animal Health; Desoto, KS, USA) and shade provision affected cattle mobility and other measures of performance, physiology, and carcass quality of finishing steers.[59] Overall, the investigators found that feeding zilpaterol hydrochloride (8.33 mg/kg dry matter for the last 21 days on feed [DOF] with a 3-day withdrawal period) had minimal impact on cattle mobility and suggested that mobility may be exacerbated as cattle gain weight, are transported, and stand on concrete at the packing plant, regardless of feeding zilpaterol hydrochloride. Similarly, other unpublished studies found minimal impacts on feedlot cattle mobility when BAAs were fed (BAA treatment diet included zilpaterol hydrochloride at 6.76 g/ton for the last 20 DOF with a 3-day to 4-day withdrawal period).[60,61] Another study by Woiwode and Grandin[62] assessed the welfare of cattle fed zilpaterol hydrochloride (81.6 mg/head/day for 20 days with a 4 to 6 day withdrawal period) at the feedyard and found no differences in mobility. However, cattle were not observed at the packing plant. Two studies by Hagenmaier and colleagues[63,64] used physiologic measures and the NAMI Mobility Scoring System[30] to investigate if high-stress handling and ractopamine hydrochloride (Optaflexx; Elanco Animal Health, Greenfield, IN, USA) negatively affected fed cattle mobility, FCS, and physiologic responses. Collectively, these studies found that ractopamine (fed at 400 mg/head/day for 35 to 36 days[63] or 28 days[64]) did not adversely affect mobility at the feedlot. However, abnormal mobility scores increased across all treatment groups following transport and lairage at the slaughter facility. The investigators also reported that, although hormonal responses were altered in ractopamine-fed cattle following high-stress handling and transportation, metabolic acidosis (a precursor for FCS) can be developed in cattle exposed to high-stress handling regardless of ractopamine inclusion, emphasizing the importance of handling intensity on cattle welfare. Other factors to consider that may contribute to impaired mobility and FCS include breed, extreme weather conditions, sorting cattle by mixed body weights before transport, higher body weights, handling practices during loading and unloading, distances cattle have to walk before loading or after unloading, and transport duration and conditions, as well as cattle footing throughout the feedyard, slaughter facility, and on trucks.[58,62,65] Altogether, it is apparent that cattle mobility is a multifactorial issue that warrants further research to evaluate multiple factors and mitigate their potential effects on mobility.

The mobility scoring systems used in the aforementioned studies have helped establish new knowledge of the complex nature of impaired mobility in finished cattle. The limitations in using these scoring systems, however, include the subjective nature of how observers apply the scores and the large number of animals required to detect differences among a population. Thus, future research evaluating factors potentially associated with impaired mobility will need to assess large populations and/or couple mobility welfare tools with objective measures, many that have already been studied extensively in the dairy cattle lameness literature and developed with FCS research. Furthermore, additional data on mobility conditions across the industry are needed to better understand and monitor the prevalence of this disease-state industry-wide. These collective approaches may help overcome limitations and provide a systematic approach to identifying and managing mobility problems.

INDUSTRY EFFORTS TO IMPROVE AND MONITOR FINISHED CATTLE MOBILITY

Immediately following the events in 2013, it became evident that there was an instantaneous vacuum of information regarding finished cattle mobility and this created a sense of urgency among industry stakeholders to work toward understanding and appropriately measuring finished cattle mobility. Within weeks of the NCBA industry meetings, data gathering efforts across the industry were launched. As previously discussed, the first step taken in gathering this data was developing and standardizing a system for mobility scoring of finished cattle that could be disseminated across the industry. There was then a need to develop programs in which this information could be captured, analyzed, and shared across the North American beef industry. One approach is the Full Value Beef Cattle Mobility Assessment program launched by Elanco Animal Health in August of 2013. In this program, trained mobility evaluators score individual cattle during the process of unloading, antemortem inspection, or lairage at packing plants using the NAMI Mobility Scoring System. Evaluators are trained to observe and identify cattle that exhibit an abnormal mobility score. Although individual cattle are evaluated, all information in this program is accumulated back to a slaughter lot level. If available, additional information is obtained on each lot of cattle, such as gender, breed type, weight, head count, transportation distance, truck wait time before unloading at the plant, and weather conditions at the feedlot of origin and packing plant. This information is then used to identify issues and trends that are observed in cattle at slaughter. Risk assessments are also conducted to determine if specific factors (eg, gender, breed, temperature, and slaughter weight) are significant and to calculate odds ratios on significant effects. As with any population data-based program, sampling rates and volume of information are important in determining what inferences and conclusions can be drawn from the information. As of December 2016, this program has collected data over the past 3.5 years on approximately 6.3 million cattle from more than 61,000 individual slaughter lots across 12 plants in 7 states and 1 Canadian province. Across all cattle evaluated in this program, 92.1% of cattle scored walked with normal mobility (mobility Score 1) and 0.5% were identified as mobility score 3 or 4. At a high level, there is a seasonal trend with the number of cattle identified as a mobility score 2 or higher increasing during the warmer months of the year and being at their lowest levels from November through March (**Fig. 1**).

In the wake of the events in 2013, large packing companies also initiated internal mobility monitoring programs at their beef processing facilities to ensure that each lot of cattle processed received a score. Thus if repetitive or severe situations of cattle immobility are observed, feedback and interaction with the supply chain could be initiated. One individual company implemented a program in which lots (ie, groups or pens) of cattle are scored using a 4-point scale (0–4), which is similar to the NAMI Mobility Scoring system and subsequently assigned a categorical score for the movement of the group: movement codes A or B. Movement code A (desirable) is assigned to lots of cattle that include individuals with a mobility score similar to that of the NAMI Mobility Scoring system of 1 or 2. Movement code B (undesirable) is assigned to groups of cattle in which 50% or more of the observed individuals within the lot are identified as NAMI mobility score 3, any instance of a NAMI mobility score 4, or a non-ambulatory animal. In this program, producers receive feedback on their lot settlement sheets, which creates an opportunity for communication and engagement between the production and packing sectors in addressing issues of cattle welfare and mobility. Currently, a universal standard for an acceptable level of mobility impairment within a lot of finished cattle at the packing facilities does not exist and thus packing companies may apply slightly different rules of reporting than those discussed in this scenario. That being said, it was recognized in the packing industry that a standardized method for mobility scoring was needed and most of internal company programs are likely based on the NAMI Mobility Scoring System.

In any process in which industry-wide data are being collected, it is important to recognize and address data collection challenges. Some of the challenges associated with large-scale cattle mobility scoring efforts are consistency and subjectivity of mobility scoring, the environment in which cattle are evaluated, and the speed at which cattle must be evaluated in commercial environments. Ongoing evaluator training and correlation is important in any subjective evaluation system, as is a thorough evaluation of the processes occurring during the handling and lairage of cattle at the location of scoring. Identifying the proper locations that are safe for the evaluator and cattle, does not affect the flow of cattle through the process, and provides an unobstructed vantage point to view individual cattle in motion is crucial to obtaining useful and reliable information. Even when all of these factors are addressed, it has become apparent through data collection experience that comparisons of cattle mobility scores across environments (eg, plants, handling facilities) can be misleading and more appropriate benchmarks focus on evaluations at common locations, under similar environmental conditions, when scored by a single evaluator.

Analysis of these data has not identified a single causative factor but rather emphasizes (1) that this is a multifactorial issue and (2) that, although individual cattle may be identified as having the same mobility score, they are likely to be exhibiting symptoms of different maladies. Thus, drawing conclusions from single day, plant, or lot events will likely lead to erroneous findings. However, these data allow the beef industry to understand trends and shifts in cattle movement at packing plants and help identify

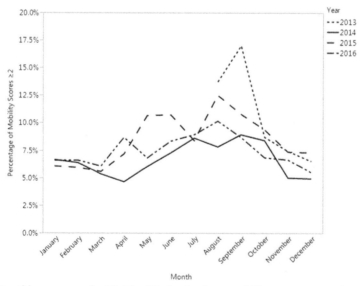

Fig. 1. Monthly averages of cattle identified as having a mobility score greater than or equal to 2 per the NAMI Mobility Scoring System (1, normal, walks easily with no apparent lameness or change in gait; 2, exhibits minor stiffness, shortness of stride, or a slight limp but keeps up with normal cattle in the group; 3, exhibits obvious stiffness, difficulty taking steps, an obvious limp or obvious discomfort and lags behind normal cattle walking as a group; 4, extremely reluctant to move even when encouraged by a handler, statue-like). The data represent information from approximately 6.3 million fed cattle from up to 12 commercial packing plants in 7 states and 1 Canadian province from August 2013 through December 2016. During the collection of the data presented, zilpaterol hydrochloride was available on the market until October 2013. BAA use cannot be tracked in this database, thus cattle observed in the data presented may or may not have been fed BAA. (*Courtesy of* and with permission from Elanco Animal Health, Greenfield, Indiana, 2017).

and address repetitive outcomes with the supply chain. This has led to conversations with feedyards, nutritionists, veterinarians, and processors working together to collaboratively identify root causes and implement changes that ultimately improve the welfare of cattle entering the food supply.

SUMMARY

Lameness is an important issue in both dairy and finished cattle because it negatively affects animal welfare and can be costly due to its impact on animal production and performance. Additionally, lameness (locomotion) scoring has become a component of on-farm assessment programs such as the FARM Program and this area is likely to grow in other cattle sectors. Although finished cattle lameness may not have been a top priority for the industry in the past, its relationship to the use of new technologies used in the industry will likely make it a focus and, therefore, area of needed research in the future.[66] The NAMI Mobility Scoring System provides an opportunity for the beef industry to use a standardized method for locomotion scoring in finished cattle as additional data collection, monitoring, analytics, and benchmarking activities are performed. The use of the NAMI system has helped establish new knowledge in the complex nature of impaired mobility in finished cattle. Future research evaluating impaired mobility will need to assess large populations and/or couple mobility scoring programs with objective measures such as those used in lameness and FCS research. Furthermore, additional data on finished cattle mobility across the industry are needed to better understand the multifactorial nature of impaired mobility, and to effectively monitor the prevalence of this disease-state industry-wide. Collectively, these efforts may help provide further insight to the welfare of finished cattle and provide a systematic approach to identifying and managing mobility problems.

ACKNOWLEDGMENTS

Authors would like to acknowledge Lora Wright and Paula Alexander, Tyson Fresh Meats, Dakota Dunes, NE, for their contributions to this publication.

REFERENCES

1. von Keyserlingk MAG, Rushen J, de Passille AM, et al. Improving dairy cattle welfare: key concepts and the role of science. J Dairy Sci 2009;92:4101–11.
2. Ventura BA, von Keyserlingk MAG, Weary DM. Animal welfare concerns and values of stakeholders within the dairy industry. J Agric Environ Ethics 2015;28:109–26.
3. Archer SC, Bell N, Huxley J. Lameness in UK dairy cows: a review of the current status. In Prac 2010;32:492–504.
4. Webster AJF, Knott L, Tarlton JF. Understanding lameness in the dairy cow. Cattle Pract 1986;13:93–8.
5. Whay H, Waterman A, Webster A. Associations between locomotion, claw lesions and nociceptive threshold in dairy heifers during pre-partum period. Vet J 1997; 154:155–61.
6. Green LE, Hedges VJ, Schukken YH, et al. The impact of clinical lameness on the milk yield of dairy cows. J Dairy Sci 2002;85:2250–6.
7. Juarez ST, Robinson PH, DePeters EJ, et al. Impact of lameness on behavior and productivity of lactating Holstein cows. Appl Anim Behav Sci 2003;83:1–14.
8. Collick DW, Ward WR, Dobson H. Association between types of lameness and fertility. Vet Rec 1989;125:103–6.

9. Melendez P, Bartolome J, Archbald LF, et al. The association between lameness, ovarian cysts and fertility in lactating dairy cows. Theriogenology 2003;59: 927–37.

10. Kossaibati MA, Esslemont RJ. The cost of production diseases in dairy herds in England. Vet J 1997;154:41–51.

11. Willshire JA, Bell NJ. An economic review of cattle lameness. Cattle Pract 2009; 17:136–41.

12. von Keyserlingk MAG, Barrientos A, Ito K, et al. Benchmarking cow comfort on North American freestall dairies: lameness, leg injuries, lying times, facility design, and management for high-production Holstein dairy cows. J Dairy Sci 2012;95:7399–408.

13. Griffin D, Perino L, Hudson D. Feedlot lameness. Animal Diseases, Neb Guide, Institute of Agriculture and Natural Resources, Cooperative Extension University of Nebraska Lincoln 1993. G93–1159A. Available at: http://www.feedbarnstore.com/animalscience/beef/g1159.pdf. Accessed January 28, 2017.

14. Terrell SP, Thomson DU, Reinhardt CD, et al. Perception of lameness management, education and effects on animal welfare of feedlot cattle by consulting nutritionists, veterinarians, and feedlot managers. Bov Pract 2014;48:53–60.

15. Fabian J, Laven PA, Whay HR. The prevalence of lameness in New Zealand dairy farms: A comparison of farmer's estimates and locomotion scoring. Vet J 2014; 201:31–8.

16. Espejo LA, Endres MI, Salfer JA. Prevalence of lameness in high-producing Holstein cows housed in freestall barns in Minnesota. J Dairy Sci 2006;89: 3052–8.

17. Tibbetts GK, Devin TM, Griffin D, et al. Effects of a single foot rot incident on weight performance of feedlot steers. Prof Anim Sci 2006;22:450–3.

18. Grandin T. Improving animal welfare: a practical approach. Wallingford (United Kingdom): CABI Publishing; 2010.

19. Grandin T. Heat stress and lameness in feedlot cattle is detrimental to welfare. 2014. Available at: http://grandin.com/heat.stress.lameness.html. Accessed January 7, 2017.

20. Manson FJ, Leaver JD. The influence of concentrate amount on locomotion and clinical lameness in dairy cattle. Anim Prod 1988;47:185–90.

21. Sprecher DJ, Hostetler DE, Kaneene JB. A lameness scoring system that uses posture and gait to predict dairy cattle reproductive performance. Theriogenology 1997;47:1179–87.

22. Winckler C, Willen S. The reliability and repeatability of a lameness scoring system for use as an indicator of welfare in dairy cattle. Acta Agriculturae Scandinavica 2001;51:103–7.

23. O'Callaghan KAO, Cripps PJ, Downham DY, et al. Subjective and objective assessment of pain and discomfort due to lameness in dairy cattle. Animal Welfare 2003;12:605–10.

24. Flower FC, Weary DM. Effect of hoof pathologies on subjective assessment of dairy cow gait. J Dairy Sci 2006;89:139–46.

25. Whay HR, Main DCJ, Green LE, et al. Assessment of the welfare of dairy cattle using animal-based measurements: direct observations and investigation of farm records. Vet Rec 2003;153:197–202.

26. Wells SJ, Trent AM, Marsh WE, et al. Prevalence and severity of lameness in lactating dairy cows in a sample of Minnesota and Wisconsin herds. J Am Vet Med Assoc 1993;202(1):78–82.

27. FARM. Farmers Assuring Responsible Management Animal Care Reference Manual, Version 3.0, Appendix C. 2016. Available at: http://nationaldairyfarm.com/sites/default/files/Version%203.0%20References%20and%20Appendices.pdf. Accessed January 28, 2017.

28. Adams AE, Lombard JE, Fossler CP, et al. Associations between housing and management practices and the prevalence of lameness, hock lesions, and thin cows on US dairy operations. J Dairy Sci 2017;100:2119–36.

29. Terrell SP. Feedlot lameness: industry perceptions, locomotion scoring, lameness morbidity, and association of locomotion score and diagnosis with case outcome in beef cattle in Great Plains feedlots. Manhattan (KS). Kansas State University; 2016.

30. Step-Up® Locomotion Scoring System. Zinpro Corporation. 2016. Available at: http://www.zinpro.com/lameness/beef/locomotion-scoring. Accessed January 2017.

31. Simon GE, Hoar BR, Tucker CB. Assessing cow welfare. Part 1: Benchmarking beef cow health and behavior, handling; and management, facilities, and producer perspectives. J Anim Sci 2016;94:3476–87.

32. NAMI. North American Meat Institute Mobility Scoring System. 2016. Available at: https://www.youtube.com/watch?v=QIsIfHCvkpg. Accessed January 2017.

33. Cima G. Cattle drug's sales suspended after lameness reports. J Am Vet Med Assoc 2013;243:1086.

34. Vance A. Tyson stops buying cattle fed popular beta-agonist. Feedstuffs. 2013. Available at: http://www.feedstuffs.com/story-tyson-stops-buying-cattle-fed-popular-beta agonist-45–101133. Accessed January 5, 2017.

35. Shearer JK, Stock ML, Van Amstel SR, et al. Assessment and management of pain associated with lameness in cattle. Vet Clin North Am Food Anim Pract 2013;29:135–56.

36. Van Nuffel A, Zwertvaegher I, Van Weyenberg S, et al. Lameness detection in dairy cows: Part 2. Use of sensors to automatically register changes in locomotion or behavior. Animals (Basel) 2015;5:861–85.

37. Whay HR. Locomotion scoring and lameness detection in dairy cattle. Practice 2002;24:444–9.

38. Telezhenko E, Bergsten C. Influence of floor type on the locomotion of dairy cows. Appl Anim Behav Sci 2005;93:183–97.

39. Van Nuffel A, Sprenger M, Tuyttens FAM, et al. Cow gait scores and kinematic gait data: can people see gait irregularities? Animal Welfare 2009;18:433–9.

40. Weary DM, Niel L, Flower C, et al. Identifying and preventing pain in animals. Appl Anim Behav Sci 2006;100:64–76.

41. Tuyttens FAM, Sprenger M, Van Nuffel A, et al. Reliability of categorical versus continuous scoring of welfare indicators: Lameness in cows as a case study. Animal Welfare 2009;18:399–405.

42. Poursaberi A, Bahr C, Pluk A, et al. Real-time automatic lameness detection based on back posture extraction in dairy cattle: Shape analysis of cow with image processing techniques. Comput Electron Agric 2010;74:110–9.

43. Rajkondawar PG, Tasch U, Lefcourt AM, et al. A system for identifying lameness in dairy cattle. Appl Eng Agric 2002;18:87–96.

44. Neveux S, Weary DM, Rushen J, et al. Hoof discomfort changes how dairy cattle distribute their body weight. J Dairy Sci 2006;89:2503–9.

45. Rushen J, Pombourcq E, de Passille AM. Validation of two measures of lameness in dairy cows. Appl Anim Behav Sci 2006;106:173–7.

46. Pastell M, Kujala M, Aisla AM, et al. Detecting cows lameness using force sensors. Comput Electron Agric 2008;64:34–8.

47. Chapinal N, de Passille AM, Rushen J. Weight distribution and gait in dairy cattle are affected by milking and late pregnancy. J Dairy Sci 2009;92:581–8.

48. Chapinal N, de Passille AM, Rushen J, et al. Automated methods for detecting lameness and measuring analgesia in dairy cattle. J Dairy Sci 2010;93:2007–13.

49. Chapinal N, de Passille AM, Rushen J, et al. Effect of analgesia during hoof trimming on gait, weight distribution, and activity of dairy cattle. J Dairy Sci 2010;93:3039–46.

50. Kotschwar JL, Coetzee JF, Anderson DE, et al. Analgesic efficacy of sodium salicylate in an amphotericin B-induced bovine synovitis-arthritis model. J Dairy Sci 2009;92:3731–43.

51. Flower FC, Sanderson DJ, Weary DM. Hoof pathologies influence kinematic measures of dairy cow gait. J Dairy Sci 2005;88:3166–73.

52. Flower FC, de Passille AM, Weary DM, et al. Softer, higher-friction flooring improves gait of cows with and without sole ulcers. J Dairy Sci 2007;90:1235–42.

53. Rajapaksha E, Tucker CB. How do cattle respond to sloped floors? An investigation using behavior and electromyograms. J Dairy Sci 2014;97:2808–15.

54. Pastell M, Tiusanen J, Hakojärvi M, et al. A wireless accelerometer system with wavelet analysis for assessing lameness in cattle. Biosyst Eng 2009;104:545–51.

55. Whay HR, Webster AJ, Waterman-Pearson AE. Role of ketoprofen in the modulation of hyperalgesia associated with lameness in dairy cattle. Vet Rec 2005;157:729–33.

56. Laven RA, Lawrence KE, Weston JF, et al. Assessment of the duration of the pain response associated with lameness in dairy cows, and the influence of treatment. N Z Vet J 2008;56:210–7.

57. Strydom PE, Frylinck L, Montgomery JL, et al. The comparison of three β agonists for growth performance, carcass characteristics and meat quality of feedlot cattle. Meat Sci 2009;81:557–64.

58. Thomson DU, Loneragan GH, Henningson JN, et al. Description of a novel fatigue syndrome of finished feedlot cattle following transportation. J Am Vet Med Assoc 2015;247:66–72.

59. Boyd BM, Shackelford SD, Hales KE, et al. Effects of shade and feeding zilpaterol hydrochloride to finishing steers on performance, carcass quality, heat stress, mobility, and body temperature. J Anim Sci 2015;93:5801–11.

60. Bernhard BC, Maxwell CL, O'Neill CF, et al. The effects of technology use in feedlot production systems on the performance, behavior and welfare of steers finishing during late summer. In: Proceedings of the Plains Nutrition Council Spring Conference, San Antonio (TX), 2014. p. 142–3. Available at: http://amarillo.tamu.edu/files/2010/10/2014-Proceedings-final.pdf. Accessed January 7, 2017.

61. Burson WC, Thompson AJ, Jennings MA, et al. Evaluation of objective and subjective mobility variables in feedlot cattle supplemented with zilpaterol hydrochloride. In: Proceedings of the Plains Nutrition Council Spring Conference, San Antonio, TX, 2014. p. 145. Available at: http://amarillo.tamu.edu/files/2010/10/2014-Proceedings-final.pdf. Accessed January 7, 2017.

62. Woiwode R, Grandin T. Field study on the effect of zilpaterol on the behavior and mobility of Brahman cross steers at a commercial feedlot. 2013. Final Report to the National Cattlemen's Beef Association.

63. Hagenmaier JA, Reinhardt CD, Bartle SJ, et al. Effect of handling intensity at the time of transport to slaughter on physiological response and carcass characteristics in beef cattle fed ractopamine hydrochloride. J Anim Sci, in press.

64. Hagenmaier JA, Reinhardt CD, Ritter MJ, et al. Effects of ractopamine hydrochloride on growth performance, carcass characteristics, and physiological response to different handling techniques. J Anim Sci, in press.

65. Frese DA, Reinhardt CD, Bartle SJ, et al. Cattle handling technique can induce fatigued cattle syndrome in cattle not fed a beta adrenergic agonist. J Anim Sci 2016;94:581–91.

66. Tucker CB, Coetzee JF, Stookey JM, et al. Beef cattle welfare in the USA: identification of priorities for future research. Anim Health Res Rev 2015;1–18.

Diagnosis and Prognosis of Common Disorders Involving the Proximal Limb

André Desrochers, DMV, MS

KEYWORDS

- Lameness • Cattle • Surgery • Fracture • Septic arthritis • Osteochondritis

KEY POINTS

- Lameness originating from the proximal limb is more challenging because it is less visible.
- Palpation of the limb combined with specific manipulations are essential to determine the affected area.
- A precise diagnosis will help the clinician to provide appropriate treatment recommendations.

 Video content accompanies this article at http://www.vetfood.theclinics.com.

It has been well known that the feet are at the origin of most lameness in cattle. Nowadays, claw trimmers, producers, and veterinarians are better trained to handle claw diseases. Unless there is an obvious visual cause to explain the lameness and feet have been checked, the affected animal is often treated empirically with antibiotics and nonsteroidal antiinflammatory drugs. A basic knowledge of the most common conditions and their prognosis might preclude the unnecessary administration of drugs avoiding the risk of residue. Moreover, a more precise diagnosis will help the veterinarian and the owner to make the best medical decision. In this article, upper leg lameness is defined as any condition involving the carpus and tarsus or above. Emphasis is on locating the origin of the lameness and using the appropriate diagnostic tools to give an accurate prognosis to the owner.

LAMENESS EXAMINATION

There are 4 steps in the determination of the cause of lameness:

- Locomotion or mobility scoring
- Hands-on examination

Disclosure Statement: The author has nothing to disclose.
Department of Clinical Sciences, Faculty of Veterinary Medicine, Université de Montréal, St-Hyacinthe, 3200 Sicotte, Quebec J2S 7C6, Canada
E-mail address: andre.desrochers@umontreal.ca

- Establish a differential according to the location of the problem
- Usage of appropriate diagnostic tools

Locomotion or Mobility Scoring

Locomotion scoring is an important objective in assessing lameness. It helps to orient the veterinarian toward the most likely cause and can also be used to evaluate improvement after treatment. It is also a great tool to make animal caretakers aware of cattle needing immediate assistance, closer attention, or simply the need for scheduling of functional claw trimming. Many scoring systems have been described in the literature. Recently, the ProAction initiative in Canada established 2 distinct scales for free stalls and tie stall barns (www.dairyfarmers.ca/proaction).[1] This grading system will be used across Canada giving producers a tool to objectively monitor the herd situation and establish benchmarks. Please (see Lily Nowell Edwards-Callaway and colleagues' article, "Mobility Scoring of Finished Cattle," in this issue) for further information on mobility scoring.

Stall lameness assessments

Gibbons and colleagues[2] validated a tie stall lameness scoring system based on 4 specific behaviors. Cows must have been standing for at least 3 minutes with the animal being quiet (not urinating or defecating) before scoring them. A cow showing at least 2 to 4 behaviors is considered lame. A trained investigator can perform the assessment in less than 30 seconds by assessing the following behaviors:

1. Assessment of foot placement while the animal is standing with the observer at 1 m behind the stall.
   a. Weight shifting: Cows are regularly shifting weight while lifting their feet completely off the ground.
   b. Uneven weight bearing: Cows are protecting the affected leg by shifting weight to the contralateral leg. The entire foot can be off the ground at some point.
   c. Edging: Cows voluntarily place one or both hind feet on the stall's edge. If both hind feet are in the gutter, it is not considered abnormal.
2. Shifting of the animal from side to side is evaluated by either moving alternatively to the right and left side of the animal or simply tapping on the hip bone on each side.
   a. Uneven movement: During the maneuver, the animal is reluctant to move. She may favor one side more than the other by moving more rapidly on that side (Videos 1 and 2).

Observation at a distance

Cattle lameness is generally obvious by observing the cow's stance. Attention should be paid to the posture of the cow, including the back, shoulders, pelvis, and major limb joints. With the animal standing, the general stance is observed first and then more specifically each limb and digit. Compare one region to the opposite side and determine if there are obvious swelling, wounds, shifting of weight, and foot posture, such as toe touching or displacement of weight bearing on the medial or lateral claw are present.

Examination of the claws reveals excess wear of the wall and sole of the healthy digit. In long-standing diseases with severe lameness, the heels are taller and the wall longer on the affected claw compared with that of the healthy claw. A dropped fetlock (ie, hyperextension of the fetlock joint) may be noticed on the sound limb because of excessive load on the flexor tendons and suspensory ligaments (**Fig. 1**). In young animals, angular limb deformities secondary to uneven weight bearing

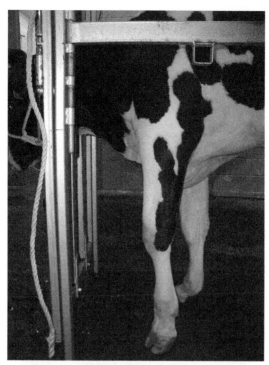

Fig. 1. Holstein bull presented for a left humeral fracture. The right front fetlock is dropped from weight shifting while protecting the fracture.

occurs rapidly with chronic lameness. When chronic lameness occurs in a hind limb, the contralateral tarsus will typically develop varus deformity (**Fig. 2**). When chronic lameness occurs in a forelimb, the carpus typically develops a valgus deformity.

Differential diagnoses for non–weight-bearing lameness should always include

- Sole abscess
- Fracture
- Major joint luxation (eg, tarsus)
- Critical weight-bearing ligament or tendon injury (eg, gastrocnemius muscle)
- Critical nerve injury (eg, radial nerve, femoral nerve, sciatic nerve)
- Septic arthritis
- Septic tenosynovitis

An acute abnormal deviation of the limb is usually related to a fracture or joint luxation. The stance and position of the limb is abnormal with nerve damage, tendon rupture, or a severe ligament injury. A dropped elbow can be caused by radial nerve injury but also from a humeral fracture, radius/ulna fracture, or septic arthritis of the elbow joint (**Fig. 3**). A rupture of the gastrocnemius muscles at the junction with their tendinous portion is reavealed by a hyperflexion of the hock and a drop calcaneus, but this must be differentiated from a fractured calcaneus or sciatic nerve paralysis (**Fig. 4**). Careful attention should be paid to muscle atrophy because this could be caused by nerve injury or disuse. Neurogenic muscle atrophy occurs very rapidly (7–10 days) and is severe. Muscle atrophy caused by disuse occurs over weeks rather than a few days. Chronic lameness of the front limb will usually bring atrophy of the

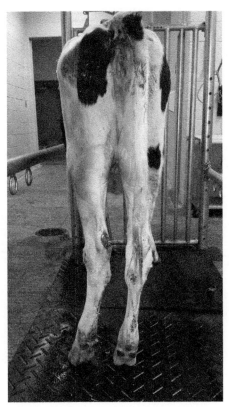

Fig. 2. A young Holstein heifer with left coxofemoral septic arthritis. The opposite hind limb has a slight varus from compensation.

triceps, biceps, and scapular muscles. The consequence of this atrophy is a more apparent shoulder with joint instability, and the animal may be falsely diagnosed with shoulder joint diseases. Similarly, atrophy of the muscles of the rear limb causes the greater trochanter of the femur to appear more pronounced or obvious, which may be misdiagnosed as a coxofemoral joint condition.

Examination of the Affected Limb

Unless an obvious lesion is apparent, the author starts by palpation of the limb from the digit working up the leg. The clinician should watch for a pain reaction and determine if swelling, deformation, crepitation, warmth, and wounds are present. A hoof tester is used to evaluate pain of the claw. Sedatives and tranquilizers should be avoided whenever it is necessary to assess responses to pain. The most common conditions and their location are summarized in **Table 1**.

Examination of long bones is performed by applying firm pressure in regions of minimal soft tissue covering (eg, medial aspect of tibia and radius, greater trochanter of femur, greater tubercle of humerus, and so forth). If the animal has an adverse response, evidenced by withdrawal, avoidance, attempts to kick the evaluator, or muscular flinching, then the opposite leg should be palpated for comparison. Most fractures are obvious, but incomplete nondisplaced fractures can be suspected if there is a painful reaction after deep palpation of the limb. Each joint should be

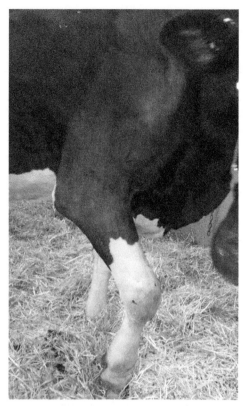

Fig. 3. A right radial nerve paralysis on an adult Holstein cow secondary to prolonged decubitus.

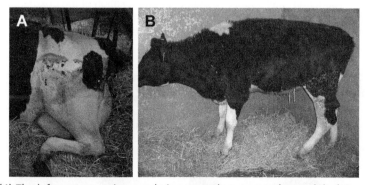

Fig. 4. (A) The left gastrocnemius muscle is ruptured on a recumbent adult dairy cow. The tarsus is abnormally flexed, and there is an obvious swelling of the gastrocnemius muscle highlighted by the clipped area. (B) A young Holstein heifer with a partial left gastrocnemius rupture. An animal with a damaged tibial branch of the sciatic nerve will have a similar stance with a dropped hock but no muscle swelling.

Table 1
Most common conditions with their location

	Sepsis	Osteochondrosis	Degenerative Joint Disease	Ligament Rupture	Luxation	Fracture	Sequestrum
Thoracic limb							
Shoulder	X	X	—	—	X	X	—
Humerus	—	—	—	—	—	X	—
Elbow	X	X	—	—	—	X	—
Radius ulna	—	X (distal physis)	—	—	—	X	X
Carpus	X	—	X	—	—	X	—
Pelvic limb							
Hip	X	—	—	X	X	X	—
Femur	—	—	—	—	—	X	—
Stifle	X	X	X	X	—	X	—
Tibia	—	X (distal physis)	—	—	—	X	X
Tarsus	X	X	X	X	X	X	—

palpated separately; complete flexion, extension, abduction, and adduction of the limb should be performed. Isolation of the shoulder and elbow or of the stifle and tarsus are difficult when flexion or extension movements are performed because these joints are united by muscle tendon units (**Fig. 5**). Nonetheless, this kind of thorough examination can be done on a cooperative animal.

Specific physical examinations are used when suspecting injury to the coxofemoral joint, cruciate ligaments, peroneus tertius, and gastrocnemius.

For the coxofemoral joint, examination requires manipulation of the rear limb that can be difficult in heavy or stubborn animals. The relative position of the greater trochanter to that of the tuber coxae and the tuber ischii is determined. The normal position of the greater trochanter is ventral to both of these bony prominences, and imaginary lines drawn between them will create a triangle (**Fig. 6**). Failure to palpate the greater trochanter may suggest a cranio-ventral luxation of the coxofemoral joint. Positioning of the greater trochanter in-line with the tuber coxae and tuber ischii suggests caudo-dorsal luxation of the coxofemoral joint or femoral head fracture (**Fig. 7**).

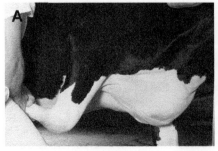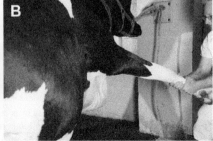

Fig. 5. (*A*) Extension of the elbow and flexion of the shoulder during the systematic lameness examination. (*B*) Abduction of the right front limb.

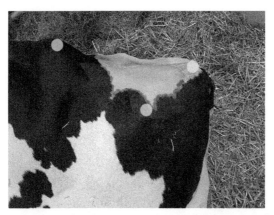

Fig. 6. The left hip of a normal Holstein cow. The dots are on the tuber coxae, greater trochanter, and ischium.

Young animals can be laid down with the affected leg uppermost. This examination is also routinely performed on downer cows. The foot or the metatarsus III/IV is grasped and the entire limb rotated while performing repeated abduction and adduction motions (**Fig. 8**). Fracture of the physis of the head of the femur (capital physeal fracture) should elicit crepitation of the hip that can be felt and occasionally heard. Coxofemoral joint luxation might elicit more crepitation with ventral luxation, excessive movement of the greater trochanter, and ease of abduction if the luxation is cranioventral (Video 3).

For gastrocnemius and peroneus tertius rupture, these structures are evaluated simultaneously. The reciprocal apparatus allows the stifle and the hock to either flex or extend simultaneously (**Figs. 9** and **10**). There is damage to this structure if one flexes while the other can be extended.

The gastrocnemius is ruptured if the stifle is extended and the hock can be flexed (see **Fig. 4**A).

The peroneus tertius is ruptured if the stifle is flexed and the hock is extended (**Fig. 11**).

With cranial cruciate ligament (CCL) rupture, typically, the stifle is swollen and painful to palpation. A drawer test can be performed with the animal standing. It is easier if the animal is bearing weight on the injured limb. The examiner stands

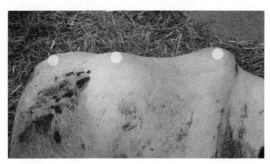

Fig. 7. An adult downer cow with a right dorsal hip luxation. Notice that the dots are aligned demonstrating the dorsal displacement of the greater trochanter.

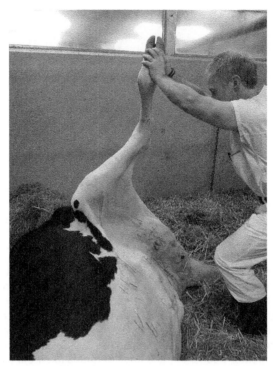

Fig. 8. Special examination of the left hip on a downer cow. The abduction is more than 90° because she had muscular damage following a fall on slippery concrete. Ventrally luxated cattle will show the same degree of abduction.

immediately behind the affected leg and places both hands on the tibial crest by encircling the limb. Then, the examiner's knee is placed on the back of the calcaneus (**Fig. 12**A). A drawer test is positive if displacement or a crepitation can be felt after firm caudal traction on the tibial crest followed by a sudden release. The anatomy and function of the rear limb of cattle is such that the tibia is already displaced cranial

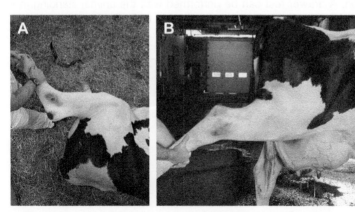

Fig. 9. (*A*) Normal peroneus tertius on a down cow. The stifle is flexed, and the tarsus stays flexed as well. (*B*) Same examination on a normal standing cow.

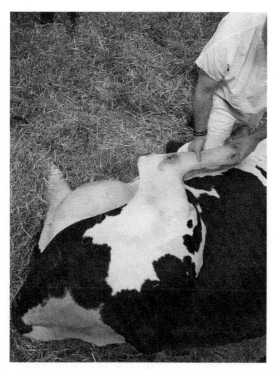

Fig. 10. A normal gastrocnemius on a recumbent cow. The stifle is partially extended while the tarsus cannot be flexed.

to the femur when the CCL is ruptured. Thus, caudal movement of the tibia is a sign of positive drawer. An alternative technique is for the examiner to stand cranial and lateral to the affected limb and place both hands on the tibial crest (see **Fig. 12**B). Then, a firm, rapid thrust is applied to the proximal tibia and the limb observed for displacement and felt for crepitus.

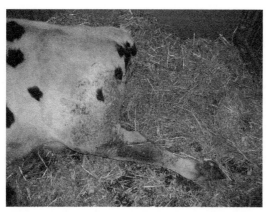

Fig. 11. A ruptured left peroneus tertius on a down cow. The stifle is flexed while the tarsus is abnormally extended.

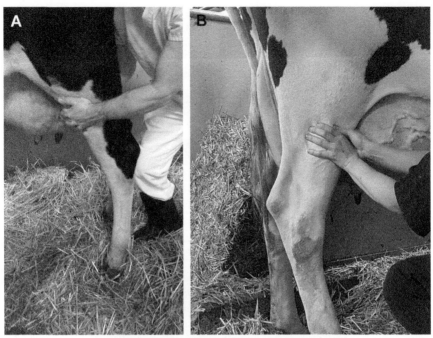

Fig. 12. Specific examination to diagnose CCL rupture. (*A*) The shoulder leans on the thigh, the knee on the calcaneum, while the hands circle the proximal tibial. The action is to pull on the tibia. (*B*) Standing in front of the stifle, both hands are firmly applied on the tibial crest, which is pushed caudally.

Usage of Appropriate Diagnostic Tools

Once the affected area is located, it is often necessary to use diagnostic tools to rule out diseases and help establish appropriate treatment and prognosis. Nowadays many diagnostic tests are available, but the author describes those that are readily available and affordable.

Synovial fluid

Arthrocentesis and subsequent cytologic and bacteriologic analyses of the synovial fluid are the complementary tests of choice for the diagnosis and the management of any joint disease. It is simple and cost-effective. Sterile technique is mandatory to avoid contamination or worse, an iatrogenic infection. Most of the joints can be done blindly just with basic knowledge of the anatomy.[3,4]

Arthrocentesis can be easily performed on a standing or lying sedated animal. The joint must always be surgically prepared. An 18- or 20-G 1.5-in needle is then inserted in specific sites related to the joint anatomy, boundaries, and communication (**Fig. 13**). If chronic septic arthritis is suspected, larger-diameter needles are suitable because of the high cellular and protein content and difficulty in aspirating the thick fibrinous synovial fluid. Gross aspects of the fluid are often enough to differentiate between a septic process (cloudy, yellow, decrease viscosity, fibrin) and the others (osteochondrosis, degenerative disease, or trauma) (**Fig. 14**).

Nuclear cell counts greater than 25,000 cells per microliter, polymorphonuclear (PMN) cell counts greater than 20,000 cells per microliter, or more than 80% PMN cells

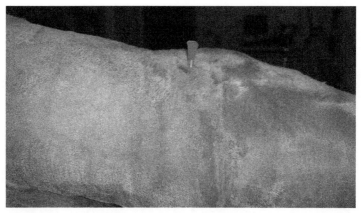

Fig. 13. Arthrocentesis of the tarsus. The needle was inserted in the tibiotarsal joint after surgical preparation.

and total proteins greater than 4.5 g/dL are compatible with a septic joint.[5,6] Microorganisms like mycoplasma can be seen on cytology but not cultured and vice versa.

Radiographic imaging
Although readily available in companion animals or among equine practitioners, it is not a routine diagnostic test in farm animals. A portable x-ray machine will allow you to examine everything from the feet up to the elbow and a portion of the stifle depending of the size of the animal. In adult cattle, a more powerful machine in a referral center is necessary to evaluate the hip and shoulder joint. Most common diseases that are evaluated with the radiographs are fracture, septic arthritis, sequestrum, and osteochondrosis (**Fig. 15**).

Ultrasound images
Soft tissues are better evaluated with ultrasound examination; however, it can be used to evaluate the musculoskeletal system.[7] In acute septic arthritis, the synovial fluid will increase in volume and echogenic (gray) material (fibrin) can be seen floating in the

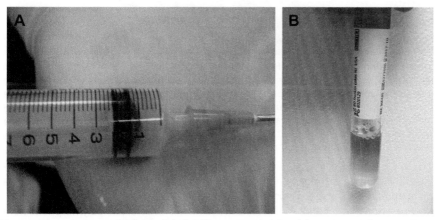

Fig. 14. Abnormal synovial fluids. (*A*) Fluid from a septic joint. (*B*) Suspicion of osteoarthritis.

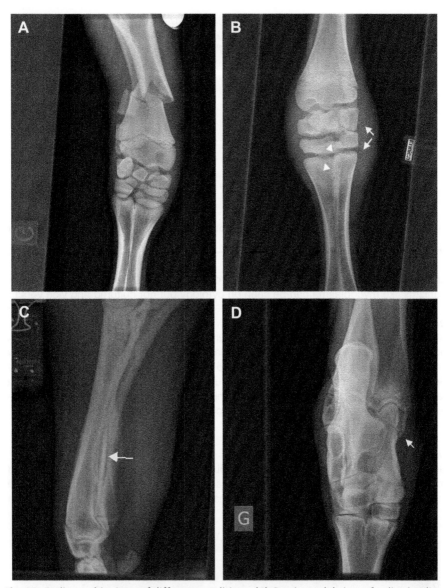

Fig. 15. Radiographic views of different conditions. (*A*) Craniocaudal view of a distal radius. There is a close complete distal transverse diaphyseal fracture of the radius and ulna with minimal displacement. (*B*) Craniocaudal view of the carpus. There are swelling and air (*arrows*) in the soft tissue surrounding the joint. The arrowheads indicate subchondral bone lysis compatible with septic arthritis. (*C*) A lateral view of the radius. The arrow shows a sequestrum at the caudal aspect of the distal radius. (*D*) Craniocaudal view of the tarsus. The arrow shows an osteochondral fragment at the distal aspect of the medial malleolus.

joint. Cartilage is anechogenic (black) because of its high content of water; but the subchondral bone is hyperechogenic (white), and lysis or a defect will change its contour. Presence and location of fibrin in the joint will help to decide which treatment should be applied to a particular animal. The author has been using ultrasound examination for all coxofemoral joint pathology. Although difficult to perform, it can be used to diagnose septic arthritis, which is often difficult to diagnose with plain radiographs. Osteochondral fragments can also be observed while scanning joints.

SPECIFIC CONDITIONS
Osteochondrosis

Osteochondrosis is a common disorder in horses and pigs but infrequently reported in cattle.[8–11] An abnormal endochondral ossification of the articular cartilage results in fragmentation of the cartilage or a subchondral cyst. It is a disease related to fast-growing animals, fed high-energy rations with mineral imbalances. Onset of the lameness is gradual, and early stages can be missed especially in large herds. Affected animals become stiffer and more reluctant to walk. Body condition is unchanged at the beginning of the disease but can deteriorate if not addressed. It might even affect fertility.[12] However, some animals do present osteochondrosis lesions at the postmortem examination without any history of lameness.[11] Affected animals are young with an average age ranging between 10 and 24 months.[13]

Osteochondrosis lesions can be located in the tarsus, stifle, atlanto-occipital joint, shoulder, elbow, and carpus.[8,10,13,14] Osteochondrosis of the stifle and tarsus is clinically easier to diagnose because the joint distention can be easily seen. Animals with clinical signs will show moderate lameness with distended joints (**Fig. 16**). Clinical diagnosis is based on the history (rapid growth) and physical examination. Lesions are often bilateral even though there are no obvious clinical signs. The joint is distended but rarely painful to palpation contrary to septic joint or osteoarthritis. Synovial fluid analysis is characterized by an abundant clear liquid with a moderately elevated nucleated cell count predominantly macrophages and lymphocytes and mild elevation of the proteins, which is compatible with degenerative joint diseases. Radiographic views of the affected joints are necessary to confirm the diagnosis and to differentiate from other joint diseases. Two types of lesions are observed: osteochondritis dissecans and subchondral bone cyst. As previously stated, more than one joint might be affected; therefore, the contralateral joint is radiographed as well. Certain radiographic lesions are difficult to differentiate from septic arthritis. A sclerotic area usually surrounds the lysis in the subchondral bone in cases of osteochondral cyst.

Osteoarthritis

This condition generally occurs as a result of either a septic process or trauma with joint instability.[12,15–17] Straight-legged, heavy-muscled animals on concrete can

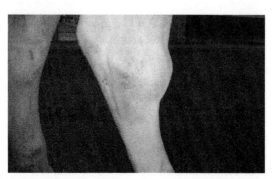

Fig. 16. A distended right tarsus on a 15-month-old Holstein heifer with osteochondrosis.

develop progressive osteoarthritis by repeated trauma to the cartilage.[15] Untreated clinical osteochondrosis may evolve toward osteoarthritis. An abnormal ratio of calcium and phosphorus was incriminated as a cause of osteoarthritis in a feedlot.[16] Osteochondrosis and osteoarthritis must be considered in any animal in a feedlot with multiple swollen joints.

Cranial Cruciate Ligament Rupture

CCL rupture is rarely reported in cattle. Therefore, it is most likely undiagnosed or ignored as a cause of hind limb upper lameness. Meniscus injury can go with CCL injury.[18,19] The rupture is caused by an acute injury or secondary to a degenerative arthritis with a progressive fraying of the ligament until rupture.[20] The cow has a lameness score of 3-4 out of 5 (being non weight bearing), and the affected stifle is significantly swollen. If the instability is severe, a popping noise can be heard while walking. Palpation of the stifle reveals severe swelling and pain. As described earlier, a drawer movement can be performed on the animal while it is standing. A drawer is considered positive if crepitation and movement are felt during the manipulation. A lateral radiographic view of the stifle while the animal is weight bearing will confirm your diagnosis (**Fig. 17**).

Coxofemoral Luxation

Most coxofemoral luxation occurred in peripartum period following a milk fever or paresis of the hind limb (obturator nerve paralysis). Other causes of luxation are accidental like mounting during estrus or slipping on a wet floor. There are 2 kinds of clinical presentation: standing or downer cows.[21] Clinical diagnosis is difficult and quite different between dorsal and ventral luxation. With dorsal luxation, there is an external

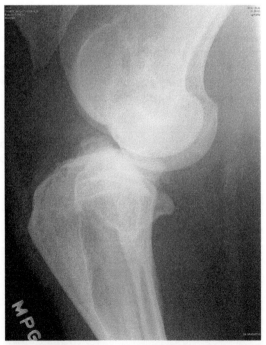

Fig. 17. Lateral view of the left stifle on a 6-year-old Holstein cow with CCL rupture. The tibial plateau is displaced cranially.

rotation of the digits and internal rotation of the hock; the greater trochanter is dorsally displaced; and crepitation can be felt while rotating the hip. Animals with ventral luxation are usually unable to stand because of concomitant muscle damage and the femoral head leaning on the pelvis. For the clinical examination, the affected leg is uppermost with the animal in lateral recumbency. If the hip is actually ventrally luxated, the limb will be flexed and impossible to extend while the trochanter cannot be seen or palpated. Abduction of the leg is equal to or greater than 90° to the other leg. A so-called subluxation is defined as an incomplete or partial luxation; the femoral head can be luxated while abducting the limb. The noise and movement engendered by the manipulation is unequivocal. The femoral head can occasionally be palpated in the obturator foramen. Femoral neck fracture or slipped capital physis should be included in the differential diagnosis.[21] Radiographic views of the hips are helpful and diagnostic but not available to most veterinarians because powerful radiographic equipment is necessary. Down cows with ventral luxation usually have a fatal prognosis because of a high probability of recurrence after reduction and concomitant nerve and extensive muscle damage.[21] Standing cows or calves usually have a dorsal luxation. The author has mostly seen calves with dorsal luxation. Nevertheless, those animals have a good prognosis if the reduction is performed within 48 hours after the beginning of clinical signs.[22,23]

Septic Arthritis

Septic arthritis is the most common cause of joint swelling in cattle. Onset of clinical signs is usually acute and severe. Lameness will vary depending of the duration and severity of the infection and the number of joints affected. During the physical examination, emphasis should be on finding the origin of the septic arthritis: trauma, pneumonia, adjacent abscess. The most common joints affected are carpus, tarsus, fetlock, and stifle (**Figs. 18** and **19**). If none of those joints seems infected, then the hip, elbow, and shoulder are investigated. Distal limb septic arthritis is often caused by a trauma, whereas proximal limb arthritis conditions are usually of systemic origin. If an animal has polyarthritis, a complete physical examination must be performed to find the origin. Typically, the animal will be severely lame (toe touching or non–weight bearing), with a swollen joint painful to the touch. If the joint is manipulated, the range of motion will be decreased and pain is easily elicited while flexing or extending the leg. Arthrocentesis will confirm the diagnosis. Arthrocentesis is performed in an area

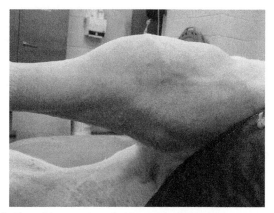

Fig. 18. A young heifer with a septic arthritis of the right stifle.

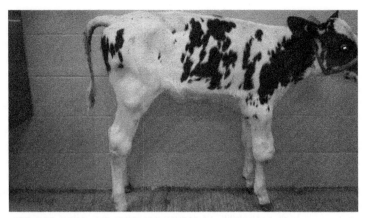

Fig. 19. A calf with septic polyarthritis caused by *Mycoplasma bovis*.

surrounding the joint where there is no wound to avoid contamination. After surgical preparation of the site, synovial fluid is withdrawn and preserved for further analysis. At that point, if there is a wound adjacent to the joint, 10 to 20 mL of a sterile solution is injected into the joint to verify the existence of a communication with the wound. Radiographic images are helpful for prognosis, especially if the duration of the disease is more than 2 weeks.

The prognosis should always be guarded unless the onset is acute and there are no bone lesions on the radiographic images. Many factors will influence the prognosis: age, joint affected, microorganism isolated, time of presentation, number of joints involved, concomitant diseases, and value of the animal.[24] If more than 2 joints are infected, it is the author's opinion that the prognosis is poor.

Patellar Luxation and Femoral Nerve Paralysis

Following dystocia, the femoral nerve or the medial femoropatellar ligament may be damaged secondary to excessive traction and hip lock.[25] Clinical signs are immediate, and the calf has difficulty rising and standing. Their stance and walking are typical. The patella is displaced laterally to the lateral ridge of the femoral trochlea. It is easy to replace the patella at its normal position; but depending of the severity or chronicity, it might stay luxated. Biomechanically, patellar luxation or femoral nerve paralysis will have the same consequences: extension of the stifle is impossible because the quadriceps have no strength. If the nerve is responsible for the patellar luxation, muscle atrophy will be observable within a week. Lack of sensation is usually present in the medial midthigh region.[25] Femoral nerve paralysis could be bilateral. The treatment is surgical, and the prognosis is guarded if only one side is affected. The goal of the surgery is to keep the patella in its anatomic position and ready to function when the quadriceps contract. It may take a few months depending on the damage. A calf with bilateral femoral nerve paralysis has a poor prognosis.[25]

Upward Fixation of the Patella

The patella becomes locked on the medial trochlear ridge; as a result, the affected leg is held in posterior extension. The fixation is usually intermittent but can become permanent.[26] In chronically affected animals, the dorsal claw walls are worn-out from excessive dragging. It is typically more frequent in *Bos indicus* bulls, but it was recently reported in 12 cows.[27,28] A desmotomy of the medial patellar tendon is the treatment of choice with a good prognosis associated with it.[27,28]

Peroneus Tertius Rupture

The peroneus tertius in cattle has muscle fibers similar to the horse. It originates from the extensor fossa of the distal femur along with the digital extensor and inserts in the area of the tarsometatarsal joint. It will rupture after hyperextension of the tarsus while the stifle remains flexed (see **Fig. 11**). This situation is often encountered when the animal slips and the limb slides backward. Its rupture renders hock flexion more difficult, and the animal might stumble having difficulty to clear the ground with its foot. Based on ultrasound findings, the rupture is more a muscle tear than a straight tendon rupture precluding any surgical options to suture it. It should not prevent the animal from standing or walking. Other than stall rest for weeks, there is no specific treatment of this condition; however, the prognosis is good.

Brachial, Radial Nerve Paralysis

While attempting to get up and stand, the cow might slide and overabduct a thoracic limb. The more dramatic consequence will be radial nerve damage. Prolonged lateral decubitus on a hard surface can also be at the origin of the damage. Typically, the elbow will drop and the carpus remains partially flexed (see **Fig. 3**). Animals with ruptured triceps, humeral or olecranon fracture will show a similar posture. Affected animals have difficulty getting up and standing, lacking strength to keep their balance. Physical examination rules out fracture. Skin pricking or pinching as well as triceps reflex confirm the diagnosis of radial nerve paralysis. Splinting at the caudal aspect of the forelimb, from the foot up to the elbow, might help the animal to stand. If there is a neurapraxia, strength will come back in less than 3 weeks. If paresis is still present after that, nerve damage is important and a prognosis is difficult to establish.

Long Bone Fractures

Humeral, femoral, tibial, and radial fractures are usually easy to diagnose but difficult to treat. Humeral fractures are the only ones that can be treated successfully with stall rest only. Internal fixation or external coaptation must be used for the other long bone fractures. Tibial and radial fractures are successfully treated with plates, pin casting, or Thomas splint. Diaphyseal femoral fractures are more frequent in calves and are usually treated with intramedullary stack pinning or interlocking nails. Femoral head fractures can be fixed with cannulated screws. Open fractures and heavy animals carry a poor prognosis. For the rest, the prognosis will vary greatly depending on the fracture configuration, age, and surgeon experience.

Femoral fractures in calves treated surgically have a prognosis of 66% to 83%.[29–31] Nichols and colleagues[30] reported fracture healing with stall rest; however, most of those animals were significantly lame. Therefore, surgical intervention was recommended.[30] Femoral capital physeal fractures in bulls treated with internal fixation have a prognosis of 70% to 75% for serviceable soundness with a better prognosis in young animals.[32,33] Most fractures in young calves occurred during delivery, and concomitant diseases significantly decreased chances of survival.[34]

Tibial and radio ulnar fractures can be treated successfully by internal fixation and external coaptation. Prognosis is extremely variable depending on type of fixation, weight, age, fracture configuration, and hospitals, ranging from 45% to 81% for tibial fractures.[34–38] Radio ulnar fractures are less frequent, but the treatment and prognosis are very similar.

Humeral fractures in cattle have been treated conservatively by stall resting or surgically with double plating of external fixation.[39–41] The radial nerve can be affected with permanent paralysis of the distal limb.

Sequestrum

Affected animals are usually moderately lame. The initial complaint is often a chronic wound nonresponsive to antibiotics and local treatment. The affected area is swollen, firm to the touch, with a draining tract. Exuberant granulation tissue might be present as well depending on its chronicity. Although osseous sequestration affects mainly the distal limbs, the tibia and radius can be affected as well[42] (see **Fig. 15C**). The definitive diagnosis of a sequestrum is made by radiographic images of the affected limb. Two orthogonal views are essential to determine the exact location and the size of the sequestrum. The treatment is usually surgical, and the prognosis is good.[42]

SUPPLEMENTARY DATA

Supplementary video related to this article can be found at http://dx.doi.org/10.1016/j.cvfa.2017.03.002.

REFERENCES

1. The Proaction Initiative. Canada, 2017. Available at: https://www.dairyfarmers.ca/proaction. Accessed April 4, 2017.
2. Gibbons J, Haley DB, Higginson Cutler J, et al. Technical note: a comparison of 2 methods of assessing lameness prevalence in tie stall herds. J Dairy Sci 2014;97:350–3.
3. Nuss K, Hecht S, Maierl J, et al. Arthrocentesis in cattle. Part 2: pelvic limb. Tierarztl Prax Ausg G Grosstiere Nutztiere 2002;30:301–7.
4. Nuss K, Hecht S, Maierl J, et al. Arthrocentesis in cattle. Part 1: thoracic limb. Tierarztl Prax Ausg G Grosstiere Nutztiere 2002;30:226–32.
5. Francoz D, Desrochers A, Latouche JS. Effect of repeated arthrocentesis and single joint lavage on cytologic evaluation of synovial fluid in 5 young calves. Can J Vet Res 2007;71:129–34.
6. Rohde C, Anderson DE, Desrochers A, et al. Synovial fluid analysis in cattle: a review of 130 cases. Vet Surg 2000;29:341–6.
7. Kofler J, Geissbuhler U, Steiner A. Diagnostic imaging in bovine orthopedics. Vet Clin North Am Food Anim Pract 2014;30:11–53, v.
8. Hill BD, Sutton RH, Thompson H. Investigation of osteochondrosis in grazing beef cattle. Aust Vet J 1998;76:171–5.
9. Jensen R, Park RD, Lauerman LH, et al. Osteochondrosis in feedlot cattle. Vet Pathol 1981;18:529–35.
10. Trostle SS, Nicoll RG, Forrest LJ, et al. Clinical and radiographic findings, treatment, and outcome in cattle with osteochondrosis: 29 cases (1986-1996). J Am Vet Med Assoc 1997;211:1566–70.
11. Weisbrode SE, Monke DR, Dodaro ST, et al. Osteochondrosis, degenerative joint disease, and vertebral osteophytosis in middle-aged bulls. J Am Vet Med Assoc 1982;181:700–5.
12. Persson Y, Soderquist L, Ekman S. Joint disorder; a contributory cause to reproductive failure in beef bulls? Acta Vet Scand 2007;49:31.
13. Dutra F, Carlsten J, Ekman S. Hind limb skeletal lesions in 12-month-old bulls of beef breeds. Zentralbl Veterinarmed A 1999;46:489–508.

14. Reiland S, Stromberg B, Olsson SE, et al. Osteochondrosis in growing bulls. Pathology, frequency and severity on different feedings. Acta Radiol Suppl 1978; 358:179–96.

15. Bargai U, Cohen R. Tarsal lameness of dairy bulls housed at two artificial insemination centers: 24 cases (1975-1987). J Am Vet Med Assoc 1992;201:1068–9.

16. Heinola T, Jukola E, Nakki P, et al. Consequences of hazardous dietary calcium deficiency for fattening bulls. Acta Vet Scand 2006;48:25.

17. Heinola T, de Grauw JC, Virkki L, et al. Bovine chronic osteoarthritis causes minimal change in synovial fluid. J Comp Pathol 2013;148:335–44.

18. Nelson DR, Huhn JC, Kneller SK. Peripheral detachment of the medial meniscus with injury to the medial collateral ligament in 50 cattle. Vet Rec 1990;127:59–60.

19. Nelson DR, Huhn JC, Kneller SK. Surgical repair of peripheral detachment of the medial meniscus in 34 cattle. Vet Rec 1990;127:571–3.

20. Huhn JC, Kneller SK, Nelson DR. Radiographic assessment of cranial cruciate ligament rupture in the dairy cow. Vet Radiol 1986;27:184–8.

21. Marchionatti E, Fecteau G, Desrochers A. Traumatic conditions of the coxofemoral joint: luxation, femoral head-neck fracture, acetabular fracture. Vet Clin North Am Food Anim Pract 2014;30:247–64, vii.

22. Larcombe MT, Malmo J. Dislocation of the coxo-femoral joint in dairy cows. Aust Vet J 1989;66:351–4.

23. Tulleners EP, Nunamaker DM, Richardson DW. Coxofemoral luxations in cattle: 22 cases (1980-1985). J Am Vet Med Assoc 1987;191:569–74.

24. Desrochers A, Francoz D. Clinical management of septic arthritis in cattle. Vet Clin North Am Food Anim Pract 2014;30:177–203, vii.

25. Healy AM. Dystocia and femoral nerve paralysis in calves. Compend Contin Educ Vet 1997;19:1299–304.

26. Pentecost R, Niehaus A. Stifle disorders: cranial cruciate ligament, meniscus, upward fixation of the patella. Vet Clin North Am Food Anim Pract 2014;30:265–81, vii-viii.

27. Baird AN, Angel KL, Moll HD, et al. Upward fixation of the patella in cattle: 38 cases (1984-1990). J Am Vet Med Assoc 1993;202:434–6.

28. Frei S, Nuss K. Intermittent upward fixation of the patella in 12 cows: A retrospective study of treatment and long-term prognosis. Schweiz Arch Tierheilkd 2015; 157:553–8 [in German].

29. Bellon J, Mulon PY. Use of a novel intramedullary nail for femoral fracture repair in calves: 25 cases (2008-2009). J Am Vet Med Assoc 2011;238:1490–6.

30. Nichols S, Anderson DE, Miesner MD, et al. Femoral diaphysis fractures in cattle: 26 cases (1994-2005). Aust Vet J 2010;88:39–44.

31. St-Jean G, DeBowes RM, Hull BL, et al. Intramedullary pinning of femoral diaphyseal fractures in neonatal calves: 12 cases (1980-1990). J Am Vet Med Assoc 1992;200:1372–6.

32. Bentley VA, Edwards RB III, Santschi EM, et al. Repair of femoral capital physeal fractures with 7.0-mm cannulated screws in cattle: 20 cases (1988-2002). J Am Vet Med Assoc 2005;227:964–9.

33. Ewoldt JMI, Hull BL, Ayars WH. Repair of femoral capital physeal fractures in 12 cattle. Vet Surg 2003;32:30–6.

34. Nuss K, Spiess A, Feist M, et al. Treatment of long bone fractures in 125 newborn calves. A retrospective study. Tierarztl Prax Ausg G Grosstiere Nutztiere 2011;39: 15–26.

35. Anderson DE, St.-Jean G, Vestweber JG, et al. Use of a Thomas splint-cast combination for stabilization of tibial fractures in cattle: 21 cases (1973-1993). Agri Pract 1994;15:16–23.

36. Martens A, Steenhaut M, Gasthuys F, et al. Conservative and surgical treatment of tibial fractures in cattle. Vet Rec 1998;143:12–6.

37. St-Jean G, Clem MF, DeBowes RM. Transfixation pinning and casting of tibial fractures in calves: five cases (1985-1989). J Am Vet Med Assoc 1991;198: 139–43.

38. Verschooten F, De Moor A, Desmet P, et al. Surgical treatment of tibial fractures in cattle. Vet Rec 1972;90:24–8.

39. Rakestraw PC, Nixon AJ, Kaderly RE, et al. Cranial approach to the humerus for repair of fractures in horses and cattle. Vet Surg 1991;20:1–8.

40. Saint-Jean G, Hull BL. Conservative treatment of a humeral fracture in a heifer. Can Vet J 1987;28:704–6.

41. Yamagishi N, Devkota B, Takahashi M. Outpatient treatment for humeral fractures in five calves. J Vet Med Sci 2014;76:1519–22.

42. Valentino LW, St Jean G, Anderson DE, et al. Osseous sequestration in cattle: 110 cases (1987-1997). J Am Vet Med Assoc 2000;217:376–83.

Traumatic Lesions of the Sole

J.K. Shearer, DVM, MS[a],*, Sarel R. van Amstel, BVSc, MMedVet[b]

KEYWORDS

- Cattle lameness • Traumatic lesions of the sole • Sole punctures • Thin soles
- Thin sole toe ulcers • Toe tip necrosis syndrome • Toe abscesses

KEY POINTS

- Perforation of the sole may occur as a consequence of the inadvertent treading on a sharp, protruding object, such as a nail or other sharp object occurring on cattle walkways.
- There are multiple foreign bodies that may become lodged within the sole, such as stones, and a variety of metallic substances, including nails, screws, and improperly discarded hypodermic needles.
- In dairy cattle, excessive wear and, on occasion, over-trimming results in thin soles and thin sole toe ulcers.
- In feedlot cattle, hyperexcitability, failure to properly bed trailers for transport, and excessive wear on concrete surfaces predisposes to a group of lesions characterized as toe tip necrosis syndrome.

INTRODUCTION

Traumatic lesions of the sole are a common cause of lameness in beef and dairy cattle. The causes vary from the inadvertent stepping on a sharp object on a concrete or other flooring surface to excessive wear on abrasive flooring surfaces that leads to thinning and separation of the sole with exposure of the underlying corium. In feedlot cattle, accelerated wear and abrasion of the sole and toe tip leads to thinning of the sole and separation of the white line in the apex of the toe, predisposing to toe abscesses.

The incidence of sole lesions due to trauma as a cause of lameness in cattle is poorly understood. Most record-keeping systems do not specifically list traumatic sole lesions as a distinct lameness condition. Instead, these lesions are captured in health records under the catchall category of sole abscesses. Labeling claw

[a] Department of Veterinary Diagnostic and Production Animal Medicine, College of Veterinary Medicine, Iowa State University, 2436 Lloyd Veterinary Medical Center, Ames, IA 50011, USA;
[b] Department of Large Animal Clinical Studies, College of Veterinary Medicine, University of Tennessee, 2407 River Dr, Knoxville, TN 37996, USA
* Corresponding author.
E-mail address: jks@iastate.edu

Vet Clin Food Anim 33 (2017) 271–281
http://dx.doi.org/10.1016/j.cvfa.2017.02.001
0749-0720/17/Published by Elsevier Inc.

lesions as sole abscesses is nearly useless as terminology for recording claw lesions, particularly when the veterinarian might want to use this information for the purpose of making management decisions to reduce lameness. A more accurate description or lesion-specific terminology for claw lesions is important and offers far greater value because strategies for control and prevention are improved when accompanied by an accurate diagnosis. For example, the underlying causes of sole ulcers are metabolic (ie, associated with enzymatic or hormonal weakening of the suspensory apparatus of P3) or physical (eg, unbalanced weightbearing from claw horn overgrowth) in nature. Sole ulcers are amenable to correction by paying closer attention to cow comfort, nutrition and feeding, and preventative foot care practices that include proper claw trimming. On the other hand, in a dairy herd experiencing multiple problems with thin soles and thin sole toe ulcers (TSTUs), attention is turned to the abrasiveness of flooring conditions or the distance cows are required to walk to and from the parlor. In feedlot cattle, lesions of the toe tip seem to bear a close relationship to abrasion-type injuries, prolonged standing during transport, and hyperexcitable cattle.

This article provides a brief description of traumatically induced conditions with specific attention to underlying causes, treatment, and prevention.

PERFORATIONS OF THE SOLE (PODODERMATITIS SEPTICA TRAUMATICA)

There are multiple objects occurring on cattle walkways capable of causing serious lesions in the sole (**Fig. 1**). Most common are stones and various metallic substances,

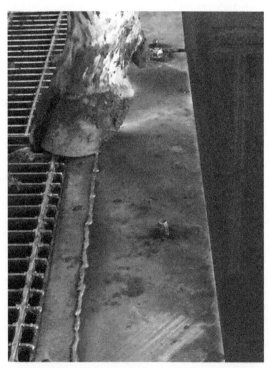

Fig. 1. The bolts used to hold down this grate in the holding area are examples of the kind of flooring conditions capable of causing serious sole injury. (*Courtesy of* Brian Pingsterhaus, Germantown, IL, USA).

including nails, screws, and hypodermic needles. Puncture-type lesions of the sole that make contact with the corium will normally create a subsolar abscess whereby purulent material rapidly accumulates between the solar corium and the sole. Initially, lameness may be mild but as the abscess develops pain increases and lameness becomes increasingly severe. Close examination of the sole reveals a dark-colored lesion in the sole consisting of necrotic horn and dirt that, when debrided with a hoof knife, discloses a tract that leads to the abscess (**Fig. 2**). Disruption of the abscess results in the discharge of a foul-smelling purulent fluid.[1–4]

PENETRATION OF THE SOLE BY FOREIGN BODIES

Foreign objects often become lodged within the horn tissue of the sole or heel (**Figs. 3 and 4**). Even though the foreign body fails to penetrate the sole, its mere presence may cause mild to moderate discomfort from localized pressure on the corium when the animal bears weight on the foot. When foreign material penetrates the sole and makes contact with the corium, development of a subsolar abscess is near certain. The penetration of a foreign body in the sole toward the apex of the claw normally induces a rapid onset of severe to nonweightbearing lameness. Lameness associated with foreign bodies that penetrate more caudally in the sub-bulbar region of the heel tends to develop more slowly and lameness may be less severe. In this case, purulent fluid associated with the lesion will migrate caudally where it underruns the heel before it is ultimately discharged at the skin-horn junction. Loose flaps of claw horn on the heel bulb are key indicators of a septic lesion in the heel region and should always be investigated to assess their connection to white line disease, sole or heel ulcer, or a lesion caused by a foreign body.[1–4]

INCIDENCE OF TRAUMATIC SOLE LESIONS

Sole lesions defined as sole punctures (foreign objects that penetrated through the sole) were 4.3% (81 per 1861) of all lameness disorders and 8.6% (81 per 946) of all claw-related lesions observed in a Florida study.[5] Incidence rate was highest during the summer months (July–September), coincident with the increase in incidence of thin soles. Thinning of the sole increases its flexibility, which alone contributes to

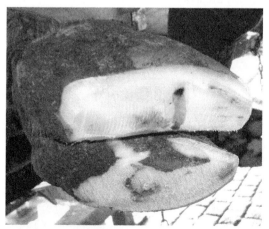

Fig. 2. Perforation of the sole caused by the remnants of a nail protruding from the flooring surface that was previously used to fasten rubber to the floor.

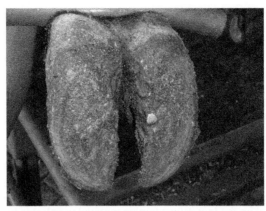

Fig. 3. A claw with a nail embedded in the sole. In this case the nail was found before it made contact with the underlying corium.

contusion of the corium and tender footedness. However, in the southeastern United States, increased amounts of rainfall combined with heat stress management procedures (ie, sprinkling and misting of cows) during the summer months results in a situation in which feet are constantly wet. The increased moisture content in hoof horn reduces its resistance to wear and presumably its resistance to penetration by foreign bodies.[5,6]

AN IMPORTANT UNDERLYING CAUSE OF SOLE LESIONS

Accelerated wear (irrespective of season) has become a predominant cause of lameness in large dairies, particularly where flooring is abrasive or the spatial layout of facilities requires cows to walk long distances. As a result, rubber has become a common addition to flooring in dairy barns. Rubberizing flooring surfaces reduces wear rates and cows naturally prefer the softer surface afforded by rubber. In addition, the compressibility of rubberized flooring surfaces improves traction and reduces injury from slips and falls. Several versions of rubber for application to floors in dairy facilities are commercially available. One of the most common noncommercial options is conveyor belting (as used by the mining industry). Although it offers a comfortable

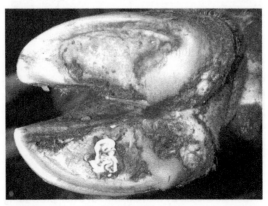

Fig. 4. A tooth that has become embedded in the sole.

walking surface, one of the drawbacks to the use of conveyor-type belting (as with other types of belting) is that it must nailed down to keep it in place, otherwise it is easily lifted by manure removal systems.[7] Problems with lameness result when the rubber becomes dislodged, exposing the nail or it's remnants above the surface of the concrete in cattle walkways. When the cow places her foot on the protruding nail, depending on length, it is apt to penetrate deeply through the sole and into deeper structures of the foot (see **Fig. 2**). This lesion is possible in any dairy where rubber is fastened down with nails. Daily examination and treatment of lame cows, ensuring an accurate diagnosis using proper terminology, and communication with responsible parties when puncture-type lesions are observed is key to control and prevention of these conditions.[8]

DIAGNOSIS OF TRAUMATIC LESIONS OF THE SOLE

The diagnosis of sole lesions (as with a sole puncture) may be determined by careful assessment of the lesion and its location on the weightbearing surface of the claw.[5,8] The presence of traumatic sole lesions may not be obvious when the foot is first examined. Proper cleaning of the claw is essential and removal of a thin layer of sole horn with a grinder will facilitate proper examination of the claw. Other helpful examination techniques include palpation of the sole surface for increase in heat compared with the remaining claws and testing for the presence of pain by tapping the sole surface with a hoof tester or the handle of a hoof knife. Pay extra attention to areas where lesions typically occur. For example, sole ulcers typically occur in zone 4, heel ulcers in zone 6, and toe ulcers in zone 5 on a claw lesion diagram (**Fig. 5**). White line lesions will typically occur in zones 1, 2, or 3 and, similar to sole ulcers, occurrence is most commonly in the lateral claw. On the other hand, lesions of the sole associated with trauma show no consistent pattern as to claw or claw zone affected, and most are associated with abscess formation and severe lameness. In cases in which the offending foreign body becomes lodged in the sole, diagnosis is quite obvious. In cases in which there is deep penetration of the sole, a pathologic fracture or sequestrum should be suspected and radiographs may be indicated.

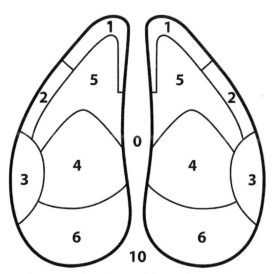

Fig. 5. Claw zones used for recording claw and foot lesions.

TREATMENT OF TRAUMATIC SOLE LESIONS

Treatment of these lesions requires the removal of the foreign object when present, accompanied by paring away of all undermined and necrotic horn around the solar lesion. This should be followed by the application of a foot block to the healthy claw. In cases in which necrosis of the corium and underlying tissue is more extensive, complications may develop, including septic osteitis of the third phalanx. In such cases, using a bone curette or loop knife, necrotic bone should be debrided until hard healthy bone is exposed. Using the bone curette or loop knife, the presence of a sequestrum can also be determined by applying pressure on the edge of the exposed bone to check for movement. The third phalanx has a great remodeling capacity and a large portion of the bone can be removed. Insufficient debridement or lack thereof may lead to persistent septic osteitis, and should be suspected when lesions do not heal properly and a persistent draining tract remains in a bed of granulation tissue on the surface of the sole. In cases in which the septic osteitis involves the apex of the third phalanx, amputation of the toe, including the abaxial and axial sections of the wall corium and the apex of P3, should be considered, making sure that the only healthy bone remains.[9] Some practitioners may elect systemic antibiotic therapy; however, there is no clear evidence of benefit to this practice.

CONTROL AND PREVENTION OF TRAUMATIC SOLE LESIONS

The control and prevention of traumatic sole lesions may be accomplished in several ways. Because nails, screws, and other construction-related materials used in repair or construction of facilities often find their way onto flooring surfaces, workers and employees should be informed or reminded of the potential for these to cause problems on cattle walkways. Be sure that used needles are properly disposed of in sharps containers. Encourage people who move cattle to and from corrals to the milking parlor to monitor floors for loose rubber and exposed nails, or screws used to hold rubber in place. Be sure all employees understand the importance of keeping alleyways and travel lanes free of foreign material that may result in foot injury. Finally, instruct trimmers to properly record these lesions and be sure that this information is communicated to managers and owners for immediate correction. Traumatic sole lesions are preventable.

LESIONS ASSOCIATED WITH EXCESSIVE WEAR ON CONCRETE

In the previous discussion of claw lesions resulting from traumatic injury, information was cited that found an association between thin soles and the incidence of lameness due to perforation and penetration of the sole by foreign bodies. However, the more common and potentially more important problems with thin soles are contusion of the solar corium and the potential for development of TSTUs.[10] These lesions are frequently misdiagnosed as white line disease. Distinguishing this lesion from a laminitis-induced toe ulcer or white line disease is important because the underlying causes and strategies to manage these conditions are very different. In feedlot cattle, a similar but slightly different lesion associated with abrasion and wear occurs in the apical white line of the toe.[11] (See Johann Kofler's article, "Pathogenesis and Treatment of Toe Lesions in Cattle Including "Non-healing" Toe Lesions," in this issue.) The following is a brief description of these lesions in the context of traumatic sole lesions.

THIN SOLES IN DAIRY CATTLE

The thin sole condition is a growing problem in confinement dairy operations throughout the United States.[5] It is particularly prevalent in confinement housing conditions in which cows may have limited relief from concrete flooring conditions. It seems to be aggravated by housing conditions and management practices that limit or discourage resting behavior. However, probably more important are housing facilities that require cows to walk long distances on abrasive flooring surfaces. Sand, despite its benefits for cow comfort in stalls, may actually contribute to claw horn wear, particularly when recycled multiple times, making sand coarser and likely more abrasive. Water is a key component of heat stress abatement strategies but the increased moisture necessary for cow cooling also softens hoof horn and reduces its resistance to wear. Indeed, it seems that although measures used to maintain performance and health during periods of intense heat stress are beneficial for cows, they may not be ideal for foot health.[5]

Foot trimming is thought to be beneficial for the purposes of maintaining balanced weightbearing and for detecting and correcting early lesions.[12] However, when feet are over-trimmed, it increases the likelihood of thin soles and TSTUs. Finally, excessive sole horn wear is commonly observed in new facilities. Freshly cured concrete creates a particularly abrasive surface as a consequence of the presence of surface aggregate that naturally forms on the flooring surface as the concrete cures. This observation has become as commonplace enough to have its own name: new concrete disease.[13]

DESCRIPTION OF THE LESION OF THIN SOLES AND THIN SOLE TOE ULCERS

Close examination of cows suffering with the thin sole problem revealed that many of those with the most severe lameness had developed a characteristic toe lesion whereby thinning of the sole lead to weakening and separation of the sole from the abaxial white line in the region of the toe.[10] Unlike white line disease in which the lesion occurs as a dark necrotic dot or defective separated area within the white line, close inspection of TSTU shows that this lesion is actually a separation of the sole in zone 5, adjacent to the junction of zones 1 and 2 on the claw zone diagram (see **Fig. 5**). Furthermore, the authors' observations indicated that thin-soled cows that develop lameness generally present with one of the following conditions: (1) thin soles that are flexible to finger pressure but do not have evidence of solar separation or ulceration, (2) thin soles that are flexible to finger pressure and have a visible separation in the epidermis and a visible ulcer (TSTU), (3) thin soles that have progressed beyond the stage of ulceration and have formed a subsolar abscess at the toe (toe abscess), and (4) thin soles that have progressed to the point of subsolar abscessation and osteitis of the third phalanx.[10] It is not uncommon to find evidence of a defect in the sole suggestive of a TSTU lesion that occurred previously and later spontaneously resolved without causing lameness (**Fig. 6**).

TREATMENT OF THIN SOLES

In herds in which thin soles and TSTU are common, it is important to be vigilant in lameness detection to remove cows for treatment as soon as they are noticed to be tender-footed (arched back, short stepping, and head down while walking). Depending on how thin the sole or how advanced the lesion, it may or may not be possible to treat affected animals with a block applied to the healthiest of the 2 claws. It is a judgment call in most cases because the healthier of the 2 claws will also be thin and may not able to support the full weight of the cow on one claw. If a block to relieve weightbearing is used, it is important that these animals are closely observed in the post-treatment period to ensure that the block does not exacerbate the lameness problem. In many cases, the only option for treatment is to move the animal to a soft surface close to the milking parlor.

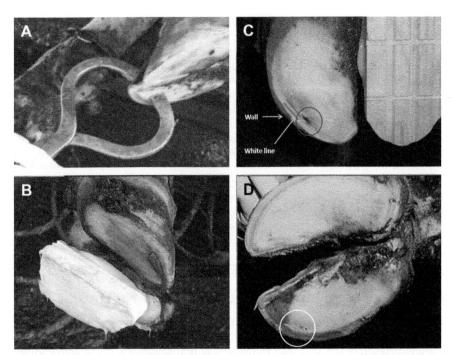

Fig. 6. (*A*) A flexible sole suggests it is thin. (*B*) A TSTU. (*C*) TSTU with a break in sole and abscess formation beneath the sole. (*D*) Separation of the sole away from the white line in the area where lesions typically occur.

Recently, low-profile foot blocks have been introduced. These lower profile blocks have shown promise as a way to elevate the most seriously affected of the 2 claws and limit wear on both. The thinner block provides sufficient weight relief to prevent additional wear while offering greater stability that seems to be better tolerated by the cow.

TRAUMA-INDUCED TOE ABSCESSES IN FEEDLOT CATTLE

The predominant causes of foot-related lameness in feedlot cattle include foot rot, digital dermatitis, injuries, and toe tip necrosis. A recent review of health records from 445,876 animals from 26 Alberta feedlots over an 8 year period (2005–2013) revealed that 22% of all cattle were treated at least once during their stay at the feedlot.[14] Of those treated 28% were identified as lame and approximately 4% of the lameness was due to toe tip necrosis. Nearly all affected were febrile with rectal body temperatures in excess of 104.5°F.[14]

Sick and colleagues[15] suggested that toe abscesses were more common in high-spirited excitable animals, animals shipped in aluminum trailers without sufficient bedding, and animals exposed to concrete surfaces. This was corroborated by Miskimins,[16] who reported that the toe abscesses he observed in Midwestern feedlots during the winter months of 1992 to 1993 were associated with excessive wear that lead to white line separation and subsequent abscess formation in the apex of the toe in rear claws. Herein lies an important distinction between the trauma-induced toe lesions observed in dairy cattle compared with those in feedlot cattle. Whereas thinning of the sole leads to separation of the sole away from the white line in dairy

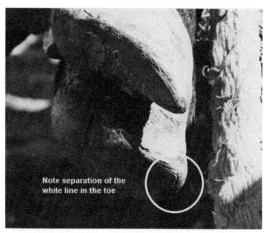

Fig. 7. Hemorrhage and separation of the white in this feedlot steer. This is believed to be a precursor to ascending infection and the toe tip necrosis syndrome.

cattle, excessive wear and thinning leads to separation of the white line in apex of the toe with subsequent abscess formation.

Recently, closer examination of these lesions has established that toe lesions in feedlot cattle are associated with multiple complications and symptoms, including septic osteitis of the third, second, and first phalanxes; and tendonitis, tenosynovitis, cellulitis, and embolic pneumonia. Because these lesions are commonly observed to occur together (much like a disease syndrome), toe abscesses and their related complications in feedlot cattle are often referred to as toe tip necrosis syndrome (TTNS).

TOE TIP NECROSIS SYNDROME IN FEEDLOT CATTLE

TTNS is described as a hind limb lameness disorder of feedlot cattle characterized by varying degrees of ulceration, abscess formation, and necrosis of the toe tip that normally develops early in the feeding period.[17] A case-control study of TTNS was conducted by Canadian researchers to assess risk factors for the condition in western Canadian feedlot cattle.[11] Cases were defined as animals having white line separation in the apical portions of affected claws with gross pathologic involvement of the third phalanx (P3). A control animal was the next animal to be necropsied that was free of gross lesions involving the P3. Researchers had access to 222 hoof samples from 16 different feedlots for study. Despite a general belief that toe lesions are often related to laminitis, researchers found no evidence of P3 rotation in TTNS cases. The most significant and consistent lesion observed was thinning of the sole in the apex of the toe and along the apical and abaxial regions of the white line in cases categorized as TTNS compared with controls. Thinning and abrasion of the white line predisposed to development of microfissures and separation within the white line, leading to the retrograde movement of organic matter and digital sepsis of P3 and deeper structures of the foot **(Fig. 7)**.[11]

IN SUMMARY

Traumatic lesions of the sole are important causes of lameness in beef and dairy cattle. Perforations of the sole, penetration of the sole by foreign bodies, and lesions caused by excessive wear or abrasion lead to TSTU in dairy cattle or TTNS in beef cattle. Prompt identification and treatment of traumatic sole lesions requires corrective trimming and the use of blocks to relieve weightbearing on injured claws. Accurate diagnosis and proper recording of claw lesions is a first step toward control and prevention of these lesions, which may necessitate greater surveillance of flooring surfaces for the presence of protruding nails and foreign bodies. In situations in which TS or TSTU are continual problems, it may be necessary to reduce the abrasiveness of flooring surfaces or apply rubber in the holding area, walkways, and exit lanes. If possible, for feedlot cattle in which TTNS is a problem, limit exposure of cattle to concrete surfaces; handle animals quietly; and, when necessary, assure that trailers are well-bedded when transporting.

REFERENCES

1. Blowey R, Weaver D. Foreign body penetration of the sole in color atlas of diseases and disorders of cattle. 3rd edition. Mosby Elsevier; 2011. p. 106–7.
2. Greenough PR. Foreign body in sole of cattle, in Merck veterinary manual, section on lameness in cattle. Available at: https://www.merckvetmanual.com/musculoskeletal-system/lameness-in-cattle/foreign-body-in-sole-of-cattle. Accessed December 24, 2016.
3. Shearer JK, van Amstel SR. Manual of foot care in cattle. 2nd edition. Atkinson (WI): WD Hoards and Sons Company, Ft; 2013. p. 1–132.
4. Shearer JK, Plummer PJ, Schleining JA. Perspectives on the treatment of claw lesions in cattle. Vet Med Res Rep 2015;6:273–92.
5. Sanders AH, Shearer JK, De Vries A. Seasonal incidence of lameness and risk factors associated with thin soles, white line disease, ulcers, and sole punctures in dairy cattle. J Dairy Sci 2009;92:3165–74.
6. van Amstel SR, Shearer JK, Palin FL. Moisture content, thickness, and lesions of sole horn associated with thin soles in dairy cattle. J Dairy Sci 2004;87(3):757–63.
7. Shearer JK, van Amstel SR. Effect of flooring and/or flooring surfaces on lameness disorders in dairy cattle. Proceedings of the Western Dairy Management Conference. Reno (NV), March 7–9, 2007. p.149–59.
8. Shearer JK, van Amstel SR, Brodersen BW. Diagnostic pathology, clinical diagnosis of foot and leg lameness in cattle. Vet Clin North Am Food Anim Pract 2012;28:535–56, edited by V. Cooper.
9. Nuss K, Kostlin R, Bohmer H. Significance of septic, traumatic ungulocoriitis (pododermatitis) at the tip of the bovine claw. Tierarztl Prax 1990;18(6):567–75.
10. van Amstel SR, Shearer JK. Clinical report: characterization of toe ulcers associated with thin soles in dairy cows. Bovine Pract 2008;42:1–8.
11. Paetsch C, Fenton K, Perrett T, et al. Prospective case-control study of toe tip necrosis syndrome (TTNS) in western Canadian feedlot cattle. Can Vet J 2017; 58(3):247–54.
12. Toussaint Raven E. Cattle foot care and claw trimming. Ipswich (United Kingdom): Farming Press; 1989. p. 24–6.
13. Cermak J. Design of slip-resistant surfaces for dairy cattle buildings. Bov Pract 1998;23:76–8.
14. Schwartzkopf-Genswein KS, Janzen E, Jelinski M, et al. Occurrence, characterization and risk factors associated with lameness within Alberta feedlots: preliminary results. Proceedings of the 4th International Symposium on Beef Cattle Welfare, Iowa State University. Ames (IA), July 16–18, 2014.
15. Sick FL, Bleeker CM, Mouw JK, et al. Toe abscesses in recently shipped feeder cattle. Vet Med Small Anim Clin 1982;77:1385–7.

16. Miskimins DW. Bovine toe abscesses. Proceedings 8th International Symposium on disorders of the ruminant digit. Banff (Alberta), June 26-29, 1994.
17. Jelinski M, Fenton K, Perrett T, et al. Epidemiology of toe tip necrosis syndrome (TTNS) of North American feedlot cattle. Can Vet J 2016;57(8):829–34.

Pathogenesis and Treatment of Sole Ulcers and White Line Disease

J.K. Shearer, DVM, MS[a],*, Sarel R. van Amstel, BVSc, MMedVet[b]

KEYWORDS

- Cattle lameness • Laminitis • Sole ulcers • White line disease • Claw lesions
- Corrective trimming • Foot blocks

KEY POINTS

- Sole ulcers and white line disease are 2 of the most common claw horn lesions in cattle.
- Laminitis refers to a weakening of the suspensory apparatus of the third phalanx that predisposes to sole ulcers and white line disease.
- Risk factors for claw horn lesions include increased metalloproteinase enzymes and peripartum hormonal activity, cow comfort, prolonged standing on hard uneven walking surfaces, horn overgrowth, and claw conformation.
- Application of an orthopedic foot block and corrective trimming form the basis for successful treatment of sole ulcers and white line disease.
- Claw lesions heal by secondary intention requiring a range of 24 to 30 days for the reepithelization of an uncomplicated lesion.

Housing of dairy cows has changed over the past 50 years. Whereas cows were housed largely in stanchions and on pasture in years past, more than 75% of cows are housed in freestalls and drylot conditions. Performance has steadily improved as cows and herds have benefited from better feeding and management. Based on US Department of Agriculture statistics, dairy herds have also continued to get larger over the same period; in fact, over the past 4 decades the average herd size has increased from 29 to more than 187 cows per farm. Out of necessity, as herds have gotten larger, concrete has become the predominant flooring system. For a land animal like the dairy cow, these changes have come at a price. Cows housed in freestalls usually have a higher percentage of lameness, which most attribute to more time spent on concrete.

The authors have nothing to disclose.
[a] Department of Veterinary Diagnostic and Production Animal Medicine, College of Veterinary Medicine, Iowa State University, 2436 Lloyd Veterinary Medical Center, Ames, IA 50011, USA;
[b] Department of Large Animal Clinical Studies, College of Veterinary Medicine, University of Tennessee, 2407 River Dr, Knoxville, TN 37996, USA
* Corresponding author.
E-mail address: jks@iastate.edu

NONINFECTIOUS DISORDERS OF THE BOVINE FOOT

The most common causes of lameness affecting the cow's digit or claw are sole ulcers, white line disease (WLD), and traumatic lesions of the sole, including thin sole toe ulcers predisposed by thinning of the sole owing to excessive wear rates or overtrimming. Some of these conditions are predisposed by metabolic disorders, including rumen acidosis and laminitis, along with other physiologic changes that occur during the transition period. Nearly all are complicated by mechanical factors that are part of life on hard flooring surfaces that contribute to lameness by encouraging claw horn overgrowth and altered weight bearing. With few exceptions, sole ulcers and WLD are the most common claw disorders in confined dairy cattle.

THE DISTINCTION BETWEEN LAMINITIS AND CORIOSIS

Laminitis is an important underlying cause of sole ulcers and WLD; however, closer observation demonstrates that far more than just the suspensory tissues of the laminar corium are involved. The term coriosis better describes the condition as an inflammatory insult affecting the coronary, laminar, perioplic, and solar regions of the corium.[1] Involvement of the coronary corium accelerates the growth of wall horn; however, altered blood flow reduces keratinization of horn cells, making hoof walls weaker and abnormally deformed. Dorsal walls are often concave, and axial and abaxial walls flatten as they reach the weight-bearing surface. Coriosis also occurs as a subclinical disorder. Horn produced under these conditions is softer and may appear yellowish or reddish in color as a consequence of poor keratinization and staining by transudates that leak into the extravascular tissues during horn formation.

Laminitis better describes the physiologic or pathologic changes occurring to the laminar corium (suspensory apparatus of P3). In contrast with the horse, laminitis in cattle is primarily a degenerative rather than inflammatory process affecting the dermal–epidermal junction and basal cell layer of the epidermis. Inflammation may be largely a secondary event occurring subsequent to an increase in interstitial tissue pressure associated with the vascular events of vasodilatation, congestion, transudation, and diapedesis occurring within the corium.[2] Furthermore, despite its common association with rumen acidosis, few studies have been able to confirm a clear link between rumen acidosis and laminitis. Instead, weakness of the suspensory tissues of the third phalanx (P3) seem to bear a closer relationship with physiologic events occurring during the peripartum period. These are described in greater detail in the sections to follow.

LAMINITIS: PHASES 1, 2, AND 3

Laminitis occurs with greatest frequency during the peripartum period; however, the incidence of claw disorders often peaks at 100 plus days in lactation. Understanding laminitis as a 3-stage process helps to explain the temporal relationship between laminitis and claw lesions.

Laminitis is described as a disorder occurring in 3 distinct but overlapping phases.[2] Phase 1 is initiated by the release of vasoactive substances that impair blood flow to the corium and requires only a matter of hours to cause significant degeneration and damage to the dermal–epidermal junction. Phase 2 is characterized by the sinking and downward displacement of P3 that leads to compression-related injury of the corium and digital cushion beneath. Injury to the solar corium and digital cushion from compression causes hemorrhage, thrombosis, and variable amounts of necrosis, similar to that observed in phase 1, but in this case the lesion is a consequence of contusion-related trauma from the sinking of P3. Phase 3 is manifested by the development of sole ulcers and WLD that occurs over a period of 8 to 12 weeks or more after the initial events in phases 1 and 2.[1,2] Phases 1 and 2 are generally subclinical conditions whereas the claw disorders that result in phase 3 are more likely to result in clinical lameness.

THE PATHOGENESIS OF SOLE ULCERS

Sole ulcers are among the most frequent causes of lameness in cattle and occur most commonly in the lateral claw of the rear foot.[3] They are frequently bilateral and have a high rate of reoccurrence. The incidence of sole ulcers in both beef and dairy cattle is variable depending on predisposing causes on individual farms including housing and nutrition, foot trimming and claw care, and genetic conformational problems such as screw claw.[4,5] These predisposing causes result in mechanical loading and/or metabolic/enzymatic changes, which directly lead to failure of the suspension system of the third phalanx resulting in vascular injury as result of compression of the corium between P3 and the sole[6] (**Figs. 1** and **2**). Disturbances in the microvasculature lead to ischemia and hypoxia. Consequently, cellular proliferation and differentiation in the basal layers of the sole epidermis are interrupted, with subsequent development of a full-thickness horn defect (ulcer) that typically occurs in zone 4 (typical sole ulcer, Rusterholtz ulcer, or pododermatitis circumscripta; **Fig. 3**), zone 6 (heel ulcer; **Fig. 4**) or zone 5 (toe ulcer; **Fig. 5**) with exposure of the underlying corium.[3,7]

The most common metabolic conditions predisposing to claw lesions include rumen acidosis, laminitis, and conditions caused by coliform bacteria such as coliform mastitis.[4,5] Endotoxin release associated with these conditions can result in the formation of vasoactive cytokines, causing vascular changes as well as activation of metalloproteinases responsible for the breakdown of collagen, a major component of the suspension system of P3.[8] Hormonal changes, specifically relaxin (or relaxin-like hormone) and estrogen in the peripartum period, may contribute to elongation and

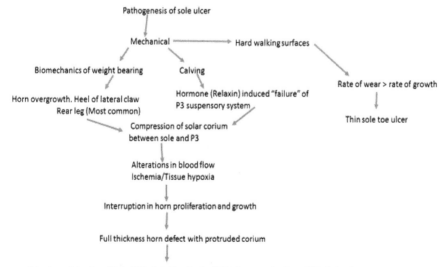

Fig. 1. Pathogenesis of sole ulceration associated with primary mechanical factors causing a full-thickness defect in the solar horn.

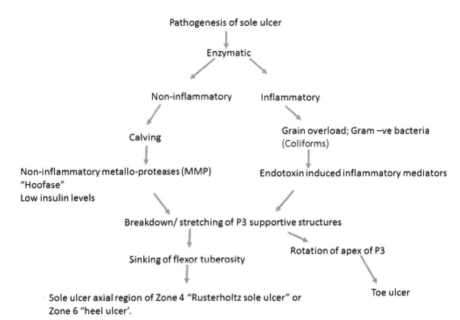

Fig. 2. Pathogenesis of sole ulceration associated with primary enzymatic/metabolic factors causing a full-thickness defect in the solar horn.

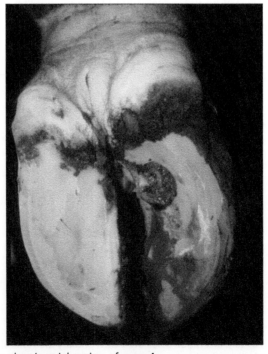

Fig. 3. Typical sole ulcer in axial region of zone 4.

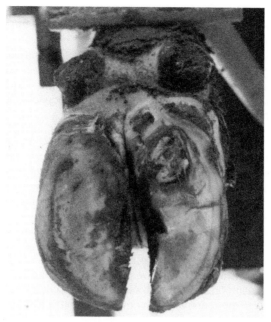

Fig. 4. Heel ulcer in zone 6.

weakening of the P3 suspension system resulting in failure. Therefore, enzyme degradation of the strong collagen fiber bundles within the laminar corium coupled with weakening of these structures by peripartum hormonal changes leads to sinking and rotation of the P3 and compressive damage of the solar and perioplic vasculature

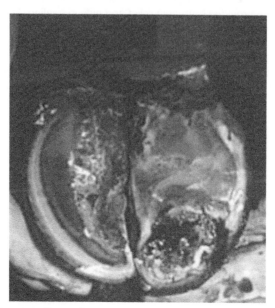

Fig. 5. Toe ulcer in apex of zone 5.

in the corium that lie beneath.[6,8] Displacement of P3 and subsequent damage to the underlying corium is compounded by mechanical loading secondary to claw horn overgrowth and unbalanced weight bearing.

In addition, hydrocortisone and prolactin, a lactogenic hormone, may also play a role in the pathogenesis; both were noted to decrease protein synthesis of bovine claw explants.[9] High levels of a 52-kD protease ("hoofase") were demonstrated in tissues after calving.[10] This finding may explain the high incidence of sole hemorrhages seen 2 to 4 months after calving.

Composition of the digital cushion may also play a role in the pathogenesis of sole and heel ulcers.[11] In heifers, the digital cushion consists primarily of loose connective tissue and a small amount of fat, primarily in the form of saturated fatty acids, whereas in older cows the digital cushion has more fat consisting mainly of monounsaturated fatty acids, which make the cushion softer, thus providing more shock absorption. This may be one of the reasons for the greater incidence of sole ulcers in heifers housed on concrete.[11]

Normal biomechanics of weight bearing may also play a role in the pathogenesis of sole ulcer formation. During normal locomotion, the lateral claws of the rear legs carry more weight as opposed to the medial claws, which results in accelerated horn growth, particularly at the heel. This overgrowth of the hind lateral claw leads to concussion of the solar corium and contributes to sole ulcer formation.[12]

Mechanical injury without primary inflammatory changes also occurs in thin-soled dairy cattle where the protective function of sole horn becomes inadequate, particularly on hard walking surfaces. The sole becomes thin and eventually results in a full-thickness defect[13] (thin sole toe ulcer; **Fig. 6**).

TREATMENT

Suggested approaches to treatment depend on the clinical presentation (**Table 1**). One of the most important treatment considerations in all cases of sole ulcer is the application of a claw block on the sound claw to relieve weight bearing from the affected claw.[3] This provides both pain relief and aids in healing. In cases of a developing ulcer characterized by hemorrhage and pain, lowering of the affected heel will transfer sufficient weight to the healthy claw for healing to take place and can be done instead of applying an orthopedic block to the sound claw (**Fig. 7**).[14]

Horn covering and surrounding the ulcer is often necrotic and under run, resulting in the entrapment of dirt. Pare loose and necrotic horn away from the ulcer at a 45° angle

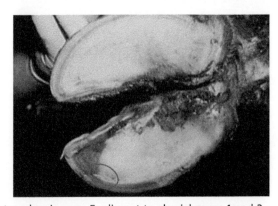

Fig. 6. Thin sole toe ulcer in zone 5 adjacent to abaxial zones 1 and 2.

Table 1
Clinical presentation and complications associated with sole ulcers

Sole Ulcer Type	Toe Ulcer, Apex Zone 5	Sole Ulcer Axial Zone 4 Heel Ulcer Zone 6	Thin Sole Toe Ulcer Zone 5 Adjacent to Abaxial Zones 1 and 2
Lameness score	Mild to severe	Moderate to non-weight bearing	Mild to severe
Postural change	Heel first foot placement	Severe swelling to above dew claws with ascending infection	Stiff, stilted, painful walk particularly if all 4 feet affected
Lesion presentation	Mainly front claw Often no visible lesion Pain response on sole tapping/hoof tester	Full-thickness horn defect Protruding corium normal or granulating Ascending tract with swelling	Sole hemorrhage Partial to complete sole thickness defect Zone 5 adjacent to abaxial zones 1 and 2
Possible complications	Subsolar separation/abscess P3 osteitis Pathologic P3 fracture/sequestrum	Granulating corium Bulbar abscess Retroarticular abscess Septic tenosynovitis Septic distal interphalangeal joint Digital dermatitis overgrowth	Subsolar separation/abscess P3 osteitis/sequestrum
Treatment	Remove loose and undermined sole and wall horn Remove sequestrum Debride P3 Apply orthopedic foot block	Remove undermined sole and granulating corium Bandage optional Lance bulbar abscess Deep digital flexor tendon resection Claw amputation Joint arthrodesis Apply orthopedic block Regional IV antibiotics	Remove loose and undermined sole Remove sequestrum Debride P3 Apply orthopedic foot block Both claws on same leg affected Place on soft surface

until a thin layer of horn remains around the circumference of the ulcer, taking care not to damage normal corium.[3,14] Protruding corium showing exuberant granulation tissue (**Fig. 8**) should be removed to the level of the thinned horn surrounding the ulcer. This usually results in a fair amount of bleeding, which justifies the use of a bandage.[14]

Because the corium is highly innervated, regional anesthesia below a tourniquet should be used in all cases involving exposed corium before the start of any corrective trimming.[14] The use of systemic antiinflammatory agents or antibiotics are usually not necessary in uncomplicated cases of sole ulceration.

THE PATHOGENESIS OF WHITE LINE DISEASE

A study of 37 dairy farms in 4 regions of England and Wales found that, of 8645 lesions causing lameness, most (92%) affected hindlimbs. Of lesions affecting hindlimbs, 65% were in the outer claw, 20% in the skin, and 14% in the inner claw. Sole ulcers (40%) and white line lesions (29%) were the predominant claw lesions observed.[15]

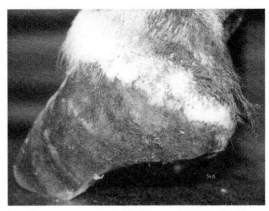

Fig. 7. Transferring weight to the sound claw by lowering the heel on the affected side.

STRUCTURE OF THE WHITE LINE

A detailed summary of the anatomy of the white line as described by Mulling is available elsewhere.[16] A portion of this discussion is provided here for purpose of describing the structure of the white line and its relationship to WLD. The white line is a 3-part structure consisting of an outer, intermediate, and inner zones that are formed by epidermal cells in the distal wall and laminar regions. Horn of the white line is produced by epidermis overlying the dermal laminae, by cap papillae on the

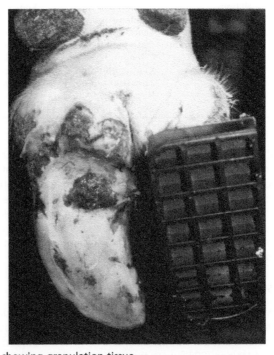

Fig. 8. Sole ulcer showing granulation tissue.

crests of the laminae, and by terminal papillae at the distal end of the dermal laminae. The dermal laminae are positioned in a proximal–distal orientation (ie, parallel to the dorsal surface of P3). At the distal end, the dermal laminae bend underneath the tip of the apex of the toe where they merge with thick terminal papillae before transitioning into rows of dermal papillae that produce the horn of the sole. The outermost region of the white line is formed in the uppermost part of the dermal laminae that lies adjacent to the wall. It consists of nonpigmented and nontubular horn. The intermediate zone of the white line consists of cap horn produced by the cap papillae and the inner zone contains tubular horn, which is formed by the epidermis of the terminal papillae.[17]

The differences in origin and, more important, in the heterogeneity of horn within each of these zones represent a point of weakness within the white line and weight-bearing surface of the claw. The strength and resistance of the white line to mechanical factors encountered on flooring surfaces is improved by the proper keratinization and cornification of horn cells within these zones.[17] In contrast, a disease such as laminitis, which disrupts blood flow to the corium, leads to the production of poorly keratinized or dyskeratotic horn that is weaker and less resistant to physical forces and the incursion of foreign material. Weakened, defective, or poor quality horn is prone to separation and colonization by bacteria and fungi, which are key factors in the pathogenesis of WLD.

THE ENTRAPMENT OF FOREIGN MATERIAL IN THE WHITE LINE

Stones and other debris on cattle walkways commonly become entrapped within the soft heterogeneous horn of the white line. Some of this may be explained by microscopic evaluation of the white line that indicates it is prone to the development of microcracks and fissures that often become infiltrated with organic matter and other foreign material on cattle walkways.[17] Once wedged within the white line, these objects are forced deeper into the white line by weight bearing and continued mechanical impact, which is a natural consequence of locomotion and placement of the foot to the floor or ground. Bacteria associated with the foreign material colonize within the white line horn, causing further decay as the infection migrates toward the vascular tissues of the corium. Upon reaching the corium, an abscess forms that causes pain and thus lameness.

When WLD is detected at this early stage, correction of the localized lesion through corrective trimming is sufficient to effect resolution (**Figs. 9–12**). If the condition is detected later in the course of the disease, it is not uncommon to find that the abscess will have migrated beneath the wall exiting at the coronet as a purulent discharge. Alternatively, the abscess may undermine the heel and become discharged at the heel bulb. The worst case scenario is that where the infectious process moves proximally to deeper structures including the distal interphalangeal joint, retroarticular space, and other deeper tissues of the foot. In this case, surgery will likely be required (see David E. Anderson and colleagues' article, "Surgical Procedures of the Distal Limb for Treatment of Sepsis in Cattle," in this issue).

FACTORS HYPOTHESIZED TO CONTRIBUTE TO WHITE LINE DISEASE

Internal forces generated during normal weight bearing are well-tolerated in normal feet; however, they may be problematic in situations where the white line has been weakened by separation and the accumulation of organic matter or other material within the white line. When weight is borne on the foot, forces extend in multiple directions (downward, medially, and laterally toward the wall) within the claw horn capsule.

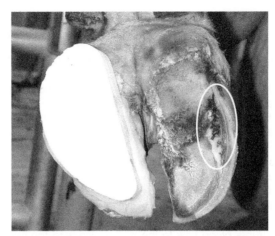

Fig. 9. White line disease in the abaxial region of the white line, block attached to the healthy claw before corrective trimming.

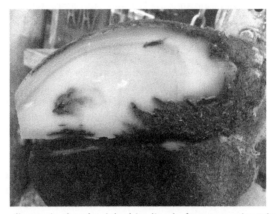

Fig. 10. White line disease in the abaxial white line before corrective trimming.

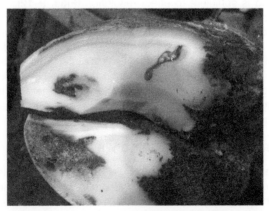

Fig. 11. Additional corrective trimming sufficient to make contact with the abscess. Careful removal of loose undermined horn is necessary to permit healing.

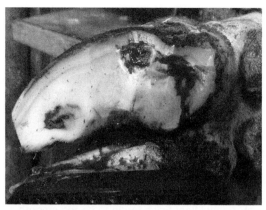

Fig. 12. Corrective trimming complete with minimal damage to the underlying corium. A block applied to the healthy claw is sufficient to permit a full recovery.

Because the abaxial heel is a common site for WLD, some have theorized that compression and expansion of the digital cushion may be one of the factors responsible for a tendency toward separation of the white line in this region.[18] The abaxial heel is also the site of heel strike during locomotion. As foreign substances become lodged within the white line, further separation, bacterial decay, and deterioration of the white line horn predisposes WLD.

Similar physical stresses to the white line may occur as a result of the confinement of animals on hard, uneven flooring surfaces. In this case, the stresses are external in nature, but their effect is not only on the white line, but also on the laminar corium (ie, suspensory apparatus) and its connection to the lamellae of the wall. The vascular architecture of the white line in these regions is particularly delicate and therefore easily disturbed.[17] Physical stresses associated with weight bearing on rough and irregular surfaces are believed to increase sheering forces on the axial and abaxial walls that are transmitted to the laminar corium. Inflammation of these tissues follows, as does an increase in lateral pressure on the wall.

Finally, mechanical stresses to the white line may occur when cattle are simply pushed laterally or medially while their feet are firmly placed on the floor. Cook describes this as a condition that occurs in milking parlor holding areas, where cattle at the rear of the pen are caught between herd mates in front and the forward movement of the crowd gate behind them. The cows turn sideways to make room for the on-coming gate. As the gate contacts the cows and pushes forward, the feet of the cows slide laterally along the floor, putting tremendous stress on the axial and abaxial walls (from comments during a presentation delivered at the Western Dairy Management Conference, 2017).[19]

RELATIONSHIP OF PROLONGED STANDING TO WHITE LINE DISEASE

Prolonged standing on hard surfaces is considered an important risk factor for lameness. Cattle are believed to be particularly susceptible to damage of the laminar corium during the transition period, when these tissues are more likely to be weakened by metabolic and hormonal factors. A possible mechanism for this is an increase in lateral (ie, outward pressure on the wall) resulting from inflammation and swelling of the dermal laminae that may contribute to white line separation.[20] It is also hypothesized that WLD may be caused by the hypostasis of blood in the distal limb associated with prolonged standing. Impaired blood flow was suggested to result in ischemia, hypoxia, necrosis, and separation of the white line in the apex of P3.[18,21–23]

FLOORING CONSIDERATIONS FOR REDUCING WHITE LINE DISEASE

Cows are land animals; therefore, concrete is certainly a less than ideal flooring surface. Beyond its hard and unforgiving nature is the fact that the way the surface of concrete is finished has significant consequences for foot and leg health. Rough finishes increase the rate of claw horn wear and are associated with a higher incidence of lameness.[24] New concrete is particularly abrasive because of the sharp edges and protruding aggregate that naturally develop as it is cures. These may be removed by dragging heavy concrete blocks or a steel scraper over the flooring surface. They may also be removed mechanically by grinding or polishing of the surface. Generally speaking, concrete finished with a wood float provides one of the best surfaces for a cow's foot. A steel float finish tends to be too smooth and may be particularly slippery when covered by manure slurry. Smooth concrete reduces wear and may contribute to claw horn overgrowth, which may require more frequent trimming of claws. Smooth surfaces are also slippery and predispose to injury, usually of the upper leg from falling. A Dutch study determined that concrete floors normally do not provide sufficient friction to support normal locomotion of dairy cattle.[25]

Grooving the surface of smooth concrete floors is generally necessary to improve traction and reduce injuries from falling. Although recommendations may vary, grooving in a parallel or diamond pattern on the floor maximizes traction and reduces slips and falls. Grooves running in a parallel direction should be three-eighths to one-half inch wide and three-eighths to one-half inch deep and spaced approximately 3 to 4 inches on center. When grooves are wider than 2 inches, the floor is less comfortable because support at the weight-bearing surface is less uniform. For the same reason, it is advised that the floor area between the grooves be kept flat also. Flooring area between grooves on a diamond pattern may be slightly wider, at 4 to 6 inches on center. The diamond pattern is considered to be particularly useful in high-traffic areas. The orientation of grooves at right angles to the direction of the manure scraper travel should be avoided.[26]

WOUND HEALING IN THE CONTEXT OF CLAW LESIONS

The objective in wound healing of claw lesions is closure of the defect that includes reconstruction of the tissues involved and the creation of new epithelium over the defect. Claw lesions that extend through the horn capsule to expose the corium heal by secondary intention with the formation of granulation tissue and eventually new epithelium. Wound healing is a dynamic and complicated process generally described in terms of 3 (some do not include hemostasis) or 4 overlapping phases including hemostasis, inflammation, proliferation, and maturation or remodeling.[27,28] An understanding of these events and what conditions may interfere with the process are useful in terms of guiding proper treatment decisions.

Hemostasis

Hemostasis is normally the first response to injury affecting the dermis or corium. In cases of acute injury, hemorrhage plays a key role in wound repair as a means to cleanse the lesion and provide the source of blood platelets for clot formation. Within minutes, platelets enter the site of injury and begin to clump, forming a clot that is later reinforced by fibrin proteins that ultimately create an insoluble blockage essential for long-term hemostasis. Coincident with the clotting process is the release of numerous cytokines and vasoactive mediators that cause vasoconstriction to reduce blood loss and also activate inflammatory cells in preparation for the second phase of the healing process.[27,28]

Inflammation

Inflammation is characterized by the movement of white blood cells from the vascular system to the site of injury. However, in acute lesions, it is often described as a process involving 2 overlapping stages: the vascular and cellular stages. The vascular stage begins with vasoconstriction of the arterioles and venules near the site of injury. After 10 minutes or so, vasoconstriction gives way to a period of vasodilatation and increased vascular permeability whereby fluids move from the blood stream into the extravascular spaces of the injured tissue. The transudation of fluid into and around the site of injury contributes to pain, heat, redness, edema, and loss of function of the affected tissues.[27,28]

The cellular stage of the inflammatory process is marked by the movement of white blood cells from the blood stream to the site of injury. Neutrophils are the predominant white cells early in the inflammatory process. Their role is the engulfment of bacteria. Neutrophils are later replaced by macrophages, which enter the site and continue to engulf residual bacteria and debride devitalized tissues.[27,28]

The Proliferative Phase

The proliferative phase begins within the first 2 to 3 days after injury and is characterized by angiogenesis, fibroplasia, granulation tissue formation, epithelialization, and tissue contraction. The predominant cell type found in lesions during the proliferative phase is the fibroblast. These cells have multiple functions, some of which are the production of ground substance and collagen (primarily collagen type III) within the wound site. With sufficient neovascularization, granulation tissue develops rapidly and fills in the defects caused by injury. Although less resistant to external factors than intact skin, it provides an early, although imperfect, barrier to injurious agents from the environment.[27,28] Any interference in the chain of events occurring during the proliferative phase is likely to result in prolonged wound healing.

The formation of new horn (ie, reepithelialization) over the exposed corium of an ulcer or white disease lesion is a primary objective in the treatment of claw disorders. Epithelialization normally occurs from the level of the basal cell layer atop the basement membrane. Keratinocytes positioned superficial to the basement membrane facilitate early repair by migrating to the surface of the intact granulation tissue bed. After a few days, keratinocytes are freed from their attachments at the wound edges and begin a slow migration toward the center of the wound. The speed of this process of reepithelialization depends on the severity and type of injury suffered. Reepithelialization of lesions is rapid when the injury is superficial (ie, such as an abrasion), and the basement membrane and basal cell layer are intact or minimally damaged. On the contrary, when a full-thickness defect of the epithelium occurs, the recovery process is prolonged because the basement membrane and basal layer are disrupted and residual keratinocytes at the site of the wound are not immediately available for recruitment to start the healing process. In these situations, reepithelialization must occur from the wound edges requiring centripetal movement of keratinocytes from the wound margins.[29]

The Maturation or Remodeling Phase

The maturation or remodeling phase is the final stage of wound healing that with lesions of the skin leads to the formation of a scar. Although the process is similar with claw lesions, the equivalent to a scar in the claw horn capsule is less obvious than would be observed in a skin lesion. This phase usually begins after a few weeks and may continue for several months.[27,28]

HEALING RATES FOR CLAW LESIONS

Although wound healing is a spontaneous and continuous process, careless trimming techniques, failure to relive weight bearing on the injured claw, or infectious conditions such as digital dermatitis may delay healing of claw lesions. Lischer and colleagues[30] evaluated healing rates on 74 cows with 105 claw lesions over a 6-month period. The mean time for the formation of a new layer of epithelium was 25 days for lesions causing slight alteration of the corium, 33 days for moderate corium alterations, and 42 days for lesions causing severe alterations of the corium. Investigators indicated that 68% of all lesions were completely covered by a solid layer of new horn at 30 days after the initial treatment.[30] Van Amstel and colleagues[31] made similar observations whereby 66% of lesions studied by these researchers were covered by a layer of new horn after 30 days. Based on these studies, one might conclude that mild-to-moderate lesions are likely to require somewhere around 21 to 30 days and more severe lesions a minimum of 40 days and potentially as long as 60 days for complete reepithelization of the lesion.

TOPICAL TREATMENT OF SOLE ULCERS AND WHITE LINE DISEASE

Topical treatments were applied to claw lesions by 59% of veterinarians and 53% of hoof trimmers. Medications most commonly used were the soluble powder forms of tetracycline or oxytetracycline (48% by veterinarians and 81% by hoof trimmers) followed by copper sulfate for veterinarians and ichthammol ointment (a sulfurous, tarry compound with mild antiseptic properties used primarily as a drawing agent) by trimmers.[32] Many assume that some form of topical treatment on claw lesions is necessary in part because claw lesions are commonly associated with secondary abscess formation. In fact, abscess formation is best managed by thorough corrective trimming alone. Removing all loose, undermined, and necrotic horn eliminates the microenvironment necessary to propagate the anaerobic organisms responsible for abscesses in claw lesions. Others believe topical therapy is necessary to counteract contamination that is unavoidable during the posttreatment period. However, topical treatment, even when combined with a wrap or bandage, does little to prevent contamination.

As described, the objective in wound healing is a rapid unimpeded reepithelialization of the lesion and anything that prolongs the inflammatory or proliferative phases of wound healing is contraindicated. The clinical indication of an interference with wound healing is the formation of exuberant granulation tissue.[28] Van Amstel and colleagues[31] found that ulcers with excessive granulation tissue healed more slowly compared with lesions free of granulation tissue. Therefore, in keeping with the tenets of the principle of "first do no harm" we take a look at some of the current options for topical treatment.

Application of caustic agents such as copper sulfate to reduce granulation tissue is contraindicated, because this application will impede healing by interfering with new cell growth from the edges of the ulcer. Similarly, oxytetracycline power should not be used directly on exposed normal corium because it seems to delay healing. A study of healing rates was conducted on 18 cows randomly divided into a treatment group treated topically with oxytetracycline soluble powder (7 cows) or copper sulfate powder (3 cows) and a bandage, and control group (8 cows), no topical treatment and a bandage. Photos of lesions at day 21 were presented to 2 independent observers who scored the lesions for the visual presence of granulation tissue and evidence of reepithelization. Based on observer scores at day 21, lesions topically treated with oxytetracycline or copper sulfate were more likely to have granulation tissue ($P > .0054$) and less likely to have evidence of reepithelization ($P > .0553$). These data suggest that the use of topical oxytetracycline or copper sulfate on claw lesions may delay healing.[33]

Topical oxytetracycline or tetracycline may be necessary if the exposed corium has become secondarily infected with digital dermatitis. Topical application of a mixture of dexamethasone added to oxytetracycline powder to form a paste applied under a bandage after resection of granulation tissue associated with protruding corium has given good results and increases the rate of healing. Apart from its antibacterial properties oxytetracycline has some antiinflammatory effects through inhibition of metalloproteinases.[34]

Other topical treatments include Solka Hoofgel, ichthammol ointment (a sulfurous, tarry compound with mild antiseptic properties used primarily as a drawing agent). Triple antibiotic ointments and silver sulfadiazine are sometimes used because of their broad spectrum of activity. Other topical products include petrolatum-based ointments, such as Aquaphor ointment (Beiersdorf Inc., Wilton, CT), white petroleum jelly, vitamin A and D ointment, which is 93.5% white petrolatum in combination with vitamins A and D and a small amount of corn oil and light mineral oil. These ointments limit surface bacterial growth and prevent dressings from sticking to wounds.[16] A product more commonly used on farms for minor skin wounds and irritation is Bag Balm (Dairy Association Co, Lyndonville, VT). It consists of 8-hydroxyquinoline sulfate 0.3% in a petroleum jelly and lanolin base. Anecdotal reports suggest that granular sugar and honey are also used as topical wound dressings on claw lesions. The theory of sugar's effectiveness in wound healing is based on its high osmolarity, which draws moisture from the wound, thus inhibiting the growth of bacteria. Sugar has also been used in infected lesions for the debridement of necrotic tissue. Honey's antibacterial benefits are likely related to its low pH, high osmolarity, and peroxide activity.[16]

USE OF BANDAGES AND WRAPS

The routine use of bandages for the treatment of sole ulcers or WLD is controversial unless used for a specific purpose such for the control of hemorrhage, treatment of digital dermatitis, or prevention of granulation tissue formation. Wraps may also be used for protection in cases where large areas of the corium have been exposed. At least 2 studies did not show any improvement in the rate of healing using bandages except for the conditions indicated.[35,36] Cases of complicated sole ulcer may require surgical intervention and other treatments, including both systemic and regional intravenous antibiotic therapy and tenovaginotomy with limited or radical resection of the deep digital flexor tendon and superficial digital flexor tendon over the whole length of the digital flexor tendon sheath with or without insertion of an indwelling drain. Arthrodesis of the distal interphalangeal joint or claw amputation may also have to be considered in such cases.[37]

SUMMARY

Sole ulcers and WLD are 2 of the most common claw horn lesions in confined dairy cattle. Predisposing causes include unbalanced weight bearing between claws and metabolic, enzymatic, and hormonal changes that result in a weakened P3 suspensory apparatus and downward displacement of P3 within the claw horn capsule. The white line is a 3-part structure that serves as the junction between the sole and the axial and abaxial wall. Because of its heterogeneous composition, this structure is vulnerable to trauma and separation that permits organic matter to become entrapped within the white line horn tissue. The colonization of bacteria and decay within the white line contributes to retrograde movement of the infection to the solar and perioplic corium where an abscess forms resulting in pain and lameness. Successful treatment requires application of an orthopedic foot block to the healthy claw and corrective trimming of the lesion. Claw lesions heal by second intention requiring a range of 24 to 30 days for the reepithelization of an uncomplicated lesion. More severe or extensive lesions may require 60 days for complete resolution. Topical treatment of claw lesions with compounds such as copper sulfate and tetracycline may delay healing and are, therefore, not advised with the exception of cases where the corium may be secondarily infected with digital dermatitis. Studies do not support the use of bandages for the routine treatment of claw lesions with the exception of situations to control hemorrhage or to provide protection for lesions where large areas of the corium are exposed.

REFERENCES

1. Blowey R, Weaver D. Color atlas of diseases and disorders of cattle. 3rd edition. London: Mosby Elsevier Ltd; 2011.
2. Ossent P, Lischer CHJ. Bovine laminitis: the lesions and their pathogenesis. Practice 1998;20:415–27.
3. Greenough PR. Pododermatitis circumscripta (ulceration of the sole) in cattle. Agri Practice 1987;1:17–22.
4. Enevoldsen C, Gröhn YT, Thysen I. Sole ulcers in dairy cattle: associations with season, cow characteristics, disease, and production. J Dairy Sci 1991;74: 1284–98.
5. Vermunt JJ, Greenough PR. Predisposing factors of laminitis in cattle. Br Vet J 1994;150:151–60.
6. Mulling CH, Lischer CHJ. New aspects on etiology and pathogenesis of laminitis in cattle. Proc Internatl Buiatrics Conference. Hanover (Germany), August 18–23, 2002:236–47.
7. Blowey RW, Watson CL, Green LE, et al. The incidence of heel ulcers in a study of lameness in five UK dairy herds. Proceedings of the XI International Symposium on Disorders of the Ruminant Digit and III International Conference on Bovine Lameness. Parma (Italy), September 3–7, 2000:163–64.
8. Lischer CJ, Ossent P, Raber M, et al. Suspensory structures and supporting tissues of the third phalanx of cows and their relevance to the development of typical sole ulcers (Rusterholtz ulcers). Vet Rec 2002;151:694–8.
9. Hendry KAK, MacCallum AJ, Knight CH, et al. Laminitis in the dairy cow: a cell biological approach. J Dairy Res 1997;64:475–86.
10. Tarlton JF, Webster AJF. A biochemical and biomechanical basis for the pathogenesis of claw horn lesions. Proceedings of the 12th International Symposium on Lameness in Ruminants. Orlando (FL), January 9–13, 2002.
11. Bicalho RC, Machado VS, Caixeta LS. Lameness in dairy cattle: a debilitating disease or a disease of debilitated cattle? A cross-sectional study of lameness prevalence and thickness of the digital cushion. J Dairy Sci 2009;92(7):3175–84.
12. Toussaint Raven E. Structure and functions (Chapter 1) and Trimming (Chapter 3). In: Toussaint Raven E, editor. Cattle foot care and claw trimming. Ipswich (United Kingdom): Farming Press; 1989. p. 24–6, 75–94.

13. Van Amstel SR, Shearer JK. Clinical report – characterization of toe ulcers associated with thin soles in dairy cows. Bovine Pract 2008;42(2):189–96.

14. Shearer JK, van Amstel SR. Functional and corrective claw trimming. In: Anderson DE, editor. Veterinary clinics of North America: food animal practice. Philadelphia: WB Saunders; 2001. p. 53–72.

15. Murray RD, Downham DY, Clarkson MJ, et al. Epidemiology of lameness in dairy cattle: description and analysis of foot lesions. Vet Rec 1996;138(24):586–91.

16. Shearer JK, Plummer PJ, Schleining JA. Perspectives on the treatment of claw lesions in cattle. Vet Med Res Rep 2015;6:273–92.

17. Mulling C. Theories on the pathogenesis of white line disease – an anatomical perspective. In: 12th International Symposium on Lameness in Ruminants. Orlando (FL), January 9–13, 2002.

18. Greenough P. Bovine laminitis and lameness, a hands on approach. 1st Edition. Saunders Ltd. Philadelphia: Saunders; 2007.

19. Cook N. A life cycle oriented approach to lameness control. Proceedings of the Western Dairy Management Conference, Reno (NV), February 28-March 2, 2017. p. 134–45.

20. Tarlton JF, Holah DE, Evans KM, et al. Biomechanical and histopathological changes in the support structures of bovine hooves around the time of first calving. Vet J 2002;163(2):196–204.

21. Paetsch CD, Jelinski MD. Toe-tip necrosis syndrome in feedlot cattle in Western Canada. In: Paper presented at: 17th International Symposium and 9th International Conference on Lameness in Ruminants, Bristol (United Kingdom); August 11-13, 2013. p. 152–3.

22. Paetsch C, Fenton K, Perrett T, et al. Prospective case-control study of toe tip necrosis syndrome (TTNS) in western Canadian feedlot cattle. Can Vet J 2017;58: 247–54.

23. Ossent P, Greenough PR, Vermunt JJ. Laminitis. In: Greenough PR, Weaver AD, editors. Lameness in cattle. 3rd edition. Philadelphia: WB Saunders; 1997. p. 277–92.

24. Wells SJ, Trent AM, Marsh WE, et al. Prevalence and severity of lameness in lactating dairy cows in a sample of Minnesota and Wisconsin herds. J Am Vet Med Assoc 1993;202:78–82.

25. Van der Tol PPJ, Metz JHM, Noordhuizen-Stassen EN, et al. Frictional forces required for unrestrained locomotion in dairy cattle. J Dairy Sci 2005;88:615–24.

26. Shearer JK. Effect of flooring and/or flooring surfaces on lameness disorders in dairy cattle. Proc. Western Dairy Herd Management Conf. Reno (NV), March 7-9, 2007. p. 1–12 Available at: http://wdmc.org/2007/shearer.pdf. Accessed December 11, 2016.

27. Stadelmann WK, Digenis AG, Tobin GR. Physiology and healing dynamics of chronic cutaneous wounds. Am J Surg 1998;176(2A Suppl):26S–38S.

28. Auer J, Stick J. Equine surgery. 2nd edition. St Louis (MO): Saunders Elsevier; 2012.

29. O'Toole EA. Extracellular matrix and keratinocyte migration. Clin Exp Dermatol 2001;26(6):525–30.

30. Lischer CJ, Dietrich-Hunkeler A, Geyer H, et al. Healing process of uncomplicated sole ulcers in dairy cows kept in tie stalls: clinical description and blood chemical investigations. Schweiz Arch Tierheilkd 2001;143(3):125–33 [in German].

31. Van Amstel SR, Shearer JK, Palin FL. Case report – clinical response to treatment of pododermatitis circumscripta (ulceration of the sole) in dairy cows. Bovine Pract 2003;37:143–50.

32. Kleinhenz KE, Plummer PJ, Danielson J, et al. Survey of veterinarians and hoof trimmers on methods applied to treat claw lesions in dairy cattle. Bovine Pract 2014;48(1):47–52.

33. Shearer JK, Plummer PJ, Schleining JA, et al. Effect of topical treatment with oxytetracycline soluble powder or copper sulfate powder on healing of claw lesions. The 18th International Symposium and 10th International Conference on Lameness in Ruminants. Valdivia (Chile), November 22–25, 2015.

34. Van Amstel SR, Shearer JK. Atypical digital dermatitis lesions. Proceedings of the International Symposium on Bovine Lameness. Rotorua (New Zealand), February 28 – March 3rd, 2011.

35. Pyman MFS. Comparison of bandaging and elevation of the claw for treatment of foot lameness in dairy cows. Aust Vet J 1997;75:132–5.

36. White ME, Glickman LT, Embree IC, et al. A randomized trial for evaluation of bandaging sole abscesses in cattle. J Am Vet Med Assoc 1981;178(4):375–7.

37. De Vecchis L. Field procedures for treatment and management of deep digital sepsis. Proceedings of the 12th International Symposium on Lameness in Ruminants. Orlando (FL), January 9–13, 2002.

Pathogenesis and Treatment of Toe Lesions in Cattle Including "Nonhealing" Toe Lesions

Johann Kofler, Dr Med Vet

KEYWORDS

- Apical white line disease • Thin sole • Toe ulcer • Toe necrosis
- Pedal bone necrosis • Digital dermatitis • Toe resection • Cattle

KEY POINTS

- Toe lesions in cattle include apical white line disease, thin soles, toe ulcers, toe necrosis, digital dermatitis–associated toe ulcers/toe necrosis, and fracture of the claw capsule and the apex of the distal phalanx.
- For anatomic reasons, the early stages of toe abnormalities (thin sole, apical white line disease, toe ulcer) are at high risk of rapidly developing into a bone infection.
- The prevalence of toe lesions differs in dairy herds and feedlots; in general, it is rather low at the animal level in feedlots and dairies, even if in singular dairy herds up to 58% of cattle can be affected; however, the herd prevalence of toe lesions can reach up to 50% in dairy herds with endemic digital dermatitis infection.
- In feedlot cattle, lameness and toe necrosis develop frequently 3 days to 3 weeks after arrival on the feedlot.
- Diagnosis of toe lesions can be made by a careful claw examination and by removing the loose horn with a hoof knife; for a definitive diagnosis of the extent of bone infection, radiography can be applied.

INTRODUCTION

The complex of disorders of the toe area in dairy and feedlot cattle includes several lesions such as apical white line disease (AWLD), thin sole, toe ulcer, toe necrosis, digital dermatitis (DD)–associated toe ulcer/toe necrosis ("nonhealing" toe ulcer/toe necrosis), and acute trauma-related lesions, such as fracture of the claw capsule and the tip of distal phalanx (P3).[1–20] Fractures of the claw capsule, and, on occasion, of

The author has nothing to disclose.
Department of Farm Animals and Veterinary Public Health, Clinic for Ruminants, University of Veterinary Medicine Vienna, Veterinaerplatz 1, Vienna A-1210, Austria
E-mail address: Johann.Kofler@vetmeduni.ac.at

the tip of P3, may lead to severe lameness and complications, such as sequestrum formation, due to the loss of blood supply.[8]

With respect to English language literature, a wide variety of different terms have been used in the past, such as "thin sole toe ulcer,"[8,17] "apical white line separation,"[12] "toe abscess,"[1,3,4,7] "toe tip necrosis,"[12] and "toe-tip necrosis syndrome" (TTNS),[10,11,18,19] all of which have contributed to a general level of confusion rather than providing clarity.

Overall, these various terms generally describe only primary lesions and different, early or advanced, stages of toe-tip abnormalities, which have a high risk of resulting in the same complication, namely a small or an extended bone infection of the tip or even large parts of P3.[5–8,10–12,16,18,20] Recently, an international harmonized terminology of bovine claw lesions was published in the *ICAR Claw Health Atlas*.[21] This atlas uses the terms "thin sole" (ie, sole horn yields, feels spongy, when finger pressure is applied), "toe ulcer" (ie, ulcer with exposed fresh or necrotic corium located at the toe), and "toe necrosis" (ie, necrosis of the tip of the toe with involvement of P3[21] caused by a bacterial infection).[6,11] In addition, an AWLD can also be the primary toe lesion.[8] These definitions of abnormalities are simple and clear with a distinct localization at the toe.

In contrast, according to Canadian researchers,[10,11,18,19] the term "toe-tip necrosis syndrome" may also include interphalangeal arthritis, osteomyelitis of the middle and proximal phalanges, flexor tendonitis, cellulitis, and the embolic spread of bacteria to the lungs, liver, and kidneys. The inclusion of abnormalities of other limb structures and even of internal organ systems within the term "TTNS" makes it very unspecific because it remains unclear whether an affected animal suffers from all of the above-mentioned abnormalities concurrently or only from an osteitis/osteomyelitis of P3. Therefore, the author proposes to use an unequivocal term such as "toe necrosis" to describe the evident abnormality of the claw, and that all complications originating from this should be reported as additional diagnoses after a thorough clinical and orthopedic examination of the animal[22] supported by diagnostic imaging procedures.[15,22–24]

Recently, toe lesions have gained more attention in the published literature following the introduction of computerized claw trimming database programs in many countries, allowing much more detailed documentation of claw lesions on hoof trimming visits.[11,25–27] Furthermore, a high herd prevalence of endemic DD infection exists in several countries today,[28–32] inevitably favoring a secondary infection of toe lesions with exposed corium with DD-associated *Treponema* spp.[14,33–38]

RELEVANT ANATOMY

After correct hoof trimming, the sole horn of Holstein Friesian cows is around 7 mm thick.[39–41] The junction of the hard claw wall and the softer sole horn is formed by the white line horn. The latter is a weak area in the horn capsule that is subject to maceration processes and to penetration by grit or stones.[39,41,42] Just beneath the claw horn is the approximately 1-mm-thick layer of corium responsible for the continual production of new keratin. Its primary role is to make the horn a pliable, insoluble, and unreactive barrier to the environment.[42] The corium is very rich in blood vessels that supply nutrients required for horn growth of around 4 to 5 mm per month. The corium is also rich in nerves that sense pain when the horn capsule is damaged. In contrast to the plantar/palmar aspect of the claw, where large fat pads are interposed between the solar corium and the surface of P3, the subcutaneous layer at the toe area (**Fig. 1**) is only 2 to 3 mm thick.[39–42] This anatomic situation at the toe makes the

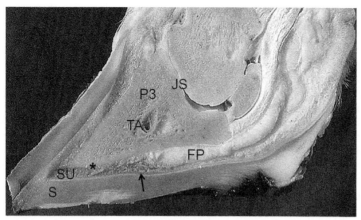

Fig. 1. Sagittal anatomic section of a healthy rear claw showing the normal sole horn (S) thickness of approximately 7 mm, the approximately 1-mm-thick layer of corium (*arrow*), the 3-mm-thick subcutaneous layer (SU) at the toe, the thicker fat pads (FP) at the plantar aspect, and the solar surface (*asterisk*) of the P3 with the terminal arch (TA) and the adjoining distal interphalangeal joint space (JS).

corium more susceptible to downward pressure of the hard P3 and upward pressure of uneven and hard surfaces on the sole as the cow walks, absorbing impact.[39] On the other hand, if the corium should become infected at the toe, the proximity of the apex of P3 (see **Fig. 1**) means that this bone is prone to become involved in the infection within a few days.[5,6,11]

The claw horn is composed of hard keratin that softens in damp conditions.[42–44] Moist keratin is more likely to abrade and become less dense as it uncoils when in a swollen, hydrated state.[43–45] If claws are continually wet, the keratin becomes softer and more easily damaged by hydraulic rupture when subjected to impacts or suddenly having to bear weight.[17,43–45] On the other hand, if claws are extremely dry, the keratin becomes very hard and brittle and can crack more easily, resulting in horn fissures.[42] The solar horn of the rear claws has a significantly higher moisture content than the fore claws.[46] Suggested reasons for this are that the fore claws have thicker soles and that rear claws are more frequently exposed to wet alleyways. This higher moisture content makes the rear claws more prone to increased wear. "Thin sole" claws have up to 21% more moisture content than normal claws under the same conditions, thought to be because the thinner soles have more immature horn exposed, which naturally has a higher water content.[43,44,46]

P3 is suspended in the horn capsule by interdigitation of dermal and epidermal laminae mainly at the wall segment.[39,41] The ventral aspect of P3 is concave, and, as a result, there are 2 points that can predispose to toe or sole ulcers if sufficient pressure is applied to the solar corium,[39,41] in particular, in cases of laminitis with sinking and/or rotation of P3.[47,48]

The arterial and venous blood supply of P3 is provided via the proper digital artery and vein entering at the axial foramen and forming the terminal arch within P3. From this loop, laminar vessels run radially to the apical, axial, and abaxial margins of P3, as clearly depicted by angiographic studies.[11,49,50] This particular vascular architecture of P3 may facilitate rapid spreading of a circumscribed apical P3 infection deeper into the bone.[11]

PREVALENCE AND INCIDENCE OF TOE LESIONS

Only a small number of reports describing the frequency of toe lesions in dairy and feedlot cattle have been published. Thin soles, defined as palpably soft soles and short dorsal wall length,[8,21,46] are a recognized problem in some dairy herds kept on grooved concrete and mastic asphalt floors.[13,51,52] An incidence of thin soles in up to 30% of cows has been recorded in individual herds.[8,46] Out of 968 and 1093 bovine patients (primarily dairy cattle) treated for orthopedic disorders at 2 referral clinics in Central Europe, 12.6%[2] and 4.8%,[5] respectively, suffered from toe ulcers and/or toe necrosis. In contrast, a mean prevalence of "nonhealing" toe necrosis of less than 2% of cows per herd and a herd prevalence of greater than 50% were reported in Dutch dairy herds,[30,53] explained by the fact that a very high percentage of Dutch herds are endemic for DD infection.

Toe ulcers have been reported as the most important claw disease in Holstein heifers on 3 dairy farms with seasonal parturition under grazing conditions in Uruguay, with a mean prevalence rate of 58.2% of heifers affected in early lactation between 15 and 60 days in milk (DIM).[54] All these heifers were required to walk approximately 6 to 8 km per day, and the problem intensified after seasonal parturition in March and April (fall) with high humidity and rainfall, and abrupt ration changes postpartum.[54] An outbreak of toe lesions was reported in a group of 150 dairy heifers in New Zealand developing AWLD, thin soles, toe ulcers, and toe necrosis resulting from excessive horn wear after having been abruptly moved from pasture onto a concrete feeding platform, resulting in lameness in 90% of these animals within 1 to 3 weeks postpartum.[9]

A prevalence of 13% for thin soles and of 20% for thin sole–induced toe ulcers has been described in a 2100-cow dairy herd.[17] The latter disorders were regarded as a consequence of sole thinning, resulting in a subsequent separation of the apical sole away from the white line and eventually leading to toe necrosis.[17] Interestingly, the highest prevalence of thin sole–induced toe ulcers, toe ulcers, and white line lesions was determined within the first 15 DIM.[17] A similar observation was made in a recent retrospective study reporting that in 50% of cows from different farms, the diagnosis of toe necrosis was made within the first 61 DIM.[16] The risk of thin sole–induced toe ulcers and all other claw lesions developing was greater in the summer; however, the risk for toe ulcers was observed to be highest in fall.[17] Last, thin soles were shown to be a statistically significant risk factor for the development of thin sole-induced ulcers, which is likely to be exacerbated by long walking distances and wet environmental conditions.[7,17,54]

In feedlot cattle, the incidence of toe necrosis can differ between feedlots, but this variability appears to be related to the management of individual lots.[12,18] Although many lots will have no animals afflicted with toe necrosis, 2 studies of 72 affected lots in North America determined that the prevalence of toe necrosis ranged from 0.5% to 1.2%[18] and from 0.01% to 3.8% of the animals affected, respectively,[11] indicating that feedlot-specific risk factors may play an important role.[18] In an outbreak of toe abscesses on 5 US feedlots occurring 3 days to 3 weeks after arrival on the lot between December and March, morbidity ranging from a few animals up to 75% of the herd, with mortality up to 7% in the worst group, has been reported.[3] In another outbreak in a feedlot with severe cases of toe abscesses, around 50% of 170 feedlot calves were affected 2 to 3 weeks after transportation.[4]

Canadian researchers reported that, from 702 confirmed cases of toe necrosis in feedlot cattle, 55% occurred in yearlings and 45% occurred in calves.[10,11,19] The mean (median) interval from arrival at feedlot to the first treatment of toe necrosis was 18.9 ± 1.7 days (12 days), and the mean (median) interval from arrival at feedlot until death was 42.7 ± 1.7 days (27.0 days). Regarding the source of the animals, 77.6% were derived from auctions, 7.5% from pastures, and 9.8% were back-grounded. A total of 75.2% were euthanized because of a lack of clinical improvement. Deaths occurred in all months of the year, but peaked in fall.[10,11,18,19]

PATHOGENESIS AND RISK FACTORS

Several hypotheses and risk factors have been suggested to play a role in the epide-miology and pathogenesis of toe lesions in feedlot and dairy cattle (**Fig. 2**), such as excessive wear of the sole horn, hypostasis associated with long transport, long walking distances, laminitis, overcrowding, excessive hoof trimming, bovine viral diar-rhea virus (BVDV) infection associated with vascular lesions and ischemic necrosis in the claws, and hematogenous infection of P3 due to embolic bacterial dis-ease.[1–13,16–20,44,50,54–56] It must also be considered that the risk factors for toe necro-sis may differ in feedlot and dairy cattle, because of varying management procedures.

Theories on Toe Lesions

Three theories on the development of toe lesions/toe necrosis are currently suggested in the literature: (1) any mechanical trauma to the claw; (2) vascular disruption to the pedal bone, due to both extrinsic and intrinsic factors; and (3) sequelae of lami-nitis.[11,50] However, some other risk factors are also thought to contribute to the devel-opment of toe lesions in general, and to toe necrosis in particular.

Excessive Wear of the Sole Horn

One hypothesis is that trauma, in the form of excessive wear of the sole associated with abrasive surfaces, such as freshly poured concrete, mastic asphalt, and metal, can cause serious damage to the horn capsule, eventually allowing bacteria to enter the apical white line or to induce other disruptions.[3,4,7,8,13,44,50,51,57,58] In a Canadian study, the sole thickness in the apical white line region was found to be significantly thinner than in healthy control animals, with a mean thickness of 3.74 mm in claws

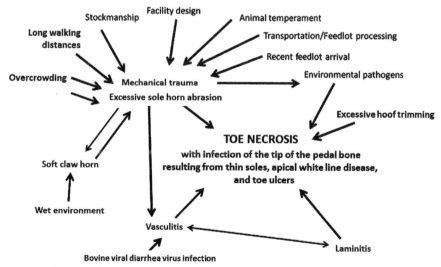

Fig. 2. Web of risk factors causing toe necrosis in feedlot and dairy cattle. (*Adapted from* Fig. 4.1 published in the thesis of C. Paetsch, 2014, p. 71; with permission).

affected by toe necrosis, and this finding strongly supports the "abrasion theory."[19] Excessive sole horn wear is particularly common in new installations where freshly hardened concrete creates a particularly abrasive surface.[8,58,59] This causative factor has become so commonplace that it has gained the name, "New Concrete Disease,"[58,59] and such problems are known to generally disappear after 6 to 9 months.[13,59] Fresh concrete forms a thin suspension of calcium hydroxide on its surface, which has a very high pH (>12). At this pH, keratin is very susceptible to degradation, and claw horn can become severely compromised. Washing new concrete with water will dilute this surface alkali, but because this is continually being produced, continuous washing is required. Washings from 3-day-old and 7-day-old concrete floors induced horn swelling of greater than 50% and greater than 33%, respectively, compared with the effect of rainwater alone.[43] In contrast, in barns with mastic asphalt floors installed in the entire traffic area, excessive sole horn wear is a continuous problem that increases over the years due to the impact of chemical, mechanical, and climatic exposure charges, leading to deterioration of the asphalt and increasing the exposure of the claw horn to coarse aggregate.[51,52] Despite this, this floor type is not uncommon in Central European dairy farms.[13,51,52]

Several investigators have reported the development of severe lameness in feedlot cattle between 3 days and 3 to 4 weeks after arrival on the lot, resulting from abrasion and trauma to the claw during transportation and processing of feedlot cattle.[1,3,4,10–12,18,55] The claws of these animals showed excessive wear in the toe tip and separation of the wall and sole at the apical white line associated with an infection of P3.[1,3,4,18,60] The investigators postulated that common risk factors for disease development were transportation in an aluminum trailer with minimal bedding or cattle being maintained and handled on concrete surfaces. Therefore, standing for long periods of time during transport, sudden turning and movement during transportation, and processing of cattle seen especially in hyperexcitable animals can lead to excessive abrasion and rasping of the hoof horn, which can damage the apical white line, allowing for impaction of fecal material.[1,3,4,7,11,18,60] Furthermore, it was hypothesized that soft hooves due to wet conditions, combined with hyperexcitable behavior, may put animals at a higher risk of traumatic injuries to the toe during processing or hauling.[3,7,8,11] Most cattle with toe necrosis were found to have come from a livestock auction, and the study determined that auction-derived and grass-fed animals were more likely to be discharged earlier due to toe necrosis than ranch-direct and backgrounded animals.[11] Grass-fed cattle have softer horn in the claw that predisposes to injury, whereas auction-derived cattle spend more time on hard abrasive concrete surfaces during transportation and processing times at the feedlot. Both of these scenarios can contribute to a disruption of claw soundness. A combination of damage to the claw and the impact of hard surfaces on this lesion allows pathologic processes to progress more rapidly.[11]

Despite dairy cattle often being confined for most of their lifetime on concrete floors in the barn, in milking parlors, and in sheds, only a small number of reports of toe tip lesions have been published.[2,5,6,16] An outbreak of toe lesions was reported in 90% of 150 dairy heifers in New Zealand developing after they were abruptly moved from pasture onto a concrete holding yard within 1 to 3 weeks.[9] Other investigators have described apical necrosis of P3 as a complication of toe ulcers observed in dairy cows, calves, and breeding bulls.[2,5,6,16] These investigators reported that traumatic injuries, excessive hoof trimming, and laminitis accounted for most toe ulcers and apical necrosis of P3. Dairy cattle can be afflicted by the same clinical signs of toe necrosis as seen in beef cattle, even though different names have been used to describe these toe lesions.[9,11,16] Furthermore, thin soles and their consequences, such as AWLD, toe ulcer, and toe necrosis, in dairy cattle on pasture year round are likely to be exacerbated by long walking distances and wet environmental conditions.[7,17,54]

Hypostasis Associated with Long Transports

A second theory postulates that toe necrosis could be initiated due to vascular and/or physiologic disturbances of P3.[11,20,50] The proper digital artery passes through the axial foramen as it forms the terminal arch. The location of this axial foramen is below the level of the coronary band. Because walking aids blood circulation and passive movement of the arteriovenous anastomoses, it is suggested that prolonged standing time in auction yards or livestock trailers could result in hypostasis of blood in the distal limb.[11,47,50] Because the distal limb relies on blood flow through the arteriovenous anastomoses while the animal is standing, this flow could be impaired, leading to ischemia, hypoxia, and subsequent aseptic necrosis of the apex of P3[11,50] followed by rupture of the white line with clinical signs following 10 to 13 days later.[1,3,4,55,60]

Furthermore, it has been speculated that BVDV might cause vascular lesions and ischemic necrosis in the claws and may predispose some animals to toe necrosis; however, a causative role of BVDV infection remains unclear.[10,11,18,19] The BVD virus is known to cause vasculitis, thereby reducing blood perfusion. A decreased integrity of the vasculature in the claw could allow for corium disruption permitting environmental pathogens to transverse the corium resulting in P3 osteitis, which could be further supported by the immunosuppressive effect of the BVDV infection.[11,19] These investigators determined a significantly higher risk for toe necrosis among feedlot cattle infected with BVDV and having vascular lesions in the heart and lungs than in healthy control animals.[12,19] They hypothesized that a hematogenous infection of P3 due to embolic bacterial disease had taken place in the infected feedlot cattle.[10–12,18]

Excessive Hoof Trimming of Sole Horn

Even "iatrogenic" causes, for example, excessive or incorrect hoof trimming, can lead to weakening and damage of the horn capsule.[11] Excessive hoof trimming of the sole horn has been reported as a causative factor for the development of thin soles, AWLD, toe ulcers, and toe necrosis[2,5–7,40,41,61] developing 1 to 3 weeks after the initial damage.[5,16,61] In a retrospective study of 53 head of cattle (mainly dairy cattle) with toe ulcers and toe necrosis, excessive hoof trimming and/or perforation of the sole/dorsal wall during hoof trimming 1 to 3 weeks previously could be elicited as causative factors in 49.0% of cases, by evaluating the clinical history of the animal and assessing the still visible traces of the grinding disc.[5] Similar observations, with excessive hoof trimming of the sole horn and/or extreme shortening of the dorsal wall length, were assessed as causative for toe necrosis in around 23% of cattle in other studies.[2,16] Inexperienced hoof trimmers, who do not adhere to the guidelines for proper trimming, tend to overtrim the horn sole especially when using a grinding disc and/or when farm-specific conditions (long walking distances, highly abrasive floors, young animals) are not considered.[7,13,40,41] This problem is common for those hoof trimmers who trim every claw of every cow in the same way, without considering the age of the cow, toe length, and sole thickness before trimming.[40,41] It was obvious in these reports that all the cows with apical bone infection on 3 claws per cow, and most of the cases with the problem on 2 claws per cow, were caused by incorrect hoof trimming.[2,5,6,16]

Laminitis

Another theory is that toe necrosis is a consequence of laminitis. Laminitis, by definition, can be a subclinical, subacute, acute, or chronic degeneration of the laminae of

the claw that results in pedal bone rotation and sinking.[47,48,50,62] It has been speculated that a rapid switch to a high grain ration upon arrival at the feedlot or directly after
parturition in dairy cattle leads to a metabolic disturbance causing subacute ruminal
acidosis and subsequent laminitis, which then results in the displacement or rotation
of P3 relative to the claw capsule and penetration of the apex of P3 through the
sole.[12,47,48,50,54,62] However, such severe clinical signs of acute laminitis in dairy
and feedlot cattle are relatively rare; more frequently, a nutritionally associated pathogenesis leads to subclinical and subacute laminitis linked to an increased prevalence
of sole hemorrhages, double soles, softer and lower-quality claw horn, and osteologic
changes to the apex of P3.[48,62,63] These alterations of the sole and the white line horn,
and osteopathic changes to the apex of P3,[48,54,63–65] may make cattle more prone to
the above-mentioned mechanical-, transport-, and hypostasis-related factors.

Secondary Infection of the Toe Corium with Treponema spp in Herds with Endemic Digital Dermatitis Infection

An increasing herd prevalence of DD has been reported recently in many dairy herds
all over the world, leading to a higher number of secondary infections with *Treponema*
spp in cases of toe and other claw horn lesions associated with an exposed corium.
Today, between 15% and 90% of the herds in many countries have been reported
to harbor an endemic DD infection, meaning that a secondary infection with DD is
much more likely nowadays compared with 10 to 15 years ago.[28–32,53] Claw horn lesions at the toe exhibiting a secondary infection with *Treponema* spp are often called
"non-healing" toe ulcers/toe necrosis.[17,30,33–38,53,66,67] However, a more appropriate
term would appear to be "digital dermatitis–associated" toe ulcers/toe necrosis,[14]
as all of these lesions can be successfully treated if an appropriate therapy is
applied.[14,36] These DD-associated toe ulcers/toe necrosis have also been encountered in pasture-based cattle farming systems.[37,54,68,69] As causative factors for
horn capsule damage at the toe, a combination of the following aspects can be
assumed: "normal" (although rather thin) soles of pastured cows, the long walking distances from pasture to the milking parlor, poor cow tracks, and long periods of standing on hard concrete surfaces with overcrowding in the parlor holding area.[7,11,54,70,71]

The reported osteologic changes to the apex of P3 in cases of "nonhealing" toe ul-
cers/toe necrosis[64,65] may be explained by the fact that, in such cases, the chronic DD
inflammation of the corium persisted for several months and in some cases for more
than one year, creating alterations of the adjoining bony tissue without an obvious
bone infection, or that these osteolytic changes can be interpreted as a long-term
result of repeated laminitis bouts.[47,48,63] The tip of P3 may be atrophied, but is not
necessarily infected in cases of "nonhealing" toe ulcers/necrosis.[15,16]

Other Risk Factors

Overcrowding, poorly designed stalls, insufficient bedding, and poor stockmanship
can all contribute to excessive horn loss,[7,13] in particular, when they are associated
with some of the above-mentioned risk factors.

When the nutrient supply to keratin-forming cells is compromised or completely
altered, inferior keratinized tissue is produced, increasing the susceptibility to the
development of claw disorders independent of genuine causative factors (see earlier
discussion). Calcium, zinc, copper, manganese, cobalt, selenium, vitamins A, D, and
E, and biotin all play important roles in the production and maintenance of healthy keratinized tissues.[42,72–75] Increasing the bioavailability of the above-mentioned trace
minerals improves their utilization and thus contributes to an improved integrity of
both the skin and the claw horn.[42,72–75] Supplementation of the diet with a

combination of complex trace minerals has been reported to reduce the incidence of white line separation, sole hemorrhages, double soles, sole ulcers, and DD.[74,75]

It has been speculated that corkscrew claws may also predispose to toe ulcers/toe necrosis due to an outer-to-inner twist of the claw and subsequent internal rotation of P3 and the corium. This resulting rotation may cause the corium to be in abnormally close proximity to the weight-bearing surface in claw zones 1 (white line at the toe) and 2 (abaxial white line).[7,8] However, this assumption is not evidence based, and it is the personal experience of the author that many cases of DD-associated toe necrosis, the development and final diagnosis of which may take more than 6 months, are frequently associated with a corkscrew claw deformation. Therefore, corkscrew claws can be interpreted as a long-term consequence of the painful, DD-associated toe ulcer/toe necrosis rather than a risk factor in itself.[16]

CLINICAL SIGNS AND DIAGNOSIS

Cattle suffering from toe lesions exhibit a mild to severe lameness, primarily in the rear limbs, with the affected lateral claw, in particular, leading to an obvious abduction of the cow's limb while both standing and walking.[1–5,7,9,16,55] However, lameness can also be observed in the forelimbs, affecting either lateral or medial claws. In the latter case, affected cattle demonstrate a characteristic cross-legged stance of the forelimbs.[11,76] One of the hallmark signs of toe lesions in their early stages is lameness with no swelling of the coronet and/or the bulbs of the heel of the distal limb.[1–5]

The diagnosis of toe lesions (AWLD, thin sole, toe ulcer, and toe necrosis involving the tip of P3) can be easily made in many cases by a thorough clinical examination after careful cleaning and diagnostic trimming of the claws (**Figs. 3–7**A).[22,40,76] Closer examination often reveals that the toe tip of the claw is worn, rounded off (see

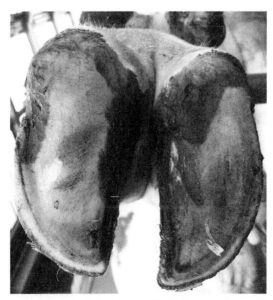

Fig. 3. Plantar view of the claws of the left rear limb of a cow from a freestall system barn with mastic asphalt floor: the sole horn shows severe abrasions and the sole is so thin (1 mm) on the toe of the lateral claw that the inflamed and damaged corium shines through; in addition, a small white line separation can be noted axially at the toe.

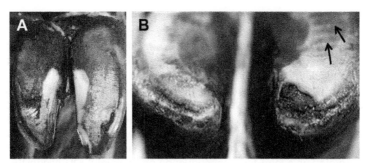

Fig. 4. Plantar views of the rear claws of 2 cows (*A*, *B*) showing excessively trimmed sole horn with hemorrhages in the white line horn and a white line separation dorsoabaxial (claw zone 2) on the lateral claw (*A*), and an apical white line separation on both claws with a toe ulcer on the lateral claw (*B*). The sole horn is about 2 mm thick, and traces of the grinding disc can still be seen on the sole surface (*arrows*).

Fig. 3; **Fig. 8**A), and associated with an excessively short dorsal wall length (<7 cm) in many cases (see **Figs. 7**A and 8B). Such a meticulous examination allows the detection of thin soles that are flexible to finger pressure, and even small areas of separation of the horn sole from the wall within the apical white line or toe ulcers can become visible (see **Figs. 3–4**B). Finger pressure and the pressure of a hoof tester can be used to assess a painful reaction, which will be observed in cases of apparent inflammation.[2,8,11,13,15,22,76] In the case of thin soles, the exact sole horn thickness can be determined in vivo by ultrasonographic measurement using a 7.5-MHz linear (rectal) probe. Even the underlying subcutaneous layer and plantar/palmar bone contour of P3 can be imaged (**Fig. 9**) ultrasonographically.[77,78]

Small tracks or cracks located in claw zone 1 and claw zone 5 (the apex of the sole)[8] are a frequent pathway of infection.[2,5,55,61] The use of a probe that can be inserted into such tracks enables further information to be obtained as to the extent and depth of the lesion and a possible involvement of P3 if hard bone surface is probed.[5,11,22,76] It is suggested that an ascending infection and subsequent involvement of P3 can occur quite rapidly in this anatomic area because of the approximately

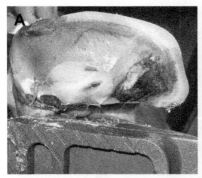
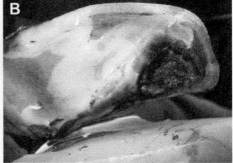

Fig. 5. Plantar views of the lateral rear claw of a cow exhibiting toe necrosis with double sole after partial removal of loose horn (*A*), and intraoperative view of the same claw after complete removal of all loose horn and the infected, necrotic corium at the toe (*B*). Now the discolored brown surface of the tip of P3 can be seen. A block has been already attached to the adjacent claw in preparation for the planned treatment.

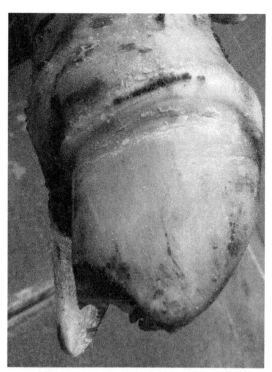

Fig. 6. Lateral view of the lateral rear claw of a cow showing a fracture at the tip of the claw with exposed corium and P3, in addition to an obvious swelling of the dorsal and abaxial coronet clearly indicating a bone infection. The medial claw had been prepared for attaching a block.

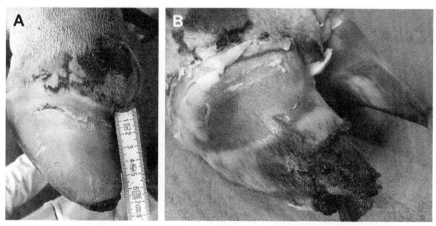

Fig. 7. Lateral view (*A*) of a lateral rear claw of a Simmental cow exhibiting toe necrosis, an excessively short dorsal wall length of about 6.5 cm and a severe swelling, and a decubital wound to the skin of the dorsal coronet. The lateral pathoanatomical view (*B*) after thermal exungulation of the claws at necropsy shows the extent of the severe toe necrosis with necrotic corium and bone infection to around the dorsal half of P3. Similar findings were observed on the 2 claws of the contralateral limb; as such, the cow was euthanized on welfare grounds. In this case, incorrect hoof trimming could be identified as the causative factor.

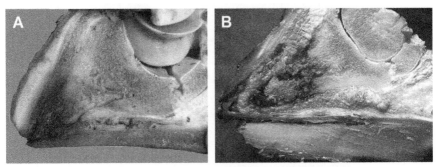

Fig. 8. Sagittal necropsy sections of 2 lateral rear claws amputated at the midlevel of phalanx media showing severe toe necrosis/bone infection to around the dorsal third reaching already to the terminal arch (*A*) and involving more than the half of P3 (*B*). The causative factor was considerable abrasion of the dorsal wall and the apical sole horn in a young heifer (*A*) after transition from a deep straw bedding yard to a barn with a mastic asphalt floor; (*B*) excessive shortening of the dorsal wall length by an inexperienced hoof trimmer. A large underrun sole, with a thick sole horn, can also be noted.

2- to 3-mm thin layer of corium and subcutaneous tissue (see **Figs. 1** and **8A**).[2,5,6,16] This observation has been confirmed by studies revealing that the prediction of toe necrosis based on the presence of AWLD was statistically significant in feedlot cattle.[12]

The clinical signs of toe lesions vary widely depending on their severity, thin soles versus toe necrosis, the number of claws involved, and the causative factors.[5,7,16] In some cases, a marked lameness in one single limb is observed; in other cases, when claws of 2 or more limbs are involved, the animals are primarily recumbent, and severely stilted limb movements are observed while standing and walking, which could be assumed, at first glance, to be a "neurologic" disorder.[5]

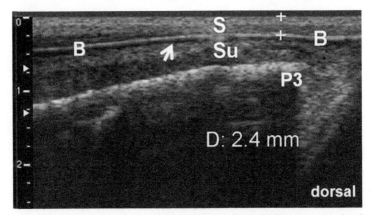

Fig. 9. Longitudinal sonogram of the middle and dorsal weight-bearing area (at the toe) of a lateral rear claw showing a 2.4-mm (distance from + to +) thin sole horn layer (S) in a 5-year-old Simmental cow housed on mastic asphalt floor. The thin echogenic line indicates the sole horn/corium border (B). Furthermore, the very thin, anechoic corium layer (*arrow*), the less echogenic, reticular patterned subcutaneous layer (Su), and the clearly outlined, hyperechoic solar surface of the P3 ending at the tip of P3 are clearly imaged.

In a recent study by the author, 57.6% of cases of toe necrosis were diagnosed in the lateral rear claws (see **Figs. 3–8**; **Figs. 10–14**),[16] and similar results have also been reported by others.[2,5,46,79] This finding can be explained by the higher biomechanical load on lateral rear claws,[80,81] by the higher moisture content of rear claws (and of thin soled claws in general) compared with fore claws and to claws with a physiologic sole horn thickness, and finally, by the fact that softer claws are more prone to abrasion.[46,82]

As the condition progresses over a period of days, an obvious soft tissue swelling can be determined, commonly at the dorsal coronet. This sign, in combination with an evident toe lesion, is a clinical hallmark sign (see **Figs. 6** and **7A**) for the involvement of P3.[3,7,16,76] In the author's personal experience, there is only one exception when a moderate or severe local swelling of the dorsal coronet is not necessarily associated with P3 infection, and this is when prolonged cases of DD-associated toe ulcers have been in existence for several months.

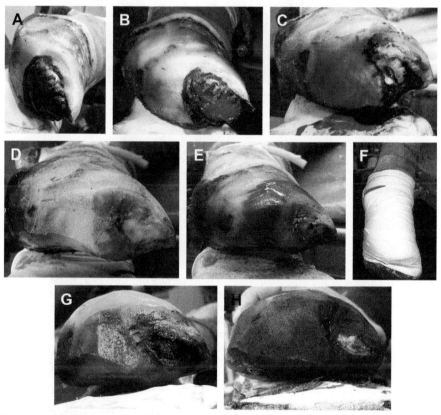

Fig. 10. Views of a "nonhealing" (DD-associated) toe ulcer of a lateral rear claw in a Limousin breeding bull after cleaning and hoof trimming (*A, B*). Intraoperative views after removal of all infected soft tissues (*C, D*) showing now a clean wound surface. In the background, the yellow elastic tourniquet (*B–E*) can be seen; this was used for the application of local anesthesia. Topical application of tetracycline spray (*E*) and a protecting bandage (*F*). Healing status 8 days (*G*) and 23 days (*H*) after surgical treatment demonstrate very good progress with respect to cornification. On the medial claw, a wooden block is attached.

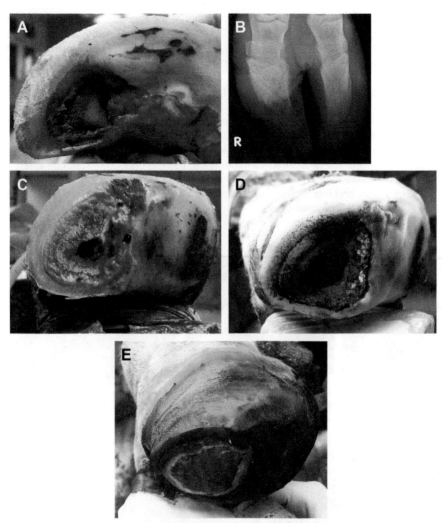

Fig. 11. Plantar view of the exposed discolored bone surface of P3 (*A*) of a lateral rear claw in a cow; corresponding dorsoplantar radiograph showing severe osteolysis of the dorsal third of P3 (*B*). Intraoperative view after resection of the infected part of P3 using a disc with steel knives mounted on an angle grinder showing the clean, vital bone surface (*C*). Healing status 4 days (*D*) and 20 days postoperatively (*E*), showing the differing amount of granulation tissue that covers the bone completely after 20 days. Even some new horn production on the wound margins can be noted. On the medial claw, a block is attached to remove the weight-bearing load from the wound.

When the loose horn around the toe lesion is removed with a hoof knife, the underlying tissues exhibit either hematoma, dry or wet black material, and/or a purulent exudate (see **Figs. 4, 5** and **10**A, B), and in advanced cases, the discolored (yellow, brown, or black) surface of the tip of P3 (see **Figs. 5**B and **11**A) can be visually identified.[2–5,16,61]

In advanced stages of toe necrosis, complications can develop, such as a purulent arthritis of the distal interphalangeal joint indicated clinically by a moderate to severe

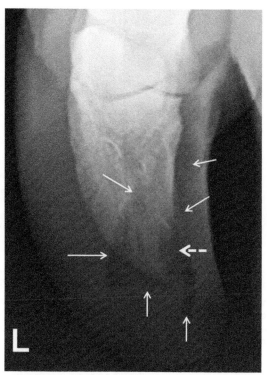

Fig. 12. Dorsoplantar radiographic view of the left lateral rear claw showing a slight osteolysis of the axial tip of the pedal bone (*broken arrow*). In addition, a sharply demarcated radiolucent gas pocket can be noted, located between the sole horn and the pedal bone contour (bordered by the *arrows*).

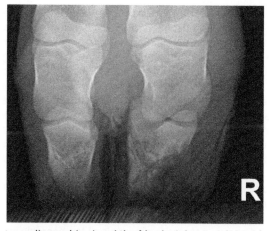

Fig. 13. Dorsoplantar radiographic view (*A*) of both right rear claws of a 6-month-old calf showing toe necrosis and an obvious severe osteolysis involving more than the half of P3 on the lateral claw, caused by trauma.

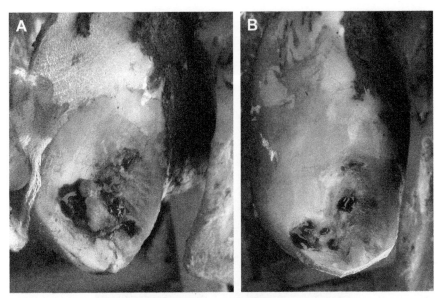

Fig. 14. Plantar views of a "nonhealing" (DD-associated) toe ulcer of a lateral rear claw after removal of most of the loose horn around the lesion (*A*), and after complete surgical removal of the infected corium layer (*B*). The surface of the wound looks clean and free of any infected tissue.

circular swelling of the coronet around the claw.[3,5,6,16] Furthermore, venous embolization of bacteria can result in a septic thrombosis of the distal limb veins, and hematogenous embolization with abscessation in the lungs, liver, and the heart, associated with elevated rectal temperature, reduced appetite, and emaciation.[1,3–5,7,10,11,18]

If radiography is available, the degree of involvement of P3 can be visualized and assessed. Dorsoplantar/dorsopalmar and oblique lateromedial projections, or lateromedial projections using an interdigital plate, are considered to be the most informative views.[5,16,23] Radiographic signs in cases of P3 infection can range from a slight osteolysis of the apical margin of P3 to extensive osteolytic changes of a quarter to a half or more of P3 (see **Figs. 11**B, **12**, and **13**). Depending on the presence of loose sole horn and double soles, sharply demarcated radiolucent areas may be perceived between the sole horn and plantar/palmar P3 contour, indicating gas pockets (see **Fig. 12**). Even pathologic fractures of the apex of P3 can be assessed based on the progressed stage of infection and caused by persistent leverage forces.[2,5,11,16,61] Previous studies have shown that the size of the visible lesion at the toe does not correspond with the extent of the radiographically assessed bone infection.[5,11] Similar radiographic alterations of P3 as described here (ie, in apical pedal bone necrosis due to bacterial infection) were reported in a cow with squamous cell carcinoma affecting almost the entire P3.[83] In this case, however, visible lesions of the horn capsule were absent.

Using radiography enables the extent of bone infection to be categorically determined, which facilitates the choice of adequate surgical treatment.[15,16,23] However, many bovine practitioners do not generally have easy access to a mobile radiographic unit.[23] As mentioned above, a tentative diagnosis of toe necrosis involving P3 can be made solely based on a thorough clinical examination that determines the presence of a toe lesion in combination with a marked swelling of the dorsal coronet (see **Figs. 3–7,**

10) and obvious lameness. Furthermore, in patients with a unilateral affliction where the owner explicitly insists on treatment, a definitive final diagnosis can be made intra-operatively (see **Fig. 5**).[16,84]

Culture swabs taken from the surface of the infected apex of P3 in 79 cases in feedlot cattle revealed that *Escherichia coli*, *Trueperella pyogenes*, and *Streptococcus* spp accounted for a total of 66% of the isolates.[11] A similar bacterial flora with frequent mixed infections has also been reported in several other studies of toe necrosis of feedlot and dairy cattle[3,5,19] from farms without endemic DD infection.

The clinical verification of a secondary infection of a toe ulcer/toe necrosis with *Treponema* spp (DD-associated toe ulcer/necrosis) can be based on the herd's history (presence of an endemic DD infection) and the veterinarian's olfactory senses, noticing the same characteristic pungent smell as can be found in classical DD skin lesions.[14,35] Confirmation of such a *Treponema* spp infection of the toe lesion can be achieved using qualitative and quantitative polymerase chain reaction to detect DD-associated *Treponema* spp–DNA from corium samples.[30,35,85]

TREATMENT

Decision making for the treatment of cattle suffering from toe lesions is based on careful evaluation of the soles of all claws, by examination of the coronet and the distal limb for swelling and cellulitis, and by checking the rectal temperature and other vital parameters of the animal.[3,5,8,22,76] Toe lesions can be expected to have a good prognosis if they are diagnosed at an early stage or if only one claw is affected without spread of a bacterial infection to the internal organs. However, cattle have a poor prognosis when 2 or more claws present with toe ulcers and/or toe necrosis with bone infection.[2–5,8,10,11,15,16,18,54] Early treatment of toe lesions is imperative[3,54] for improving the prognosis and simplifying treatment. Management of individual cattle exhibiting toe lesions depends not only on the severity of the condition and the number of affected claws but also on the stage of lactation, pregnancy status, age of the animal, and the presence of any concurrent disease of other organ systems.[5,8,11,15,16] Culling should be considered in cases of nonpregnant older cows, in late lactation with a low milk yield, and in all cattle with toe necrosis involving 2 or more claws.[8,16]

The first aim in treating claws exhibiting toe lesions is to determine whether the sole horn of the adjacent claw is thick enough to support the weight of that limb if fitted with a conventional block of adequate thickness (see **Figs. 5**, **10**, and **11C–E**) to relieve the damaged claw from weight bearing.[2,5,8,13,86] If it is determined that neither claw can support the weight of the respective limb in cases of thin soles, then neither claw should be fitted with a block and the animal should be housed separately from the herd but very close to the milking parlor, in a soft bedded area with relatively "soft" (ie, avoiding concrete) floor surfaces.[8] An alternative to housing in a special recovery stall is a grassy area or dry lot close to the parlor that limits the distance the animal must walk on hard or abrasive surfaces during the period of time required for recuperation and horn growth.[1,8,13] A novel alternative system to protect thin soles can be the application of approximately 5-mm thin soft plastic blocs (Accu-sole; Comfort Hoof Care Inc, Baraboo, WI, USA) or soft rubber pads using a very thin layer of glue (Walkease; Shoof International Ltd, Cambridge, New Zealand) to the healthier of the 2 "thin-soled" claws[8,15,87] instead of the conventional hard wooden or hard plastic blocks.

In cases where the condition has progressed to a toe ulcer, subsolar abscess, or toe necrosis with infection of the tip of P3, additional corrective trimming, removal of all loose horn, and thorough debridement procedures are necessary.[8,16] For these measures, the application of local anesthesia is mandatory. The preferred choice is the use of a retrograde intravenous regional anesthesia after application of an elastic tourniquet at mid-metatarsus/metacarpus level (see **Fig. 10**D, E) and subsequent intravenous injection of 10 to 15 mL procaine-hydrochloride or lidocaine, depending on local licensing laws.[2,5,16,88,89] In cases of toe ulcers and subsolar abscesses without involvement of deeper structures, all loose and undermined sole and wall horn must be carefully removed by thinning out the horn margins around the lesion (see **Figs. 5**, **10**A–E, and **14**), without causing damage to the adjacent corium.[8,40,41]

In contrast, in cases with a DD-associated toe ulcer/toe necrosis in herds endemically infected with DD,[33–38,66,67] several investigators recommend carefully debriding all *Treponema* spp–infected corium,[14,15] in addition to the sole and wall horn, using a sharp hoof knife or scalpel blade (see **Figs. 10**A–E and **14**) under local anesthesia to allow a complete healing of these alleged "nonhealing" toe lesions. In both cases, the wound is rinsed with 0.9% saline solution and dried with cotton gauze and silver spray (Agro Chemica Aloxan-Silberspray; Agradi BV, Den Bosch, The Netherlands), or a tetracycline spray (preferred in cases of DD-associated toe ulcer/toe necrosis) can be applied topically with or without a bandage (see **Fig. 10**E, F). The adjustment of weight bearing, by means of a block on the adjacent healthy claw, is vital for pain management as well as for subsequent recovery of the horn-forming tissue of the epidermis.[8,86]

The exclusive administration of antimicrobial or anti-inflammatory medications without topical treatment including careful debridement in cases of toe necrosis with or without a secondary DD infection has been shown in several studies to result in very limited or no improvement.[1,11,19] This experience is not surprising as, in many cases of obvious AWLD, toe ulcers, and subsolar abscesses, the infection has already reached the tip of P3, resulting in varying degrees of bone infection.[2,5,84] Therefore, and in accordance with the basic rules of surgery, every infected wound must be completely debrided of all necrotic and infected tissue until healthy tissue layers are reached.[15,16,84,90]

The main objective of treatment of toe necrosis/infection of the tip of P3 is the complete removal of all infected bone and soft tissue. Several surgical techniques have been described, such as aggressive debridement of the infected bone using a hammer, chisel, and curette,[5] debridement using a Forstner drill under continuous flushing with 0.9% saline solution,[2,15,84] the resection of the apex of the claw using a wire saw,[15,61,79,84] or resection of the apex of the claw using a rotating disc equipped with steel knives mounted on an angle grinder.[16,79] The final option is the amputation of the affected claw in toto in cases where the P3 infection has reached the subchondral area (see **Fig. 8**A, B) of the joint or has already penetrated the distal interphalangeal joint, resulting in a purulent arthritis.[2,5,15,16,84,91,92] Recently, "nonhealing" claw horn lesions including "nonhealing" toe ulcers/toe necrosis have been considered indications for claw amputation by some clinicians.[15,35,91,92] In the author's experience over the last 4 years, none of the "nonhealing" toe ulcers/toe necrosis cases encountered required claw amputation in toto. All of these cases were successfully treated by aggressive surgical debridement of the infected soft tissue or by resection of the tip of P3.[16] Therefore, the author's recommendation is that the surgeon should first completely remove all infected tissue to enable an accurate impression of the extent of these "nonhealing" toe ulcers/toe necrosis cases to be made and then make the final decision intraoperatively whether to preserve the claw or to continue with entire claw amputation.

For the treatment of P3 infection, patients should be restrained in a hoof trimming crush or on a hoof trimming table, and sedation using xylazine or detomidine is recommended.[88] All other claws must be examined, and, if necessary, hoof trimming should be carried out. At the very least, a block will have to be attached to the sound adjacent claw, and the dirty superficial layers of sole and wall horn (1–2 mm) of the affected claw will be removed with a grinding disc (see **Figs. 5, 10**A, B, **11**A, and **14**A) to create a clean surface.[15,16,84] After application of a retrograde intravenous regional anesthesia,[88,89] the surgeon can begin the procedure using one of the above-mentioned resection techniques.

Over recent years, the resection of the tip of the claw using an aluminum disc equipped with 7 steel knives (DL-disc, 10 cm diameter; Demotec, Demel, Nidderau, Germany) mounted on an angle grinder[16,79] has become increasingly common.[16,53] Such discs are routinely used for hoof trimming[40]; however, for use as a "surgical instrument," the disc should be carefully cleaned and disinfected in 70% ethanol solution before being mounted on the angle grinder.[16] The resection procedure is simple: the rotating disc is pressed steadily against the tip of the claw and all the tissues (horn, corium and bone) will be removed at this level so that the resection surface reveals completely healthy bone structure (see **Fig. 11**C; **Fig. 15**A, B).[16] For the success of all these resection techniques of the tip of P3, it is essential to completely remove all the infected bone tissue. For this reason, several investigators recommended resecting not only the visibly discolored bone tissue but also an additional 2- to 3-mm-thick layer of bone with a healthy appearance to ensure that no infected bone residue is left in place.[5,15,16,84]

Regardless of the surgical technique applied for the treatment of toe necrosis/pedal bone necrosis, once the surgical procedure is complete, as described above, the wound is flushed and dried with sterile gauze, a tetracycline spray may be administered before the wound is covered with a sterile wound dressing, gauze, or polyurethane-soft foam (eg, Ligasano wound dressing; Ligamed Medical Products, Ötztal, Austria), and a pressure bandage is applied up to the level of mid-metatarsus/metacarpus to prevent bleeding after removal of the tourniquet.[5,15,16,84,90]

In cases of bone resection and amputation, it is recommended to administer systemic antibiotic treatment and nonsteroidal anti-inflammatory drugs for 3 to 5 days.[2,5,15,16,79,84,88] The bandage should be changed 3 to 5 days postoperatively, and later, at intervals of around 7 days until the wound is completely covered with healthy granulation tissue (see **Figs. 10**G, H and **11**D, E).[2,5,15,16,79,84,88] Furthermore, to allow undisturbed healing, it should be ensured that the block attached to the adjacent claw will be in place for the entire recovery period of approximately 5 to 8 weeks.[2,5,15,16,79,84,86]

If the above-mentioned surgical methods for treating toe ulcers and toe necrosis are performed in cattle with a secondary DD infection of the lesions in herds endemically infected with DD (DD-associated toe ulcer/toe necrosis), several investigators strongly recommended covering these surgical wounds with a bandage until they are completely reepithelialized with new horn to protect the exposed corium from recontamination with *Treponema* spp.[5,14,84,93]

A good success rate of 81.5% has been reported for the surgical treatment of apical pedal bone necrosis using one of the above-described resection techniques of the tip of P3 in cattle with only one involved claw.[16] Similar favorable results were reported by others after a strong case selection for treatment.[2,79,94] Cornification of the surgical wound usually requires 5 to 8 weeks depending on their size.[15,16] However, it must be noted that between 15%[16] and 30% to 40% of the cattle in these studies[2,5] were culled immediately after diagnosis because they were suffering from toe necrosis and other severe and deep claw disorders in 2 or more claws each. A mean postsurgical lifespan of around 24 to 26.6 months has been reported for cattle treated with resection of the tip of P3, with some of these cattle still alive at completion of these retrospective studies.[2,16]

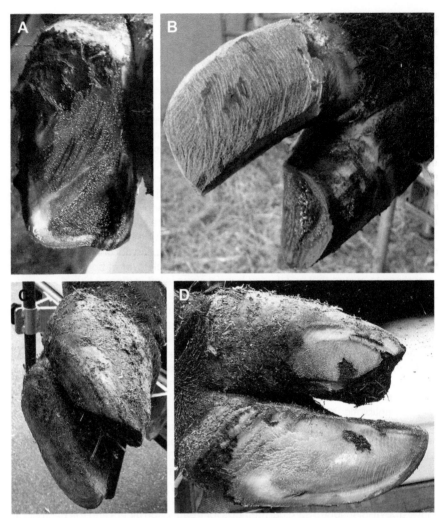

Fig. 15. Plantar view 10 days after resection of the tip of P3 of a medial rear claw due to a pedal bone necrosis caused by an apical white line lesion in a 5-year-old Aberdeen Angus breeding bull (*A*). A fine layer of granulation tissue covers the bone surface, after topical application of tetracycline spray (*B*). After 35 days, the bull exhibited no more lameness; the views taken 90 days postoperatively (*C, D*) when a corrective hoof trimming procedure had been carried out show a complete and thick cornification of the resection site.

An interesting novel alternative for the treatment of toe ulcers and toe necrosis is the application of photodynamic therapy (PDT) using a diode laser.[68] The resulting energy transfer generates a reactive oxygen species cascade promoting selective death of the relevant microorganisms without the need for antibiotics, thereby preventing the development of antimicrobial resistance.[68] After careful diagnostic claw trimming and thorough cleaning of the lesion, a topical photosensitizer (methylene blue) is applied to the wound and left for 5 minutes. PDT is then initiated using a diode laser (660 nm) at 8 J/irradiated point, and a protective bandage is applied to protect the lesion and prevent contamination. PDT is continued twice a week followed by a protective bandage until complete cornification of the lesion occurs. In this case report, the mean total wound healing time was 30 days and occurred after 8 irradiations.[68]

It is evident that there are differences in the treatment options of toe necrosis for dairy farms where cows are kept indoors compared with pasture-based dairy farms or feedlots. On many dairy farms, even large ones, good conditions exist for surgical treatment, even of severe cases requiring resection of the tip of P3, blocking, and bandaging or amputation of the claw in toto because they are often equipped with recovery stalls.[15,84,95] However, in feedlot and pasture-based dairy systems, the treatment of severe toe lesions causing lameness scores of 4 and 5 may not be practical because often there is no confinement area available at all or lame animals cannot be separated from the herd and pastured close to the milking parlor.[18,54] In such circumstances, locomotion scoring must be implemented to identify cattle showing mild signs of lameness, and treatment has to focus on mild cases of toe lesions that can be successfully treated by removal of all loose horn using step 4 of functional hoof trimming and the removal of load-bearing from the involved area by retaining the heel height of the adjacent claw as high as possible, or by blocking of the partner claw, if conditions allow.[40,41,54]

PREVENTION

In general, the main focus should be on the prevention of toe lesions, in particular of toe necrosis, by regular hoof trimming twice or 3 times a year, depending on individual farm circumstances; by regular weekly or fortnightly locomotion scoring of the herd by experienced personnel to identify cattle showing mild lameness; by prompt claw examination of cattle detected to be lame; and by correct and adequate therapeutic trimming and topical treatment of mild lesions by trained hoof trimmers or veterinarians.[40,41,96] Correct lesion identification and documentation of underlying causes are important for appropriate lameness prevention strategies in large dairy herds.[8,25–27] In addition, feedlot personnel should be trained to recognize early lameness and lesions that could be successfully treated to reduce the number of nonresponding lame cattle.[11]

The mechanical abrasiveness of new concrete can be reduced in several ways.[7] It has been recommended that concrete finished with a wood float in combination with grooving provides one of the best surfaces for cattle claws.[7] Grooves should be 12 mm wide and 10 mm deep and placed 5 to 7.5 cm apart and should run in the same direction as the manure scraper.[7] Sharp edges and protruding aggregate in new concrete floors that naturally develop as it cures may be removed by dragging heavy concrete blocks or a steel scraper over the flooring surface or by grinding or polishing of the surface.[58] An alternative "emergency" option is the spreading of dry manure in new corrals and transfer lanes in dry lots.[7]

One way to reduce the excessive mechanical abrasion of new concrete in freestall barns was assessed by incorporating rubber mats along feed alleys and in walkways to and from the milking parlor.[7,58] Observation of cattle behavior indicated that cattle prefer the softer surface offered by rubber flooring.[58,97] A recent California study evaluated the effects of rubber flooring on the development of claw lesions, locomotion scores, clinical lameness, and rates of hoof growth and wear in multiparous cows and suggested that the rubber flooring system was beneficial to hoof health.[98] Cows on rubber flooring had decreased rates of horn wear compared with cows kept on concrete.[98] Other investigators even described a beneficial effect of the installation of rubber mats,[51,97] decreasing the prevalence of lameness from 66.9% to

32.6%, and the incidence of thin soles in first lactation animals from 21.8% before the installation of rubber to only 4% thereafter.[8,58] The installation of rubber mats on the loading platform of transport vehicles could also be beneficial in preventing excessive hoof horn abrasion during transport in feedlot cattle.

It is likely that the principal causes of excess hoof horn wear in several studies of cattle were prolonged contact times with concrete, combined with the agitated nature of heifers and feedlot cattle, and extremely wet conditions underfoot.[3,9,11,54] This combination leads to the recommendation, in particular for heifers and feedlot cattle, that management of transport is improved to avoid excessive abrasion and trauma by handling cattle as quietly as possible, by sorting and processing cattle on dirt or deep sand, and by repairing or replacing damaged concrete surfaces and walking tracks.[9,54,70]

The most important causal factor of seasonality of thin soles is most likely to be the wet environment created by humidity and cow-cooling systems, although other effects of heat stress may contribute.[17,58] Decreasing the moisture content by creating dry flooring areas and by improving the quality of cubicles can decrease sole horn abrasion.[46]

Further preventive measures, in particular in those herds with an endemic DD infection, to be installed are hoof baths using licensed hoof bath solutions. It is imperative for the success of foot bathing to use the "ideal" hoof bath length of 3 to 3.6 m and width of 0.5 m,[99] the correct concentration of hoof bath solution, and adequate intervals depending on seasonal variable risk factors, and to replace the hoof bath solution after every 300 cattle.[99]

In a well-managed herd, cows suffering from prolonged toe necrosis and exhibiting a lameness score of 4 or 5 should never be observed.

SUMMARY

As the most important risk factor for toe lesions, in particular for toe necrosis, excessive wear of the sole horn caused by various conditions could be identified for both feedlot and dairy cattle.

Other risk factors that may play a role in the epidemiology and pathogenesis of toe necrosis in feedlot and dairy cattle include hypostasis associated with long transport periods, laminitis, excessive hoof trimming, overcrowding, and BVDV infection associated with vascular lesions and ischemic necrosis in the claws.

Depending on the presence of an endemic DD infection in the herd, toe necrosis with pedal bone infection can be associated with a secondary *Treponema* spp infection. However, such an infection is not necessarily always present in cases of toe necrosis.

Early recognition of toe lesions is imperative because it facilitates treatment and enables a successful outcome.

The focus should be on prevention of toe necrosis, in particular in feedlot and pasture-based cattle, because it is difficult to provide adequate treatment of advanced lesions in those production systems.

ACKNOWLEDGMENTS

The author thanks Claire Firth, MVM, MSc, BSc Vetmeduni Vienna, for language assistance.

REFERENCES

1. Sick FL, Bleeker CM, Mouw JK, et al. Toe abscesses in recently shipped feeder cattle. Vet Med Small Anim Clin 1982;77:1385–7.

2. Nuss K, Köstlin RG, Böhmer H, et al. The significance of corium infection -ungulocoriitis septica –at the toe of the bovine claw. Tieraerztl Prax 1990;18:567–75 [in German].

3. Miskimins DW. Bovine toe abscesses. Paper presented at: 8th International Symposium on Disorders of the Ruminant Digit. Banff (Canada), June 26–30, 1994. p. 54–7.

4. Miskimins DW. Update on toe abscesses in feedlot cattle. Paper presented at: 12th International Symposium on Lameness in Ruminants. Orlando (FL), January 9–13, 2002. p. 448–9.

5. Kofler J. Clinical study of toe ulcer and necrosis of the apex of the distal phalanx in 53 cattle. Vet J 1999;157:139–47.

6. Kofler J, Alton K, Licka T. Necrosis of the apex of the distal phalanx in cattle - postmortem, histological and bacteriological findings. Wien Tieraerztl Mschr 1999;86:192–200 [in German].

7. Van Amstel SR, Shearer JK. Toe abscess: a serious cause of lameness in the U.S. dairy industry. Paper presented at: 11th International Symposium on Disorders of the Ruminant Digit and 3rd International Conference on Lameness. Parma (Italy), September 3–7, 2000. p. 212–4.

8. Shearer JK, Van Amstel SR. Toe lesions in dairy cattle. Paper presented at: 46th Florida Dairy Production Conference. Gainesville (FL), April 28, 2009. p. 47–55.

9. Mason WA, Laven LJ, Laven RA. An outbreak of toe ulcers, sole ulcers and white line disease in a group of dairy heifers immediately after calving. N Z Vet J 2012; 60:76–81.

10. Paetsch CD, Jelinski MD. Toe-tip necrosis syndrome in feedlot cattle in Western Canada. In: Paper presented at: 17th International Symposium and 9th International Conference on Lameness in Ruminants. Bristol (United Kingdom), August 11–13, 2013. p.152–3.

11. Paetsch CD. Epidemiology of toe tip necrosis syndrome in Western Canadian feedlot cattle. Thesis Veterinary Medicine. Saskatoon (Canada): University of Saskatchewan; 2014.

12. Gyan LA, Paetsch CD, Jelinski MD, et al. The lesions of toe tip necrosis in southern Alberta feedlot cattle provide insight into the pathogenesis of the disease. Can Vet J 2015;56:1134–9.

13. Kofler J. Thin soles as a cause of lameness in cattle – etiology, complications and measures. Klauentierpraxis 2015;23:5–13 [in German].

14. Kofler J, Glonegger-Reichert J, Dietrich J, et al. A simple surgical treatment for digital dermatitis-associated white line lesions and sole ulcers. Vet J 2015;204: 229–31.

15. Nuss K. Surgery of the distal limb. Vet Clin Food Anim 2016;32:753–75.

16. Kofler J, Osová A, Altenbrunner-Martinek B, et al. Necrosis of the apex of pedal bone (toe necrosis) – surgical treatment techniques and outcome in 30 cattle. Wien Tieraerztl Mschr 2017;104:131–42 [in German].

17. Sanders AH, Shearer JK, De Vries A. Seasonal incidence of lameness and risk factors associated with thin soles, white line disease, ulcers, and sole punctures in dairy cattle. J Dairy Sci 2009;92:3165–74.

18. Jelinski MD, Fenton K, Perrett T, et al. Epidemiology of toe tip necrosis syndrome (TNNS) involving North American feedlot cattle. Can Vet J 2016;57:829–34.

19. Paetsch CD, Fenton K, Perrett T, et al. Prospective case control study of toe tip necrosis syndrome (TTNS) in western Canadian feedlot cattle. Can Vet J 2017; 58:247–54.

20. Greenough PR. White line disease at the toe (toe ulcer). In: Greenough PR, Weaver AD, editors. Lameness in cattle. 3rd edition. Philadelphia: WB Saunders; 1997. p. 107–9.

21. Egger-Danner C, Nielsen P, Fiedler A, et al. ICAR Claw Health Atlas 2015. Available at: www.icar.org/Documents/ICAR_Claw_Health_Atlas.pdf. Accessed December 6, 2016.

22. Shearer JK, Van Amstel SR, Brodersen BW. Clinical diagnosis of foot and leg lameness in cattle. Vet Clin Food Anim 2012;28:535–56.

23. Kofler J, Geissbühler U, Steiner A. Diagnostic imaging in bovine orthopedics. Vet Clin Food Anim 2014;30:11–53.

24. Kofler J, Franz S, Flöck M, et al. Diagnostic Imaging in Bovine Medicine. Paper presented at: 29th World Buiatrics Congress. Dublin (Ireland), July 5–8, 2016. p. 77–9.

25. Wenz JR, Giebel SK. Retrospective evaluation of health event data recording on 50 dairies using Dairy Comp 305. J Dairy Sci 2012;95:4699–706.

26. Kofler J. Computerised claw trimming database programs – the basis for monitoring hoof health in dairy herds. Vet J 2013;198:358–61.

27. Kofler J, Pesenhofer R, Landl G, et al. Monitoring of dairy cow claw health status in 15 herds using the computerized documentation program Claw Manager and digital parameters. Tieraerztl Prax 2013;41(G):31–44 [in German].

28. Cramer G, Lissemore KD, Guard CL, et al. Herd- and cow-level prevalence of foot lesions in Ontario dairy cattle. J Dairy Sci 2008;91:3888–95.

29. Hulek M, Sommerfeld-Stur I, Kofler J. Prevalence of digital dermatitis in first lactation cows assessed at breeding cattle auctions. Vet J 2010;183:161–5.

30. Holzhauer M. Non-healing white-line lesions: prevalence, causing organisms and risk factors. Paper presented at: 17th Symposium and 9th Conference of Lameness in Ruminants. Bristol (United Kingdom), August 11–14, 2013. p. 51.

31. Refaai W, Van Aert M, Ab Del-Al AM, et al. Infectious diseases causing lameness in cattle with a main emphasis on digital dermatitis (Mortellaro disease). Livestock Sci 2013;156:53–63.

32. Becker J, Steiner A, Kohler S, et al. Lameness and foot lesions in Swiss dairy cows: I. Prevalence. Schweiz Arch Tierheilkd 2014;156(2):71–8.

33. Atkinson O. Non-healing hoof lesions in dairy cows. Vet Rec 2011;169:561–2.

34. Blowey RW. Non-healing hoof lesions in dairy cows. Vet Rec 2011;169:534.

35. Evans NJ, Blowey RW, Timofte D, et al. Association between bovine digital dermatitis treponemes and a range of "non-healing" bovine hoof disorders. Vet Rec 2011;168:214–7.

36. Nouri M, Ashrafi-Helan J. Observations on healing process of wall ulcers with concurrent digital dermatitis in 52 cattle: gross and light microscopic pathology. Anim Vet Sci 2013;1:60–5.

37. Acevedo JP, Chesterton RN, Hurtado CS. Bovine Digital Dermatitis and non-healing lesions and toe necrosis in grazing dairy herds in Chile. Paper resented at: 17th International Symposium and 9th International Conference on Lameness in Ruminants. Bristol (United Kingdom), August 11–14, 2013. p. 157–8.

38. Starke A, Müller H, Wippermann W, et al. Complicated toe lesions in cattle – treatment and post-surgical care. Paper presented at: 17th Symposium and 9th Conference of Lameness in Ruminants. Bristol (United Kingdom), August 11–14, 2013. p. 126.

39. Maierl J, Mülling CKW. Funktionelle Anatomie. In: Fiedler A, Maierl J, Nuss K, editors. Erkrankungen der Klauen und Zehen des Rindes. Stuttgart (Germany): Schattauer; 2004. p. 1–28.

40. Kofler J. Functional hoof trimming in cattle. In: Litzke L-F, Rau B, editors. Der Huf. 6th edition. Stuttgart (Germany): Enke Verlag in MVS Medizinverlage; 2012. p. 325–53 [in German].
41. Shearer JK, Van Amstel SR. Anatomy of the bovine foot & Claw trimming and knife sharpening. In: Shearer JK, Van Amstel SR, editors. Manual of foot care in cattle. 2nd edition. Fort Atkinson (WI): WD Hoards & Sons Company; 2013. p. 17–23, 24–44.
42. Tomlinson DJ, Mülling CH, Fakler TM. Invited review: formation of keratins in the bovine claw: roles of hormones, minerals, and vitamins in functional claw integrity. J Dairy Sci 2004;87:797–809.
43. Gregory N, Craggs L, Hobson N, et al. Softening of cattle hoof soles and swelling of heel horn by environmental agents. Food Chem Toxicol 2006;44:1223–7.
44. Shakespeare AS. Inadequate thickness of the weight-bearing surface of claws in ruminants. J S Afr Vet Assoc 2009;80:247–53.
45. Bonser RHC, Farrent JW, Taylor AM. Assessing the frictional and abrasion-resisting properties of hooves and claws. Biosyst Eng 2003;86:253–6.
46. Van Amstel SR, Shearer JK, Palin FL. Moisture content, thickness and lesions of the sole horn associated with thin soles in dairy cattle. J Dairy Sci 2004;87: 757–63.
47. Ossent P, Greenough PR, Vermunt JJ. Laminitis. In: Greenough PR, Weaver AD, editors. Lameness in cattle. 3rd edition. Philadelphia: WB Saunders; 1997. p. 277–92.
48. Ossent P, Lischer CJ. Bovine laminitis: the lesions and their pathogenesis. In Pract 1998;20:415–27.
49. Boosman B, Nemeth F, Gruys E, et al. Arteriographical and pathological changes in chronic laminitis in dairy cattle. Vet Q 1989;11:144–55.
50. Greenough PR. Bovine laminitis and lameness: a hands-on approach. New York: Saunders Elsevier; 2007. p. 1–7, 8–28, 36–54, 84–106.
51. Telezhenko E, Bergsten C, Magnusson M. Nilsson. Effect of different flooring systems on claw conformation of dairy cows. J Dairy Sci 2009;92:2625–33.
52. Steiner B, Van Caenegem L, Schellenberg K. Durability of mastic asphalt floors in cattle housing. Agrarforschung 2008;15:536–41 [in German].
53. Holzhauer M. Practical intervention toe necrosis. Paper presented at: 17th Symposium and 9th Conference of Lameness in Ruminants. Bristol (United Kingdom), August 11–14, 2013. p. 154.
54. Acuña R, Scarsi R. Toe ulcer: the most important disease in first calving Holstein cows under grazing conditions. Paper presented at: 12th International Symposium on Lameness in Ruminants. Orlando (FL), January 9–13, 2002. p. 276–9.
55. Dewes HF. Transit-related lameness in a group of Jersey heifers. N Z Vet J 1979; 27:45.
56. Griffin D. Feedlot diseases. Vet Clin North Am Food Anim Pract 1998;14:199–230.
57. Frank A, Opsomer G, De Kruif A, et al. Frictional interactions between bovine claw and concrete floor. Biosyst Eng 2007;96:565–80.
58. Shearer JK, Van Amstel SR. Effect of flooring and flooring surfaces on lameness disorders in dairy cattle. Paper presented at: Western Dairy Management Conference. Reno (NV), March 7–9, 2007. p. 148–59. Available at: http://articles.extension.org/pages/11339/effect-of-flooring-and-flooring-surfaces-on-lameness-disorders-in-dairy-cattle. Accessed December 6, 2016.
59. Hahn MV, McDaniel BT, Wilk JC. Rates of hoof growth and wear in Holstein cattle. J Dairy Sci 1986;69:2148–56.

60. Smith DR, Brodersen BW. Lesions of the hoof wall, sole, and skin associated with osteomyelitis of the distal third phalanx (toe abscess) and other secondary foot lesions in feedlot cattle. Paper presented at: Conference for Research Workers in Animal Disease 1998. Abstract 45. Chicago (IL), November 9–10, 1998.

61. Thompson PN. Osteitis and fracture of the third phalanges following routine hoof trimming in a dairy cow. Paper presented at: 9th International Symposium on Disorders of the Ruminant digit 1996. Jerusalem (Israel), April 11–14, 1996. p. 51.

62. Nocek JE. Bovine acidosis: implications on laminitis. J Dairy Sci 1997;80: 1005–28.

63. Greenough PR, Vermunt JJ, McKinnon JJ, et al. Laminitis-like changes in the claws of feedlot cattle. Can Vet J 1990;31:202–8.

64. Blowey R, Burgess J, Inman B, et al. Bone density changes in bovine toe necrosis. Vet Rec 2013;172(6):164.

65. Atkinson O, Wright T. Bone density changes in bovine toe necrosis. Vet Rec 2013; 169:297–8.

66. Minini S, Crowhurst F, De Nicolás J, et al. Toe necrosis and non-healing hoof lesions in commercial dairy herds in Argentina. Paper presented at: 17th International Symposium and 9th International Conference on Lameness in Ruminants. Bristol (United Kingdom), August 11–14, 2013. p. 166–7.

67. Rimoldi G, Pineda M, Hall S, et al. An outbreak of toe-tip necrosis in Angus feedlot cattle. Paper presented at: 18th International Symposium and 10th Conference on Lameness in Ruminants. Valdivia (Chile), November 22–25, 2015. p. 169.

68. Sellera FP, Gargano RG, Azedo MR, et al. Antimicrobial photodynamic therapy as an adjuvant treatment of toe ulcer in cattle. Europ Inter J Sci Technol 2013;2(10): 98–104.

69. Pofcher E, Montecchia J, De Iraola J, et al. Determination of lameness prevalence in dairy cows and lesion type in dairy herds from Buenos Aires province Argentina. Paper presented at: 18th International Symposium and 10th Conference on Lameness in Ruminants. Valdivia (Chile), November 22–25, 2015. p. 158.

70. Chesterton RN, Pfeiffer DU, Morris RS, et al. Environmental and behavioral factors affecting the prevalence of foot lameness in New Zealand dairy herds – a case control study. N Z Vet J 1989;37:135–42.

71. Cook NB, Nordlund KV. The influence of the environment on dairy cow behavior, claw health and herd lameness dynamics. Vet J 2009;179:360–9.

72. Sugg JL, Brown AH Jr, Perkins JL, et al. Performance traits, hoof mineral composition, and hoof characteristics of bulls in a 112-day postweaning feedlot performance test. Am J Vet Res 1996;57(3):291–5.

73. Mülling CKW, Bragulla HH, Reese S, et al. How structures in bovine hoof epidermis are influenced by nutritional factors. Anat Histol Embryol 1999;28: 103–8.

74. Nocek JE, Johnson AB, Socha MT. Digital characteristics in commercial dairy herds fed metal-specific amino acid complexes. J Dairy Sci 2000;83:1553–72.

75. Gomez A, Bernardoni N, Rieman J, et al. A randomized trial to evaluate the effect of a trace mineral premix on the incidence of active digital dermatitis lesions in cattle. J Dairy Sci 2014;97:6211–22.

76. Kofler J. Orthopedic examination procedure. In: Baumgartner W, editor. Klinische Propädeutik der Haus- und Heimtiere. 7th edition. Wien (Berlin): Parey; 2014. p. 216–81 [in German].

77. Kofler J, Kuebber P, Henninger W. Ultrasonographic imaging and thickness measurement of the sole horn and the underlying soft tissue layer in bovine claws. Vet J 1999;157:322–31.

78. Van Amstel SR, Palin FL, Rohrbach BW, et al. Ultrasound measurement of sole horn thickness in trimmed claws of dairy cows. J Am Vet Med Assoc 2003;223: 492–4.

79. Müller KE. Resection of the toe tip in cattle. Prakt Tierarzt 1991;12:1112–3 [in German].

80. Van Der Tol PPJ, Metz JHM, Noordhuizen-Stassen EN, et al. The pressure distribution under the bovine claw during square standing on a flat substrate. J Dairy Sci 2002;85:1476–81.

81. Nuss K, Paulus N. Measurements of claw dimensions in cows before and after functional trimming: a post-mortem study. Vet J 2006;172:284–92.

82. Borderas TF, Pawluczuk B, De Passille AM, et al. Claw hardness of dairy cows: relationship to water content and claw lesions. J Dairy Sci 2004;87:2085–93.

83. Alton K, Kofler J. Squamous cell carcinoma of the distal phalanx in a cow. Wien Tieraerztl Mschr 1998;86:192–200 [in German].

84. Nuss K. Surgery of claws and digits – resection of the tip of the pedal bone. In: Fiedler A, Maierl J, Nuss K, editors. Erkrankungen der Klauen und Zehen des Rindes. 2nd edition. Stuttgart (Germany): Schattauer; 2004. p. 141–3 [in German].

85. Sykora S, Kofler J, Glonegger-Reichert J, et al. Treponema DNA in 'non-healing' versus common bovine sole ulcers and white line disease. Vet J 2015;205: 417–20.

86. Nuss K, Fiedler A. Aftercare - blocks. In: Fiedler A, Maierl J, Nuss K, editors. Erkrankungen der Klauen und Zehen des Rindes. 2nd edition. Stuttgart (Germany): Schattauer; 2004. p. 169–83.

87. Maierl J, Fiedler A, Döpfer D, et al. Wedge-shaped blocks, wood and flexible, advance a good locomotion performance. Paper presented at: 17th International Symposium & 9th International Conference on Lameness in Ruminants. Bristol (United Kingdom), August 11–13, 2013. p. 144–5.

88. Shearer JK, Stock ML, Van Amstel SR, et al. Assessment and management of pain associated with lameness in cattle. Vet Clin Food Anim 2013;29:135–56.

89. Edmondson MA. Local, regional, and spinal anesthesia in ruminants. Vet Clin Food Anim 2016;32:535–52.

90. Kofler J, Martinek B, Reinoehl-DeSouza C. Treatment of infected wounds and abscesses in bovine limbs with Ligasano®-Polyurethane-soft foam dressing material. Berlin Muench Tieraerztl Wschr 2004;117:428–38 [in German].

91. Pedersen SL. Milk production and survival following digit amputation in dairy cattle. Cattle Pract 2007;15(3):256–60.

92. Blowey RW. Changing indications for digit amputation in cattle. Vet Rec 2011;169: 236–72.

93. Klawitter M, Döpfer D, Braden T, et al. To bandage or not bandage - the curative effect of bandaging digital dermatitis lesions. Paper presented at: 29th World Buiatrics Congress. Dublin (Ireland), July 5–8, 2016. p. 174.

94. Holzhauer M. Toe necrosis, risk factors and a practical surgical intervention to a save cow's life. Paper presented at: 29th World Buiatrics Congress. Dublin (Ireland), July 5–8, 2016. p. 218.

95. Raundal PM, Forkman B, Andersen PH, et al. Lame cows benefit from being housed in recovery pens. Paper presented at: 18th Symposium on Diseases of the Bovine Digit and 10th International Conference on Lameness in Ruminants. Valdivia (Chile), November 22–25, 2015. p. 153.

96. Groenevelt M, Main DCJ, Tisdall D, et al. Measuring the response to therapeutic foot trimming in dairy cows with fortnightly lameness scoring. Vet J 2014;201: 283–8.
97. Platz S, Ahrens F, Bahrs E, et al. Association between floor type and behavior, skin lesions, and claw dimensions in group-housing fattening bulls. Prev Vet Med 2007;80:209–21.
98. Vanegas J, Overton M, Berry SL, et al. Effect of rubber flooring on claw health in lactating dairy cows housed in free-stall barns. J Dairy Sci 2006;89:4251–8.
99. Cook NB, Rieman J, Gomez A, et al. Observations on the design and use of footbaths for the control of infectious hoof disease in dairy cattle. Vet J 2012;193: 669–73.

Surgical Procedures of the Distal Limb for Treatment of Sepsis in Cattle

David E. Anderson, DVM, MS[a],*, André Desrochers, DMV, MS[b],
Sarel R. van Amstel, BVSc, MMedVet[a]

KEYWORDS

- Bovine • Digital surgery • Septic arthritis • Septic tendonitis • Pedal osteitis
- Retrobulbar abscess

KEY POINTS

- With a thorough knowledge of the anatomy of the foot, and basic surgical instruments, digit surgery can be performed in field situations.
- Sepsis of the distal interphalangeal and proximal interphalangeal joints should be treated surgically because conservative treatment is often ineffective.
- Most of the diseases described in this article are chronic and often the animals have been suffering for some time.
- Perioperative analgesia is important to alleviate the pain of those animals. All those procedures should be performed under local or regional anesthesia.

INTRODUCTION

Claw diseases in cattle are a common cause of debilitating lameness, which result in lost production, expense of treatment, and premature culling. When trauma or infection result in compromise of the joints, bones, tendons/tendon sheaths, or ligaments, surgical treatment may be required in order for the animal to be returned to soundness, productivity, and longevity. Surgical digital diseases include septic arthritis of the distal and proximal interphalangeal (PIP) joints, flexor tendon injury, septic tenosynovitis, and pedal osteomyelitis. Most digital surgical conditions are manageable under field conditions. Postoperative care, in some cases, is demanding and may limit the extent to which producers are willing to commit to treatments. Postoperative treatment most often includes wound care, antimicrobial therapy, pain management using

Disclosure: The authors have nothing to disclose.
[a] Department of Large Animal Clinical Sciences, College of Veterinary Medicine, University of Tennessee Institute of Agriculture, 2407 River Drive, Knoxville, TN 37996, USA; [b] Department of Clinical Sciences, Faculty of Veterinary Medicine, Université de Montréal, St-Hyacynthe, Québec J2S 7C6, Canada
* Corresponding author.
E-mail address: dander48@utk.edu

antiinflammatory drugs, and variable periods of restricted exercise. Treatment of musculoskeletal diseases often requires prolonged drug therapy; this necessitates that veterinarians and producers be cautious regarding drug residue contamination of meat and milk from animals treated for musculoskeletal diseases. Accurate withholding times have not been established for drugs administered repeatedly, for prolonged periods of time, and in disease states. Readers are advised to seek professional advice (eg, www.farad.org) regarding meat and milk withholding times in these cases.

SEPSIS OF THE BONE AND JOINTS OF THE FOOT
Sepsis of the Joints, Bone, Tendons and Tissues of the Distal Limb

Knowledge and understanding of the digital anatomy is essential before performing surgeries.[1-3] Sepsis of the distal interphalangeal (DIP) joint is caused mainly by extension of sole diseases, such as sole ulcers or abscesses and white line disease. A penetrating foreign body in the interdigital space or foot rot also is often implicated in sepsis of the DIP joint. In dairy cattle, the origin of DIP sepsis is most likely sole ulcers. In beef cattle, the cause is often unknown but interdigital trauma and foot rot are often suspected. The distal sesamoid bone and its bursa, the tendinous portion of the deep digital flexor (DDF) muscle, the tendon sheath of the DDF muscle, and the superficial digital flexor (SDF) muscles are in close relationship and solar infection can rapidly spread to these structures. The history of affected cattle is often typical: they have history of chronic lameness being treated unsuccessfully for foot rot or sole ulcer. Severity of the lameness is variable depending on the extent of infection and the chronicity of the disease.

The hallmarks of DIP infection are a swollen and painful coronary band with a draining tract either at the proximal aspect of the coronary band or under the sole (**Fig. 1**). A swollen heel suggests infection of the distal sesamoid bone and its bursa and the digital cushion pad, and a fistulous tract may be present at the heel skin junction. Cattle with deep sepsis of the digit show clinical signs of pain when the heel is palpated or the digit is extended. The tendinous portion of the DDF tendon (DDFT) might rupture if the necrotic process is severe, and the digit affected will tilt upward.

Radiographic evaluation of the DIP joint is helpful to determine the extent and duration of the process. Usually the lesions are not subtle because of the chronicity of the infection. Radiographic views of a DIP joint with chronic septic arthritis show an increased joint space because of subchondral bone lysis (**Fig. 2**). Distal and proximal periosteal proliferation is present. The distal sesamoid bone may show lysis of its articular surface or may be destroyed completely. The PIP joint also might be involved in

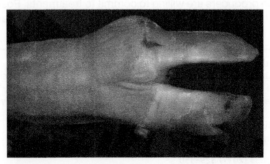

Fig. 1. Swelling localized along the lateral aspect of the coronary band indicating septic arthritis of the DIP joint (uppermost digit).

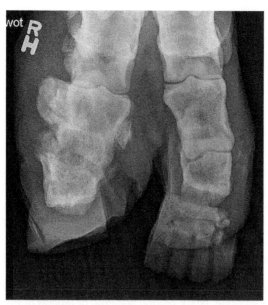

Fig. 2. Dorsal plantar radiograph. Note widening of the joint space associated with the DIP joint (left digit).

the process. If a fistulous tract is present, communication with the DIP joint is confirmed with the insertion of a sterile probe into the tract. Ultrasonography was investigated as a diagnostic method for DIP joint sepsis. Compared with the partner sound claw, the dorsal pouch of the infected DIP joint was larger. With a linear probe applied longitudinally on the dorsal aspect of the digit, it was determined that the infected joint had a dorsal pouch greater than 6 mm.[4]

Conservative treatment with systemic antibiotics and a wooden block applied to the sound claw is often ineffective because of the chronicity of the infection on presentation. Surgery is therefore the treatment of choice to provide debridement and drainage of the DIP joint. The 2 surgical options are the resection of the joint with its necrotic tissues and digit amputation.[5–11]

Ankylosis of the Distal Interphalangeal Joint

The techniques for resection of the DIP joint differ by surgical approach. Choice of a technique should be based on the anatomic structure infected and the location of existing draining tracts.[12–14] Intact ligaments and tendons should be preserved, when possible, to keep the affected digit stable during the ankylosis process. However, if necrosis of the tendon and/or tendon sheath is present, then extensive surgical exposure might be necessary.

Surgery is designed to provide drainage, debridement, and removal of articular cartilage from the DIP joint resulting in ankylosis. The surgery can be performed with the patient under sedation and intravenous regional anesthesia or regional nerve block (**Fig. 3**). Cattle are restrained in a foot-trimming chute or in lateral recumbency with the affected leg uppermost. The plantar or palmar portion of the sole and the heel should be pared away until the sole is thin enough that it can be indented easily. In severe and extensive infection of the DIP joint originating from a solar lesion, the distal sesamoid bone and the joint can be felt through the wound and the sole already

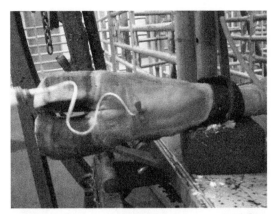

Fig. 3. Intravenous regional anesthesia being administered before surgery on the foot.

can be indented easily. The distal limb is prepared surgically. Three techniques are in common use: (1) solar approach, (2) bulbar approach, (3) abaxial approach to the joint.[15–18] The solar and plantar approaches are used most often when the heel bulb, distal sesamoid bone, flexor tendon sheaths, or tendon of the DDF muscle are affected in addition to sepsis of the DIP joint. The abaxial approach is used most often when the flexor tendons, heel, and sole are unaffected.

In the solar approach, an elliptical incision is made around the necrotic area at the sole and heel junction (**Fig. 4**). The width of the incision should be close to the axial and abaxial white line. The proximal portion of the elliptical incision joins just before crossing the coronary band, avoiding cutting a wedge out of it. Depending of the extent of infection, the elliptical incision is extended proximal as far as needed. The incision can be extended proximal to the accessory digit by making the incision axial to the accessory digit.[3,13,14] The tendinous portion of the DDF muscle is cut from its insertion on the distal phalanx and resected proximally 2 to 3 cm or more if necrotic. The distal sesamoid bone is then exposed. If the sesamoid bone is necrotic, it can easily be removed with a rongeur. If not, the 2 collateral ligaments and the distal

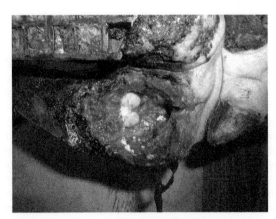

Fig. 4. Solar approach to the DIP joint with excision of the navicular bone and deep digital flexor tendon.

ligaments are resected with a scalpel blade. The DIP joint should be exposed at this point. All necrotic tissue should be removed to speed up healing. Debridement of the joint from the solar wound can be performed with a curette, a hoof knife, or with a 5-mm to 13-mm drill bit. The drill exits through the dorsal wall, 1 cm distal to the coronary band. Some investigators prefer to exit proximal to the coronary band.[15] Wherever the drill bit exits, damage to the coronary corium must be avoided so as to not compromise future horn production. Even after the joint is drilled, necrotic tissue may still be present and it has to be curetted thoroughly. Copious lavage is performed with isotonic solution. If the tendon sheath or the tendinous portion of the SDF muscle is infected and necrotic, the incision can be extended 2 to 3 cm proximally up to the accessory digit, allowing further debridement and drainage. A wooden block is attached to the sole using polymethyl methacrylate cement on the healthy digit of the affected limb. The wound is bandaged and lavage performed every other day, if possible. It is the authors' opinion that the infected digit should not be wired to the parent digit for immobilization purposes. By attaching the digits, the infected digit will be constantly moving, increasing the pain because of the movement and delaying the ankylosis process. Systemic antibiotics are given for 10 to 14 days depending on adjacent soft tissue infection. Nonsteroidal antiinflammatory drugs are given as needed for the first few days postoperatively. This technique provides good visualization of the DIP joint, excellent drainage, and a good long-term prognosis. Variations of the solar approach are described in the literature. Some are more invasive, with deep dissection of the plantar or palmar aspect of the digit, and other techniques consist only in providing drainage of the joint by drilling a hole through the joint. The extent of the infection should determine the technique to be used.

A bulbar approach is favored when the sole is intact, as is often observed in beef cattle. A horizontal incision around the circumference of the heel 1 cm distal to the skin horn junction is made (**Fig. 5**).[5] A wedge of hypodermic tissue and tendon is resected, providing visualization of the distal sesamoid bone. The sesamoid bone is resected, as described earlier, and the digit is extended to provide exposure of the DIP joint. After debridement and lavage of the joint, the incision either can be sutured and bandaged or left open for further treatment. A wooden block is applied with polymethyl methacrylate cement on the healthy digit of the affected limb. This technique provides better visualization of the DIP joint without invading the tendon sheath

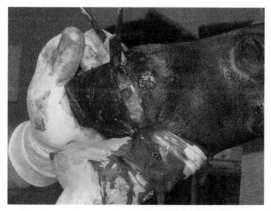

Fig. 5. Bulbar approach by making an incision along the margin of the heel bulb and pastern.

when it is not necessary. Recently, Bicalho and colleagues[15] described a modification of the technique in which the incision is proximal to the coronary band. If the DDFT is necrotic and the tendon sheath infected, then a second incision is made over the tendon through the tendon sheath, proximally to the accessory digits. First, the distal portion of the DDFT is pushed proximally into the tendon sheath, then it is grabbed and pulled by the proximal incision. A rubber drain is passed through the incisions and attached on the abaxial aspect of the digit and the proximal incision is sutured. Cattle were extremely lame for 2 weeks but were sound within 5 months.[15] The investigators have been using the bulbar approach for resection of the DIP joint in nonseptic processes (degenerative joint disease of the DIP joint and laceration), avoiding disruption of the intact solar surface and decreasing the chance of infection.[16]

The abaxial approach uses an orthopedic drill, with a 6-mm to 12-mm drill bit, to create a tunnel through the abaxial wall of the claw at the level of the DIP joint. The drill is passed through the DIP joint and exited through the dorsoaxial interdigital space distal to the coronary band. The entry site for the drill bit is estimated at the intersection of 2 imaginary lines, one drawn parallel to the coronary band approximately one-third the distance from the coronary band to the sole and the other line drawn perpendicular to the coronary band approximately half the distance from the heel bulb to the dorsal wall (**Fig. 6**). This approach is easy to perform, but the exit site of the drill bit is difficult to control, especially if the animal is not well restrained. Debridement of the cartilage and necrotic bone also is difficult to assess. The defect in the claw wall remains open to facilitate drainage. The authors have not observed specific claw wall complications of this technique, but cattle should be confined to a small area with excellent footing during the early stages of healing.

Zulauf and colleagues[17] proposed an alternative to this method. They performed a precise abaxial wall excision using a fine rotating burr. A wall segment measuring approximately 15 × 40 mm was removed and the proximal margin of the defect was approximately 1 cm distal to the coronary band. This technique provides a large, rectangular defect through which the DIP joint is accessed.

Abaxial Excision of the Navicular Bone (Distal Sesamoid Bone) and Distal Interphalangeal Joint Ankylosis

The main disadvantages of the approaches to the DIP joint through the abaxial wall are that the joint is difficult to assess for debridement and the navicular bone cannot be

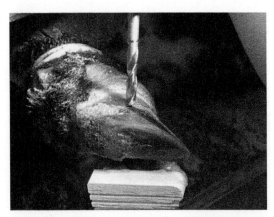

Fig. 6. Placement of a drill bit for abaxial approach to the DIP joint. Note placement of a wooden walking block on the opposite, normal digit before surgery.

accessed for resection. A modification of the abaxial approach allows better access to the joint and navicular bone for the purpose of resection. This modified abaxial approach is suitable if septic inflammation of the DIP joint and navicular bone is caused by lesions entering through the interdigital space, such as foot rot or traumatic penetrating lesions of the foot in the area of the coronary band. It is less suitable for lesions of the sole, such as sole ulcer. Advantages of this approach include good access and visual control for complete resection of both the DIP joint and navicular bone.

In the modified abaxial approach, a window 2 × 2 cm is cut into the abaxial hoof wall of the affected claw, 0.5 cm cranial to the abaxial groove and immediately below the coronary band (**Fig. 7**). The abaxial hoof wall cuts can be made with the aid of a Dremel tool with a circular diamond disc. The cuts are deepened with a scalpel until bone is reached. Alternatively, a hoof grinder may be used to thin the horn of the abaxial wall immediately dorsal to the abaxial groove and distal to the coronary band. Using a small periosteal elevator, the articulation between the navicular bone and the caudal articular surface of P2 as well as the articular surface of P3 are exposed. The proximal suspensory ligament and impar ligament of the navicular bone are transected. This technique is used in order to maintain the integrity of the deep flexor tendon and its insertion to P3. Once freed, the navicular bone can be removed by grasping it with a towel clamp and lifting it through the opening while cutting any residual attachments. The cavity is then flushed with 0.9% saline and inspected for any remaining bone fragments. This approach allows access to the caudal articular surface of the DIP joint. Using a drill bit, the articular surface of the DIP joint is debrided. In this technique, placement and angle of the drill are facilitated by removal of the navicular bone. If total resection is required, the drill should be angled such that it will emerge through the dorsal hoof wall just below the coronary band axial or abaxial to the extensor process

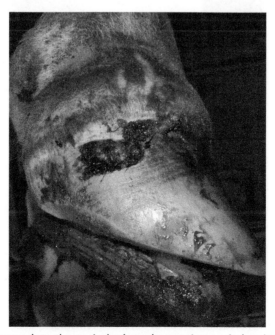

Fig. 7. Abaxial approach to the navicular bone by creating a window in the abaxial hoof wall.

of P3. Using a bone curette, the joint is further debrided in order to remove all remaining chondral and subchondral bone, followed by flushing the space with an antiseptic solution. A Penrose drain is placed to maintain patency and allow drainage.

Ultimately, complete ankylosis of the DIP joint is desired. Bony fusion of the joint is most likely to provide pain-free ambulation and return to normal activity and productive use (**Fig. 8**).

Digit amputation

Digit amputation has been used successfully to treat pedal osteitis, luxation or fracture of the distal phalanx, deep sepsis of the digit, and septic arthritis of the DIP or PIP joint (**Fig. 9**). The advantages are that it is a rapid and inexpensive procedure, all the infected tissues are resected, and cattle usually return rapidly to their previous level of production.[5–7] The disadvantages are that expected production life might be reduced, heavy animals are reported to do poorly, and cosmetic result is poor. The production life of cattle that have a digit amputated depends on which digit was

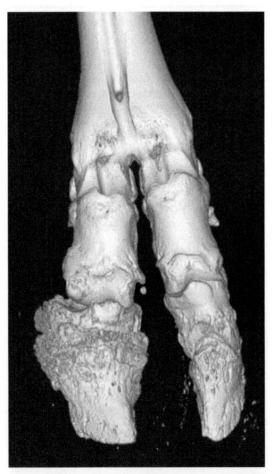

Fig. 8. Three-dimensional reconstruction of computed tomography image of the distal limb of an Angus bull 2 years after abaxial approach for resection of the navicular bone and DIP joint.

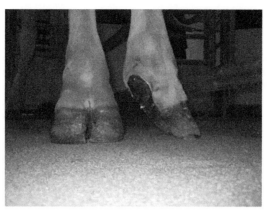

Fig. 9. Healing digit amputation wound.

removed, the weight of the animal, and the type of housing. Production longevity of cattle after digit amputation ranges between 10 and 27 months.[6,8,9] Cattle weighing more than 680 kg that have a digit amputated have a short production life.[6] Recently, Starke[9] showed no significant difference in survival time between digit amputation (27.2 months) and joint resection (21.2 months) in bulls. However, the survival time in dairy cattle affected with DIP joint sepsis treated by amputation was 13.5 months compared with 10.9 months for the joint resection group, but the results were not statistically significant.[10] Bicalho and colleagues[11] compared amputation and arthrodesis of the DIP joint in a control study on lactating cows. The failure rate, defined as culled in less than 60 days of milking after the surgery, was 44.9% compared with 0% for the arthrodesis group. Milk yield was higher for cattle that underwent arthrodesis compared with the amputation group. The investigators concluded that arthrodesis was preferred to amputation.

Digit amputation through the distal aspect of the proximal phalanx is the most common technique, but the site of amputation should be chosen based on the location and extent of the infection. Digit amputation is readily performed and usually provides a wide resection and effective drainage of the affected digit and the flexor tendon sheath. The wound is further away from the ground compared with a low amputation, preventing ulceration. However, a low amputation provides more digital stability because the interdigital cruciate ligament can be preserved. Disarticulation or amputation through the joint is an easy technique to do in field situation.[11] If the cartilage of the phalanx is left intact after disarticulation, coverage by granulation tissue might be delayed and cystlike lesion might form as well.[12]

The distal limb is prepared surgically and intravenous regional anesthesia is administered. For the proximal amputation technique, the interdigital skin is incised to the level of the PIP joint or the very distal aspect of the proximal phalanx axially. A Gigli wire is inserted in the interdigital space with an angle of 45° to the proximal digit abaxially. An assistant can hold the digit to provide more stability when the cut is performed. The cut should go through the distal portion of the proximal phalanx. The interdigital fat and all remaining necrotic tissues are removed. Digital vessels are ligated with absorbable suture as needed. The wound is lavaged and dried. A semiocclusive dressing (eg, Telfa pad) is applied on the distal portion of the proximal phalanx, and multiple layers of gauze are put over it and wrapped with adhesive bandage. The bandage is changed 24 hours after the surgery and then changed again every 4 to

5 days as needed. Ideally, bandages are continued until the surface of the bone is covered with granulation tissue. A broad-spectrum, systemic antibiotic is administered for 5 to 10 days after the surgery. It should be remembered that antibiotics never replace good surgical principles and adequate postoperative hygiene. Bulls can return to breeding 3 to 4 months after the surgery. A skin flap could be preserved to cover the stump by continuing the interdigital incision distal and abaxial at the palmar and dorsal aspect of the digit and along the proximal aspect of the coronary band.[13] Although this technique provides a superior cosmetic result and decreases subsequent care of the stump, it may prevent adequate drainage and extension of the infection. This technique is recommended for a nonseptic process of the digit (pedal fracture, digit luxation) or distal sepsis without extensive soft tissue infection (pedal osteitis). If skin flap is elected in the presence of infection, the distal portion of the incision should be left opened for drainage.

Proximal Interphalangeal Joint Infection

Septic arthritis of the PIP joint is secondary to a direct trauma, adjacent infection, or from systemic infection in young animals.[18]

Affected animals are often minimally weight-bearing lame and have a fistulous tract with necrotic tissue exiting the skin on the abaxial aspect of the pastern joint midway between the coronary band and fetlock joint. Diagnosis is based on physical examination, probing the lesion, or radiographic imaging of the digit. This condition should be treated surgically with extensive debridement of the joint or amputation. Choice of surgical technique is based on the extent of the infection. If infection is limited to the PIP joint, resection of the joint is preferred. However, if the flexor tendon sheath and DIP joint are also infected, then high amputation has to be considered. The existing wound or draining tract is used to access the joint. Arthrotomies should always be performed in such a manner so as to avoid tendons and major blood vessels; this is most easily accomplished on the abaxial or dorsal aspect of the limb. The joint should be debrided with a bone curette until hard bone can be felt. The joint is lavaged copiously, as needed, and the wound protected from environmental contamination until the arthrotomy sites are filled with sound granulation tissue. This approach often requires wound management for 7 to 10 days. In general, the prognosis for PIP joint infection is considered good if no other synovial structures are involved.[18]

TOE ABSCESS AND PEDAL OSTEITIS

Pedal osteomyelitis is defined as a septic process of the distal phalanx (P3; **Fig. 10**). Pedal osteitis results, most often, from exposure of the pedal bone by trauma (eg,

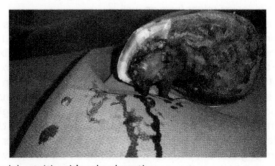

Fig. 10. Severe pedal osteitis with sole ulceration.

penetrating foreign body) or by extension of infection resulting from ulceration of the sole, abscessation of the white line, infection of the soft tissues (eg, foot rot), or sepsis of the DIP joint. The incidence of pedal osteitis increases in cattle housed or managed in facilities with extensive concrete flooring, rocky terrain, and conditions favoring development of subclinical laminitis. Cattle recently placed in a feedlot fight around a feed bunk, and their hind digits slip on the concrete floor, causing severe abrasion at the toe region, white line separation, and secondary infection. Overtrimming with a grinding disc is also a cause of apical necrosis, as described by Kofler[19] (for more information please see Johann Kofler's article, "Pathogenesis and Treatment of Toe Lesions in Cattle including "Non-healing" Toe Lesions," in this issue).

A preoperative radiograph is helpful to evaluate the extent of the infection. The DIP joint as well as the flexor tendon sheath should be examined. The surgical approach is based on the adjacent structures involved. The sole, infected corium, and the distal phalanx are debrided with a curette and rongeur until sound hard bone is felt. Detached claw wall from the corium should not be left in place and subtotal resection is often necessary to provide better healing and improve locomotion. Hoof nippers can be used to remove the affected apical portion of the claw.[3] Lavage is performed and the wound is bandaged. A wooden block is applied on the healthy digit of the affected limb. Bandaging and lavage should be continued until the infection is controlled and granulation tissue covers the distal phalanx. The DIP joint also can become infected by spread of bacteria from the surrounding tissues into the joint space. The infected joint can be either resected or amputated, as previously described. The approach for joint resection might differ depending on the location of the pedal lesion.

TENDON DISORDERS

Survey estimation of the incidence of lameness in dairy herds in the United States, Canada, and the United Kingdom reveal that tendon disorders are not a common cause of lameness when considered as a primary diagnosis.[20–22] However, one study indicated tendon involvement in 21% of limb lesions.[23] Another study reported that muscle and/or tendon lesions accounted for 74% of upper limb injuries in the forelimb and 7.8% in the hind limb.[24] Tendon injuries causing loss of the animal or a decreased level of production result in significant economic loss to cattle producers. Acquired tendon disorders include septic tendinitis, laceration, avulsion, rupture, and septic tenosynovitis. Dairy breeds, feedlot cattle, and cattle maintained in confinement housing most commonly are affected, and the incidence of lameness in dairy herds ranges widely. Lesions in dairy cattle occur most frequently during the early lactation period and in first-lactation heifers, and may occur more frequently during the spring and summer. However, based on these studies, lameness caused solely by tendon injury seems uncommon in cattle. Therefore, information regarding acquired tendon disorders in ruminants is limited. In this context, several disorders involving the tendons, as the primary lesions or as secondary lesions, are discussed.

TENDON LACERATION

Flexor tendon lacerations can be managed successfully in cattle by tenorrhaphy and external coaptation or by external coaptation alone. Economic costs associated with treatment and prolonged convalescence should be discussed with the owner before attempting therapy. Also, the owner's expectation for long-term productivity should include the likelihood of persistent lameness.

Options for treatment of tendon laceration in cattle include stall rest, use of a wooden or rubber block on the healthy digit, cast application, tenorrhaphy, and corrective farriery. The location of the lesion, individual tendon involvement, and concurrent injuries are important factors for treatment selection.[25] Stall confinement may be adequate for incomplete lacerations and partial disruption of the gastrocnemius muscle or tendon. Application of a wooden block is useful when disruption of the branches of the DDFTs (III or IV) to a single digit are affected. A full-limb or half-limb cast may be indicated for injuries disrupting the flexor tendons to both digits of the same limb. Stall rest, use of a wooden block, and external coaptation of the limb result in healing of the tendon by second intention (fibroplasia) and scar tissue formation. Flexor tendon laceration located distal to the hock may be treated with application of a cast including the foot and extending to the level of the hock but not spanning the hock.[26,27] The fetlock may be flexed during casting to release tension from the tendons and allow closer apposition of the tendon ends. Alternatively, the limb may be cast in a normal, standing position. The authors recommend that the cast be maintained for 3 to 4 weeks longer than when a flexed-fetlock cast is used. The fetlock must be lightly padded on the dorsal and palmar/plantar aspect to protect the limb from pressure-induced cast sores (ulcerations). Laceration of the calcaneal tendon may be treated with application of a cast including the foot and extending to the proximal tibia (level of the tibial crest). The portion of the cast spanning the hock must be thicker than the remainder of the cast to prevent breakage of the cast at this point. Reinforcing splints may provide a stronger construct, and if used should be placed on the tension and compression sides of the limb. Thomas splints may be used to stabilize gastrocnemius muscle-tendon disruption, but in our experience the results have been poor. We prefer to use a full-limb cast when the disruption is close to the calcaneus.

Suture repair (tenorrhaphy) of transected tendons in addition to external coaptation achieves a more mature scar and a stronger scar-tendon unit more rapidly than does healing by second intention. The Superficial digital flexor tendon (SDP tendon), DDFT, and suspensory ligament (SL) divide distally in cattle to provide 1 main branch to each digit. The bodies of the tendons in the metacarpal and metatarsal regions are wide and thin and present a challenge for anchorage of tendon sutures. In our clinical experience, the 3-loop pulley suture pattern provides superior suture holding power in damaged flexor tendons of cattle. However, we have not observed a clinically significant advantage using tenorrhaphy and external coaptation compared with external coaptation alone. Subtle benefits of tenorrhaphy may not be observed in cattle because they are not required to perform maximal exercise. Nylon, polydioxanone and polyglyconate are the most common suture materials used for tendon repair. Note that no suture material, or any suture pattern currently in use, can provide adequate breaking strength to allow ambulation without external coaptation.

Cast immobilization has been advocated for a minimum of 4 to 5 weeks based on biomechanical studies of tendon healing and on clinical observations. Supportive farrier care has also been recommended after cast removal. At present, the authors recommend external coaptation be maintained for a minimum of 60 days after complete transection of flexor tendons. After cast removal, a block may be used to elevate the heel and stall confinement should be continued for 4 weeks after cast removal. Elevation of the heel in the range of 40° to 70° decreases tendon strain in the DDFT but not in the SDF tendon or the SL in horses. Heel elevation after cast removal is not required when a standing-conformation cast has been used.

The prognosis for tendon rupture in cattle is considered good for injuries involving the SDF tendon alone. In our experience, the prognosis for survival and for long-term productivity of cattle with traumatic rupture of the digital flexor tendons (SDF and/or DDF and/or SL) is fair to good. Ultrasonography examination of the healing tendon may provide valuable information regarding treatment and prognosis. The prognosis for production soundness after disruption of the extensor tendons is considered excellent.

TENOSYNOVITIS (TENOVAGINITIS)

Pathologic lesions occur most commonly in the digital flexor tendon sheath.[28] The digital flexor tendon sheath originates from a point 6 to 8 cm proximal to the fetlock and extends distally to a point immediately distal to the coronary band. The tendon sheath is confined on its palmar/plantar surface by the palmar/plantar annular ligament of the fetlock, the palmar/plantar digital annular ligament (distal to the accessory digits or dewclaw), and the distal interdigital ligaments (proximal to the heel bulbs). Inflammation of the digital tendon sheath should be suspected when focal swelling of the palmar/plantar aspect of the pastern is observed concurrent with focal swelling extending proximally from the level of the dewclaws.

Locomotion score of affected animals varies from 3 to 5 out of 5 depending of the origin. Two forms of tenosynovitis have been recognized in cattle: aseptic (traumatic, secondary synovitis, idiopathic) and septic (direct extension, iatrogenic, hematogenous). Adhesions between the tendon and tendon sheath may result from sustained trauma or inflammation. Restrictive adhesions may cause recurrent pain and lead to decreased productive soundness. The authors have successfully treated various cattle affected with aseptic tenosynovitis using nonsteroidal antiinflammatory drugs, warm-water hydrotherapy (30 minutes, 2–3 times per day for 10–14 days), tendon sheath drainage and lavage (1 L of 0.9% saline or lactated Ringer solution, once), pressure bandages (changed every 2 days for 7–10 days), and/or intrathecal sodium hyaluronate (20 mg, once).[29] Selection of treatment is based on severity, location of the involved tendon sheath, and economic constraints.

SEPTIC TENDON AND TENDON SHEATH

Septic tendinitis is most commonly associated with extension of deep digital sepsis from white line infection or subsolar abscess involving the DDF tendon.[30,31] Avulsion of the DDF from its insertion on the flexor tuberosity of the distal phalanx (P3) may result if sufficient necrosis of the tendon or underlying bone occurs. Septic tendinitis also may occur when degloving injuries involve the flexor or extensor tendons of the distal limbs. Degloving wounds are often associated with injury from wire fencing, farm machinery, metal siding on buildings, trailer accidents, and dog attacks (**Fig. 11**). Treatment includes thorough surgical debridement, lavage, daily wound management, and systemic antibiotic and antiinflammatory medication. Antibiotic selection should be based on results of microbial culture and sensitivity. In the authors' experience, *Trueperella pyogenes*, *Escherichia coli*, *Bacteroides* spp, and *Bacteriaceae* are the most commonly involved bacteria. For empiric therapy, gram-positive and anaerobic spectrum antibiotics are the treatments of choice when microbial cultures are not performed. If DDFT involvement is confined to a single digit, a wooden or rubber block (claw block) may be applied to the solar surface of the healthy digit to improve comfort and ambulation. The authors recommend that these animals be maintained in a restricted environment (stall or small pen) during convalescence (6–8 weeks). Also, the claw block should be removed before the animal is turned out to pasture to prevent damage to the tendons and ligaments of the healthy digit. Prognosis for septic tendinitis is good for superficial wounds. Deep wounds causing

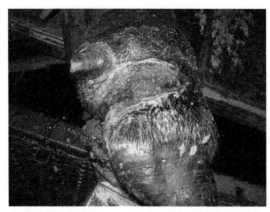

Fig. 11. Pastern laceration with extension into flexor tendon sheath resulting in septic tenosynovitis.

extensive tissue necrosis or sepsis of adjacent synovial cavities (joints, tendon sheaths) warrant a more guarded prognosis.

Septic tenosynovitis is most frequently diagnosed in the digital flexor tendon sheath but also commonly occurs in the tendon sheath of the extensor carpi radialis muscle. Sepsis of the tendon sheath typically occurs as a result of extension of local sepsis (such as with sole ulcer, a septic DIP joint, a septic navicular bursa or podotrochleosis, or a heel bulb abscess) or by direct inoculation (via penetrating wounds, foreign bodies, or iatrogenic trauma from farm implements such as a pitchfork or front-end loader).[30–32] Septic tenosynovitis caused by hematogenous translocation of bacteria (septicemia) is rare. Clinical signs include lameness (moderate weight bearing to non–weight bearing), recumbency, decreased milk production, and decreased feed intake. When standing, affected cattle may be reluctant to walk or may walk with the limb abducted or adducted to shift weight to the unaffected digit. Purulent effusion of the tendon sheath results in swelling proximal to the accessory digits (dewclaws). Swelling in the pastern region is limited by the annular ligament of the fetlock, the digital annular ligament, and the proximal interdigital ligaments. The lateral portion of the hind limb tendon sheath are more frequently affected. Diagnosis of septic tenosynovitis may include physical examination, synovial fluid collection for cytologic evaluation and culture, and radiography. Insertion of a blunt probe through the wound or injection of contrast material into the wound may facilitate diagnosis of septic tenosynovitis.

Treatment of septic tenosynovitis should include management of the inciting disease and of the infected tendon sheath. Each digital branch of the DDFT has its own tendon sheath, but the two sheaths communicate near their proximal extent. Septic tenosynovitis does not commonly occur in both tendon sheaths concurrently. The excessive fibrinous response to intrathecal sepsis, typical of cattle, may serve to localize infection to a single digital tendon sheath. Medical management alone (systemic antibiotics, hydrotherapy, protective bandages) is unlikely to be effective because of the severity of the inciting disease and the excessive fibrin deposition within the tendon sheath. This relationship was shown for septic arthritis in cattle when medical treatment successfully resolved the infection in 43% of affected cattle and surgical treatment resolved the infection in 73% of affected cattle.[33] Antibiotics cannot effectively penetrate fibrin foci to achieve therapeutic concentrations.[34]

Effective treatment of septic tenosynovitis involves surgical debridement and lavage of the affected tendon sheath (in valuable breeding animals) or digit amputation (in commercial cattle or cattle intended for salvage).

Several techniques may be used for surgical debridement, drainage, and lavage of the tendon sheath. Surgical exploration of the tendon sheath provides optimal access for thorough debridement of the tendon sheath and tendon. Exploration is performed by incising the sheath beginning at its origin proximal to the accessory digits and extending distally to a point approximately 2 cm proximal to the coronary band. After debridement and lavage of the sheath, the sheath may be closed primarily or an indwelling Penrose drain, exiting proximally and distally, may be used to facilitate drainage after surgery (**Fig. 12**). The Penrose drain is removed approximately 5 days after surgery and a bandage is maintained for an additional 5 days after the drain is removed. However, this technique is associated with extensive tissue damage and risk of injury to the neurovascular supply to the distal limb. Dehiscence of the surgical wound is another potential complication because of the high motion occurring in the palmar/plantar aspect of the fetlock. The authors do not recommend this technique for routine use. The tendon sheath is better left open if the tendons are necrotic and need to be resected.

In our experience, the treatment of choice for septic tenosynovitis without necrotic tendinitis in cattle is surgical implantation of an active lavage system using a multifenestrated silicone rubber drain (Snyder Hemovac, Zimmer, Dover, OH). This procedure is best performed with the animal sedated and restrained in lateral recumbency on a tilt table. Intravenous regional anesthesia (lidocaine 2%, 20 mL) is administered distal to a tourniquet before surgery. The authors routinely administer sodium or potassium penicillin (1 million units) distal to the tourniquet after the anesthetic has been instilled. Before surgery, a wooden block is applied to the healthy digit to improve comfort and ambulation during the convalescent period. A needle is inserted in the tendon sheath to verify correct location. A 14-gauge needle is inserted into the tendon sheath proximally and distally to guide optimal placement of the stab incisions. Then, limited debridement is performed through a stab incision placed into the proximal aspect of the tendon sheath and a second stab incision is placed into the distal tendon sheath. A large, curved forceps or clamp (Rochester-Carmalt forceps) is inserted from proximal to distal within the tendon sheath. The instrument is used to

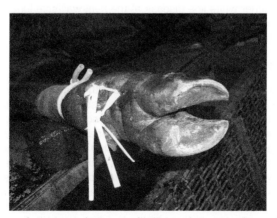

Fig. 12. Placement of Penrose drains to facilitate drainage after minimally invasive tenovaginotomy.

grasp the proximal tubing of the drain, and the drain is pulled through the tendon sheath. The drain is then sutured into place and the excess fenestrated portion of the drain is discarded. Drainage and lavage are performed by high-pressure infusion of sterile, isotonic electrolyte solutions into the drain and allowing the fluid to exit distally around the end of the drain. The authors use a 60-mL syringe and 3-way stop-cock to achieve high-pressure lavage. The distal end of the drain is sutured to occlude the lumen and force the fluids to exit the drain into the tendon sheath. The drain is su-tured to the skin proximally and distally and maintained under a sterile bandage be-tween flushings. High-pressure lavage is performed once daily for 5 to 7 days, using 1 to 2 L of saline or lactated Ringer solution. Crystalline antibiotic solutions may be instilled into the drain and tendon sheath after each lavage or when the drain is removed. Many veterinarians add antiseptic chemicals (such as povidone-iodine or chlorhexidine) to lavage fluids. However, research has shown that povidone-iodine (concentration >0.2%) and chlorhexidine (concentration >0.05%) induce significant synovitis[35–37] and may exacerbate intrathecal disease. No significant benefit was observed with use of 0.1% povidone-iodine solution based on bacterial cultures and histologic evaluation in in-vivo experimental models of septic arthritis in horses.

Optimally, the drain should be cultured at the time of removal and the results compared with initial microbial cultures. Systemic antibiotics and antiinflammatory medication are administered concurrently. A possible complication with this technique is ascending infection of the tendon sheath, and a limitation of this technique is the higher costs associated with placement of the lavage system and daily wound and bandage management. In our experience, a good to excellent prognosis for long-term productive soundness may be given with this technique.

Digit amputation proximal to the middle phalanx provides ventral drainage of puru-lent material and fibrin from the tendon sheath. Immediate relief from pain and swelling may be noted after surgery. Antibiotics should be administered for 7 to 10 days after surgery, but may be omitted if early salvage is performed. This treatment limits the productive longevity of the animal.

RETROARTICULAR AND BULBAR ABSCESSES

Lesions affecting the heel include retroarticular and bulbar abscesses, which are distinct different entities causing swelling and pain of the heel bulb, resulting in mod-erate to severe lameness. In most cases, both bulbar and retroarticular abscesses are complications of either white line disease at the heel/wall/sole junction, septic pedal osteitis resulting from sole ulcer in the axial region of the sole near the sole/heel junc-tion (Rusterholtz ulcer), or traumatic injury.[38,39]

BULBAR ABSCESS

In cases in which bulbar abscess is associated with white line disease or sole ulcer, separation of the horn of the abaxial wall or sole dissects caudally to cause infection in the heel retinaculum. The heel is swollen, painful, soft, fluctuant, and warm on palpa-tion. There may be a discharging tract at the coronary band in the region of the heel. Lameness is variable but affected animals are often only moderately lame.

Diagnosis is based on ultrasonography examination of the swollen heel bulb, which usually shows a walled-off cavity containing a heterogeneous fluid as seen with puru-lent exudates. The presence of puss on needle aspirate confirms a diagnosis of a bulbar abscess. Treatment consists of lancing the abscess through the caudal aspect of the heel bulb. Some skin adjacent to the incision should be removed in order to create an open cavity, which facilitates effective flushing and healing. In addition, all loose and undermined abaxial wall and sole horn should be trimmed. An orthopedic block to relieve weight is placed on the opposite claw. The abscess cavity should be cleaned and monitored for progressive healing, which occurs through the formation of a healthy, even granulation bed (**Fig. 13**).

RETROARTICULAR ABSCESS

Retroarticular abscess is typically located between distal aspect of P2, the DDFT, navicular bone, and the joint capsule of the DIP joint.[37,39] It results from an ascending infection caused by extension of infection from septic pedal osteitis caused by sole ulcer or white line disease.[39] Because of the close proximity of the retroarticular abscess with the DDFT, avulsion of the tendon from its insertion to the third phalanx may occur, resulting in hyperextension of the toe.[37,39] Swelling of the heel is usually firm, nonfluctuant, and painful, and may be confined to the heel or may spread up the digit to above the dewclaws, which is an indication that the digital flexor tendon sheath may be affected.[39] In such cases a fluctuant swelling is present above the dewclaws. In addition, the suppurative inflammation of the structures in the palmar/plantar aspect of the heel may or may not be associated with septic changes within the DIP joint. Animals with concurrent infection of the DIP joint are severely lame.[10]

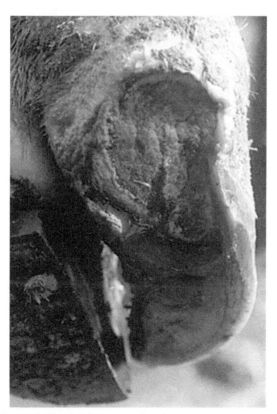

Fig. 13. Bulbar abscess following lancing and debridement. Healing with smooth, even granulation bed.

Diagnosis is based on clinical signs and the presence of an ascending tract, confirmed by insertion of a probe, into the deep structures of the heel after removal of loose and undermined horn associated with a sole ulcer or white line lesion (**Fig. 14**). On ultrasonography examination, a cavity with heterogeneous content can be visualized adjacent to the DDFT (**Fig. 15**) as well as fluid accumulation within the tendon sheath. Gas may be detected radiographically immediately caudal to the DIP joint.[37,39] In addition, changes within the DIP joint indicating septic arthritis, such as widening of the joint space with chondral and subchondral bone lysis, may be present. However, retroarticular abscessation is not consistently associated with septic changes of the DIP joint.

Treatment consists of surgical drainage, which is done as follows. After administration of local intravenous anesthesia, the affected digit is aseptically prepared for the surgical procedure. A blunt probe such as a teat cannula is passed into the sinus tract in order to determine both the depth and direction of the tract. A wedge-shaped incision is made from the proximal end of the probe to the level of the lesion (see **Fig. 2**). The incision is made to the level of the probe. Incised tissues include the skin, subcutaneous fibroelastic pad (retinaculum), and both the heel and the solar corium in cases of complicated sole ulcer, the digital cushion and the tendon sheath. Removal of a wedge of these tissues should expose the deep flexor tendon (which is often necrotic and avulsed), the navicular bursa, and navicular bone. The DDFT is resected at a level where the tendon appears normal but usually at the level where the annular ligament DDFT emerges through the ring made by the superficial digital flexor tendon.

Using a curette, the abscess cavity is debrided of remaining necrotic material taking care not to enter the DIP, PIP, or fetlock joints. The entire abscess capsule is removed down to the sole ulcer site. The navicular bone should be examined for signs of osteolysis and any necrotic bone removed. After completing the debridement, no cracks or crevices should remain that would retard or prevent healing from taking place because of persistent infection.

The tendon sheath should be flushed using a dilute povidone-iodine solution. The cavity is packed with gauze soaked in saline or a weak povidone-iodine solution and a pressure bandage is applied. The bandage is removed after 4 days and then at weekly intervals. Healing usually takes place over a 5-week to 6-week period. After healing is completed, the claw block on the sound claw should be removed. The affected claw will be functional but weight bearing could be limited to the heel and

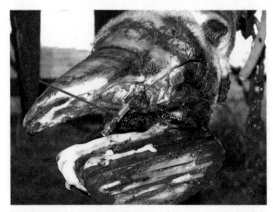

Fig. 14. Retroarticular abscess (OC/ABSCESS). Legend Teat cannula (*Solid red arrow*) Elliptical incision over heel bulb (*Broken red arrow*) DDFT.

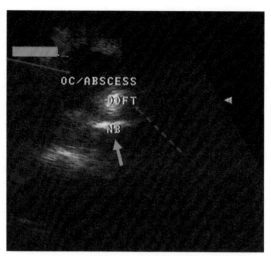

Fig. 15. Retroarticular abscess. Teat cannula (*solid red arrow*). Elliptical incision over heel bulb on DDFT (*broken red arrow*). Solid blue arrow indicates the navicular bone (NB).

heel-sole junction in some cases because of tipping of the claw resulting in shifting of the bearing surface toward the heel.[40]

ANTIBIOTIC AND ANTIINFLAMMATORY THERAPY

Treatment of cattle with antibiotic and/or antiinflammatory drugs must be instituted with consideration for potential drug efficacy, toxicity, and residues. Many drugs commonly used in food animal practice for treatment of musculoskeletal diseases are used in an extralabel manner. Veterinarians are compelled to follow strict guidelines (Animal Medicinal Drug Use Clarification Act, veterinarian-client-patient relationship) when electing to use extralabel drugs. Readers are referred to pharmacology texts and proper regulatory agencies for policies regarding the extralabel use of drugs and proper withdrawal times for meat and milk to avoid residue violations.

Optimally, selection of an appropriate antibiotic is based on in vitro microbial culture and sensitivity results. However, culturing bacteria from synovial fluid is often difficult. Therefore, empiric antibiotic selection may be elected when culture results are negative or because of economic constraints. When empiric therapy is chosen, antibiotic selection should be based on known, common pathogens involved in deep tissue sepsis in cattle and on antibiotics known to achieve adequate tissue distribution. Common pathogens isolated from septic musculoskeletal lesions in cattle include *T pyogenes*, *Streptococcus* spp, *Staphylococcus* spp, *Fusobacterium necrophorum*, *Bacteroides* spp, and coliforms.[41,42] In the authors' experience, the most common pathogens involved in septic arthritis and tenosynovitis in adult cattle are *T pyogenes* and *Escherichia coli*. In cattle with sepsis of the joints and/or bones of the distal limb, antimicrobial and antiinflammatory drug therapy is expected to require administration for periods of 10 to 14 days and occasionally up to 30 days.

The authors routinely use intra-articular or regional intravenous antibiotic infusions distal to a tourniquet as adjunct treatment of sepsis of deep tissues (eg, DIP joint sepsis, tenosynovitis, or septic cellulitis of the distal limb). This technique is used to achieve high concentrations of antibiotics in synovial spaces or peripheral tissues.

Crystalline antibiotic solutions may be infused immediately after performing local intravenous regional anesthesia. Limited scientific research is available on this practice in veterinary medicine. Intravenous administration of antimicrobial drugs distal to a tourniquet can achieve greater concentrations of drug in the target tissues if the tourniquet is maintained for a sufficient period of time for diffusion to occur.[43] The authors maintain the tourniquet in place for a minimum of 30 to 45 minutes after antibiotic infusion.

SUMMARY

With a thorough knowledge of the anatomy of the foot, and basic surgical instruments, digit surgery can be performed in field situations. Sepsis of the DIP and PIP joints should be treated surgically because conservative treatment is often ineffective. Most of the diseases described in this article are chronic and the animals often have been suffering for some time. Perioperative analgesia is important to alleviate the pain of those animals. All those procedures should be performed under local or regional anesthesia.

REFERENCES

1. Desrochers A, Anderson DE. Anatomy of the distal limb. Vet Clin North Am Food Anim Pract 2001;17:25–38.
2. Budras K-D, Habel RE. Bovine anatomy. 1st edition. Hannover (Germany): Schlütersche; 2003. p. 138.
3. Fiedler A, Maierl J, Nuss K. Erkrankungen der Klauen und Zehen des Rindes. 1st edition. Stuttgart (Germany): Schattauer; 2004. p. 216.
4. Heppelmann M, Rehage J, Kofler J, et al. Ultrasonographic diagnosis of septic arthritis of the distal interphalangeal joint in cattle. Vet J 2007;179(3):407–16.
5. Greenough PR, Ferguson JG. Alternatives to amputation. Vet Clin North Am Food Anim Pract 1985;1(1):195–203.
6. Pejsa TG, St Jean G, Hoffsis GF, et al. Digit amputation in cattle: 85 cases (1971-1990). J Am Vet Med Assoc 1993;202:981–4.
7. Desrochers A, St Jean G. Surgical management of digit disorders in cattle. Vet Clin North Am Food Anim Pract 1996;12:277–98.
8. Funk K. Late results of digit amputation in cattle. Berl Munch Tierarztl Wochenschrift 1977;90:152–6.
9. Starke A. Resection of the distal interphalangeal joint and digital amputation in 21 breeding bulls-outcome and long term follow-up. Nice (France): World Buiatric Congress; 2006.
10. Starke A, Heppelmann M, Beyerbach M, et al. Septic arthritis of the distal interphalangeal joint in cattle: comparison of digital amputation and joint resection by solar approach. Vet Surg 2007;36:350–9.
11. Bicalho RC, Cheong SH, Warnick LD, et al. The effect of digit amputation or arthrodesis surgery on culling and milk production in Holstein dairy cows. J Dairy Sci 2006;89:2596–602.
12. van Amstel SR, Shearer JK. Manual for treatment and control of lameness in cattle. 1st edition. Ames (IA): Blackwell Publishing; 2006. p. 212.
13. Nuss K. Surgery of the bovine digit. In: Anderson DE, Rings DM, editors. Current veterinary therapy 5, food animal practice. St Louis (MO): Saunders Elsevier; 2009. p. 242–61.
14. Clemente CH. Contribution to the development of tendon resection and pedal joint resection in cattle. Tierärztl Umsch 1965;20:108.

15. Bicalho RC, Cheong SH, Guard CL. Field technique for the resection of the distal interphalangeal joint and proximal resection of the deep digital flexor tendon in cows. Vet Rec 2007;160:435–9.
16. Mulon PY, Babkine M, d'Anjou MA, et al. Degenerative disease of the distal interphalangeal joint and sesamoid bone in calves: 9 cases (1995-2004). J Am Vet Med Assoc 2009;234(6):794-9.
17. Zulauf M, Jordan P, Steiner A. Fenestration of the abaxial hoof wall and implantation of gentamicin-impregnated collagen sponges for the treatment of septic arthritis of the distal interphalangeal joint in cattle. Vet Rec 2001;149:516–8.
18. Kofler J. Septic arthritis of the proximal interphalangeal (pastern) joint in cattle - clinical, radiographic, ultrasonographic findings and treatment. Berliner und Münchener tierärztliche Wochenschrift 1995;108:281–9.
19. Kofler J. Clinical study of toe ulcer and necrosis of the apex of the distal phalanx in 53 cattle. Vet J 1999;157:139–47.
20. Choquette-Levy L, Baril I, Levy M, et al. A study of foot disease of dairy cattle in Quebec. Can Vet J 1985;26:278–81.
21. Wells SJ, Trent AM, Marsh WE, et al. Prevalence and severity of lameness in lactating dairy cows in a sample of Minnesota and Wisconsin herds. J Am Vet Med Assoc 1993;02:78–82.
22. Whitaker DA, Kelly JM, Smith EJ. Incidence of lameness in dairy cows. Vet Rec 1983;13:60–2.
23. Russell AM, Rowlands GJ, Shaw SR, et al. Survey of lameness in British dairy cattle. Vet Rec 1982;111:155–60.
24. Arkins S. Lameness in dairy cows. Irish Vet J 1981;35:135–40.
25. Anderson DE, St-Jean G, Morin DE, et al. Traumatic flexor tendon injuries in 27 cattle. Vet Surg 1996;25(4):320–6.
26. Wilson DC, Vanderby R. An evaluation of six synthetic casting materials: strength of cylinders in bending. Vet Surg 1995;24:55–9.
27. Wilson DC, Vanderby R. An evaluation of fiberglass application techniques. Vet Surg 1995;24:118–21.
28. Anderson DE, St Jean G. Diagnosis and management of tendon disorders in cattle. Vet Clin North Am Food Anim Pract 1996;12(1):85–116.
29. Gaughan EM, Nixon AI, Krook LP, et al. Effects of sodium hyaluronate on tendon healing and adhesion formation in horses. Am J Vet Res 1991;52:764–73.
30. Greenough PR, MacCallum FJ, Weaver AD. Infectious diseases of deep structures. In: Greenough PR, MacCallum FJ, Weaver AD, editors. Lameness in cattle. Philadelphia: Lippincott; 1981. p. 176–96.
31. Greenough PR. Observations on some of the diseases of the bovine foot, part II. Vet Rec 1962;74:53–63.
32. Greenough PR, MacCallum FJ, Weaver AD. Diseases of muscles. In: Greenough PR, MacCallum FJ, Weaver AD, editors. Lameness in cattle. Philadelphia: Lippincott; 1981. p. 363–73.
33. Tulleners EP. Management of bovine orthopedic problems, part II: coxofemoral luxation, soft tissue problems, sepsis, and miscellaneous skull problems. Compend Cont Educ Pract Vet 1986;8:5117–23.
34. Barza M, Weinstein L. Penetration of antibiotics into fibrin loci in vivo, I: comparison of penetration of ampicillin into fibrin clots, abscesses, and interstitial fluid. J Infect Dis 1974;129:59–65.
35. Bertone AL, McIlwraith CW, Powers BE, et al. Effect of four antimicrobial lavage solutions on the tarsocrural joint of horses. Vet Surg 1986;15:305–15.

36. Wilson DC, Cooley AJ, MacWilliams PS, et al. Effects of 0.05 % chlorhexidine lavage on the tarsocrural joints of horses. Vet Surg 1994;23:442–7.

37. Smith JA, Williams RJ, Knight AP. Drug therapy for arthritis in food-producing animals. Compend Contin Educ Pract Vet 1989;11:87–94.

38. Greenough PR. Septic pododermatitis. An illustrated compendium of bovine lameness: Part 3. Mod Vet Pract Food Anim 1887;148–52.

39. Greenough PR, Ferguson JG. Alternatives to amputation. Symposium on bovine lameness and orthopedics. Vet Clin North America Food Anim Pract 1985;1(1): 195–203.

40. Heppelmann M, Kofler J, Meyer H, et al. Advances in surgical treatment of septic arthritis of the distal interphalangeal joint in cattle: a review. Vet J 2009;182: 162–75.

41. Walker RD, Richardson DC, Bryant MJ, et al. Anaerobic bacteria associated with osteomyelitis m domestic animals. J Am Vet Med Assoc 1983;182:814–6.

42. Bengtsson B, Franklin A, Luthman I, et al. Concentrations of sulphadimidine, oxytetracycline and penicillin G in serum, synovial fluid and tissue cage fluid after parenteral administration to calves. J Vet Pharmacol Ther 1989;12: 37–45.

43. Gagnon H, Ferguson JG, Papich MG, et al. Single-dose pharmacokinetics of cefazolin in bovine synovial fluid after intravenous regional injection. J Vet Pharmacol Ther 1994;17:31–7.

Corkscrew Claw

Sarel R. van Amstel, BVSc, MMedVet

KEYWORDS

- Cattle • Abnormal horn growth • Abnormal claw conformation • Genetic
- Environmental pathogenesis • Corrective trimming

KEY POINTS

- Corkscrew claw (CSC) is a conformational defect mainly seen in the outer claw of rear legs, and it is common in both beef and dairy cattle of different breeds.
- Most of the typical phenotypic changes of CSC may have both genetic and environmental components to a greater or lesser extent.
- This condition results in either expression at an early age (genetic type) or later age (environmental/acquired type).
- Heritability scores can be greatly influenced by environmental factors, particularly nutrition and body weight. This effect occurs particularly in beef cattle, in which there seems to be a high correlation between lameness and phenotypic changes associated with CSC.
- Ideal claw conformation should include a short toe; have a good width, indicating a wide bearing surface; have a steep angle of 50° to 55° for front and 45° to 50° for rear feet; have high heels; and both claws on the same leg should be the same size.

DESCRIPTION AND CLINICAL PRESENTATION

Corkscrew claw (CSC) is a well-known and common condition first reported during the 1950s in Dutch black and white cattle.[1,2] Early reports described CSC as a conformational abnormality of the digit and claws of the back leg, and it is still recognized as such.[1,2] The condition occurs primarily in the outer claw of the back leg, involving both outer claws in most cases but other claws may also be involved.[1,2] The affected outer claws are longer and narrower than the medial claw and have an inward and upward spiral rotation of the toe (**Fig. 1**). Similarly, the bearing surface of the wall, particularly at the heel and sole, is displaced inward. The animal starts to bear weight on the outer (abaxial) wall surface, particularly the caudal segment (**Fig. 2**), and the sole may become completely non–weight bearing. The inside (axial) wall is displaced dorsomedially and a fold develops in the wall.[1,2]

Other conformational defects that resemble CSC that have been reported include hooked claws in Aberdeen Angus; rolled claws in Simmental; and slipper and scissor

Department of Large Animal Clinical Studies, College of Veterinary Medicine, The University of Tennessee, 2407 River Drive, Knoxville, TN 37996, USA
E-mail address: svanamst@utk.edu

Vet Clin Food Anim 33 (2017) 351–364
http://dx.doi.org/10.1016/j.cvfa.2017.02.010
0749-0720/17/© 2017 Elsevier Inc. All rights reserved.

vetfood.theclinics.com

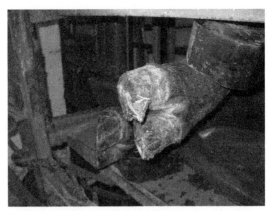

Fig. 1. CSC with spiral-shaped inward and upward rotation of the toe.

claw, which can be seen in any breed with chronic laminitis.[3] Slipper claw is usually longer than normal, the dorsal surface concave, and the horn has a dull flaky appearance.[4] Another conformational abnormality that can resemble CSC is abaxial rotation of the medial claw of the back leg, seen in heifers.[5] True screw claw is reported to be distinguishable from these abnormalities by a bony swelling present above the abaxial coronary band (**Fig. 3**).[3]

Other reported changes and signs associated with CSC (**Table 1**) that have been reported include physical and anatomic changes.

Physical

- Accelerated growth/overgrowth resulting from hyperplasia of the abaxial wall following development of a palpable periarticular exostosis incorporating the abaxial collateral ligament of the distal interphalangeal joint[3] (see **Fig. 3**).
- Sole hemorrhage.
- Separation at the non–weight-bearing part of the white line in zones 1 and 2 at the toe, which may predispose to toe abscess with pedal osteitis and pathologic fracture of the apex of the third phalanx.[6,7]
- Separation of the white line in zone 3.
- Sole ulcer in the axial part of zone 4.[7]

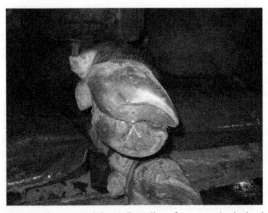

Fig. 2. Weight bearing on the outer (abaxial) wall surface, particularly the caudal segment.

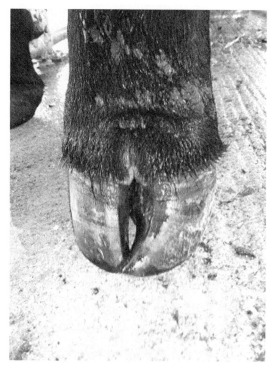

Fig. 3. Bony swelling at the abaxial coronary band.

Anatomic

- Increased blood supply to the affected claw.[8]
- The third phalanx may be abnormally long and narrow with an abaxial to axial curve[7] (**Fig. 4**).
- A deep groove has been shown to develop on the inside of the claw capsule adjacent to the white line.[7] This groove results in the sole being thinner adjacent to abaxial zones 1 and 2 of the white line.
- The dorsoplantar plane of the distal interphalangeal joint may be rotated by as much as 11°.[9]

Clinically affected animals may have a painful gait with a shortened stride or be overtly lame. The animal may have a cow-hocked stance in an attempt to displace more weight on the medial claws.[9] Animals are reluctant to move, and lose weight. Overgrowth of the affected CSC may be so severe that the medial claw can become almost non–weight bearing[7] (**Fig. 5**).

INCIDENCE AND PREVALENCE

The incidence of CSC is variable and may be influenced by differences in nutrition, management, and genetics.[10] One study involving 592 Holstein dairy cows reported an incidence of 15.7%.[11] In another study lameness associated with CSC was attributed to 18.2% of 432 lame animals.[4] In 2 studies in large herds, one evaluated claw disorders in 66 dairy herds with 2709 dry or lactating dairy cows and reported a CSC prevalence of 24.2%,[12] whereas the other reported a prevalence of 10% in 41,087 cows.[13]

Table 1
Conformation and anatomic changes reported in association with corkscrew claw and possible pathogenesis

Conformation/Anatomic Change	Possible Pathogenesis
Shallow toe angle; low heels; small claw; long, narrow claw	Genetically driven developmental changes (low heritability)
Abnormal angle of distal interphalangeal joint articular surface	Shallow toe angle; low heels; small claw; long, narrow claw plus weight bearing/body weight/walking surface
Exostosis (periosteal reaction/new bone formation) on distal phalanx	Trauma and strain on supporting structures at the level of the distal interphalangeal joint
Dilated tortuous digital artery with an increased arterial network resulting in increased vascular supply in the affected claw	Neovascularization commonly associated with laminitis Associated with development of exostosis
Overgrowth	Biomechanics of weight bearing Abaxial wall becomes part of weight bearing surface Increased blood supply
Sole hemorrhage	Overgrowth
White line disease zone 3	Overgrowth/weight bearing Dyskeratotic horn caused by laminitis
White line disease zones 1 and 2 at toe	Disintegration caused by being non–weight bearing Dyskeratotic horn caused by laminitis
Pedal osteitis ± pathologic fracture	Infection entering through white line at the toe
Sole ulcer zone 4	Overgrowth. Increased concussion Failure of caudal suspensory system of P3

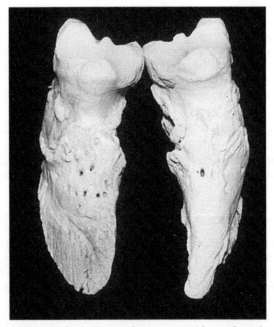

Fig. 4. The third phalanx may be longer and narrower with an abaxial to axial curve.

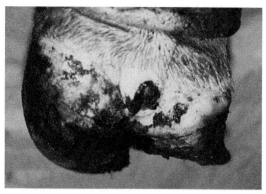

Fig. 5. Overgrowth can become so severe that the medial claw can become almost non–weight bearing.

PATHOGENESIS

The classification and proposed pathogenesis of CSC are shown in **Figs. 6** and **7** and **Table 1**. Several factors may play a role in the development of CSC.

Breed

CSC has been observed and/or reported in both beef and dairy cattle of different breeds, primarily Holstein,[3] both black and red Aberdeen Angus, Norwegian and Swedish Red cattle, Ayrshire, Finncattle, and Brown Swiss.[10,12,13] It has also been observed in the Bonsmara breed, which is one of the main beef breeds in South Africa (Dr Tony Shakespeare, University of Pretoria, South Africa, unpublished data). Note that CSC has not been observed with immobilization of more than 500 free-ranging or captive Cape buffalo (Dr Tony Shakespeare, University of Pretoria, South Africa, unpublished observations, 2012). Breed differences in the prevalence of CSC may be related to body weight, claw shape, and horn quality.[2,13]

Age

The first published reports described the condition in cattle as early as 1 year of age. Later reports mentioned 3.5 to 5 years as the age when the condition is generally first

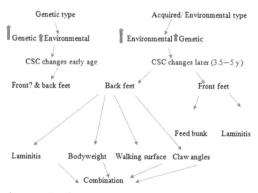

Fig. 6. Proposed pathogenesis of CSC.

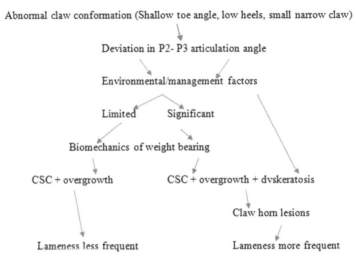

Abnormal claw conformation (Shallow toe angle, low heels, small narrow claw)

Deviation in P2- P3 articulation angle

Environmental/management factors

Limited   Significant

Biomechanics of weight bearing

CSC + overgrowth   CSC + overgrowth + dyskeratosis

Claw horn lesions

Lameness less frequent   Lameness more frequent

Fig. 7. The development of CSC.

noticed.[3,14] This age seems to imply that conformational changes associated with CSC could be primarily genetically driven if seen at a young age, whereas, if these changes develop in older cattle, they are more likely to have a larger environmental component.

Genetics

CSC has generally been regarded as a genetically heritable conformational defect, although scientific evidence to support this theory is lacking.[3] The genetic basis for this condition was partly based on research done during the 1950s on a small number of cases, which found that the angle of the articular surface of the third phalanx was statistically different when CSC was compared with the opposite normal claw.[9] It is also not clear whether this change in conformation is primarily from a genetic origin or secondary, caused by other factors.[3] Evidence that may support a possible genetic basis is that CSC has been reported to occur in cow families and in the offspring of certain bulls.[2] In addition, CSC seems to occur in association with certain heritable phenotypic traits, including a small toe angle; low heels; and long, narrow claws.[2] However, CSC heritability is generally low and is estimated to be 0.05, implying that environmental factors such as housing, lactation number, season, claw trimming, age, and body weight play important roles in the development of the phenotypic changes in CSC.[10,13,15]

Nutrition

CSC is reported to be highly correlated with laminitis and is considered to be a feed-related disease.[10,15] Claw horn changes consistent with those found in chronic laminitis are commonly seen with CSC, including multiple horizontal grooves (**Fig. 8**); vertical wall cracks; poor-quality, rough, and flaky horn; widening and discoloration of the horn of the white line; cranial rotation of the third phalanx; P3 fracture; sole ulcer in the axial part of zone 4; and white line disease[2] (S van Amstel, University of Tennessee, unpublished observations, 2016).

Some of the changes that have been regarded as being typical of CSC, such as remodeling of bone (exostosis formation) and increased vascular supply to the

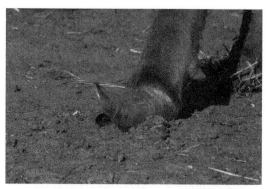

Fig. 8. CSC is highly correlated with laminitis. Note multiple horizontal grooves and poor-quality horn.

claw, have also been linked with laminitis.[7] In addition, deviation in horn growth, such as that of the abaxial wall, is also commonly seen with laminitis.[7]

Growth Rates, Weight Distribution, and Claw Angles

Growth rates of claws under fixed environmental and housing conditions are different between and within claws in the same animal.[16] This study showed that the caudal segment of the abaxial wall grew on average 40% faster than the cranial segment.[16] The same study also showed that growth rates of the caudal segment of the abaxial wall of animals with CSC were faster than those of normal claws.[16] High horn production leads to incomplete keratinization, thus producing a softer horn.[17] In addition, the abaxial white line is at its widest where it ends at the wall/heel junction and does not have a strong tubular structure, which normally provides structural strength to horn.[17] These factors could potentially predispose the abaxial segment of the wall to deviate with weight bearing, particularly in the presence of other factors, such as high body weight, hard walking surfaces, and laminitis. Laminitic horn grows fast; has a high moisture content; and keratinization within horn cells is reduced, resulting in soft, flexible horn that is more predisposed to an abaxial to axial deviation in horn growth.[16]

Another factor that may influence the development of CSC is weight distribution within the claw. There is a correlation between toe angle and heel height and weight distribution within the claw.[18] A shallow toe angle correlates with low heels, resulting in redistribution of weight bearing more toward the heel.[18] This condition may predispose to axial deviation of the outside wall, particularly the outer claw of the back foot because it bears more weight during both standing and walking relative to the inside claw.[2,19,20] This increased load bearing results in activation of mechanoreceptors with the production of epidermal growth factor, resulting in accelerated growth.[19] Animals with small and longer, narrower claws are reported to be more likely to develop CSC[2,5] (**Fig. 9**).

Other Management Factors

Walking surface

Confinement on concrete or similar hard surfaces increases the load bearing on the outer claw.[21] This load bearing can be further compounded in heavy and overconditioned animals, which may predispose to changes in claw shape.[22] Out of 73 overconditioned young bulls (<3 years of age) undergoing routine trimming in preparation for a

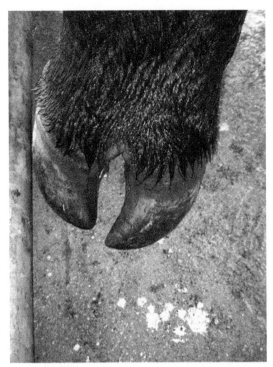

Fig. 9. Longer, small, and narrower claws are more likely to develop CSCs.

sale from a large farming operation, 35 showed typical signs of screw claw (medical records, College of Veterinary Medicine, University of Tennessee).

Feed bunk height

Bunk height has been regarded as a risk factor for development of conformation changes consistent with CSC of the medial claws of the front feet.[18,20] Unpublished data (Matthijis Schouten, University of Florida) showed that weight bearing was displaced toward the outer claw when cows were fed from a feed bunk. This finding supports bunk feeding as a risk factor for the development of CSC in the medial claw of the front legs caused by postural and weight-bearing changes. However, another study, which used pressure mats when cows were fed from a feed bunk, found no difference in the force distribution between medial and lateral claws of the front legs.[23]

Sand bedding

Unpublished data suggest that sand bedding, very soft rubber on walk ways, or other mattress materials in free stalls may be associated with the development of CSC of the medial claw (Tomlinson D, Dairy Cattle Council Meeting, Columbus, OH, 2016).

TREATMENT OF CORKSCREW CLAW
Corrective Trimming

1. The toe length of both claws is reduced by removing overgrown wall at the toe ending just on the inside of the white line (**Fig. 10**). Because of the rotation of the toe the white line at the toe is generally non–weight bearing and may even be perpendicular to the bearing surface.

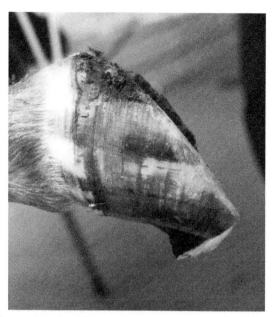

Fig. 10. Reduce the toe length of both claws to just on the inside of the white line.

2. Next the dorsal wall of the CSC is straightened to create a straight surface from the coronary band to the bearing surface (**Figs. 11** and **12**). However, watch for any hemorrhage and stop when bleeding occurs.
3. Reevaluate toe length; further reduction of the toe length may be indicated.
4. Next, reduce the overgrowth of the bearing surface, including the heel of the CSC, which in this case consists primarily of the deviated abaxial wall (see **Fig. 2**). The aim is to balance the bearing surface of the wall and the heel of the CSC with that of the opposite untrimmed claw (**Fig. 13**). However, care should be taken not to over trim the CSC because this may result in an excessively soft heel that

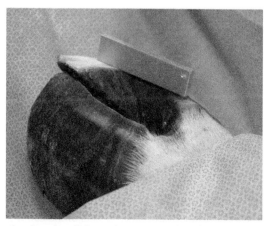

Fig. 11. Straighten the dorsal wall from the coronary band to the bearing surface.

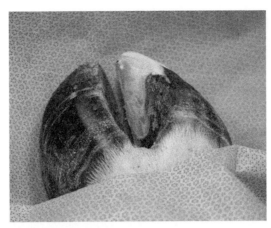

Fig. 12. Remove the curvature of the axial wall at the toe.

may be prone to bruising and/or exposure of the corium in zones 1 and 2 because of angulation of P3 with thinning of the sole (**Fig. 14**).
5. Slope the overgrown sole at the interdigital space (**Fig. 15**). In addition, remove the curve in the axial wall. The trimmed CSC is left with a narrow weight-bearing surface.
6. Trimming of the opposite claw to create a stable weight-bearing surface in that claw depends on the amount of horn removed on the bearing surface of the CSC (**Fig. 16**).
7. Further removal of loose or undermined horn may be necessary if other claw horn lesions are present, such as sole ulcer or white line disease.

Repeat trimming of CSC is done as needed but in some cases may have to be done up to 3 times per year.

SUMMARY

Most of the typical phenotypic changes of CSC may have both genetic and environmental components to a greater or lesser extent, which results in either expression at an early age (genetic type) or later age (environmental/acquired type). Heritability

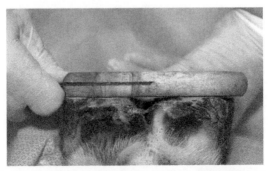

Fig. 13. Balance the bearing surface of the wall and heel of the CSC with that of the opposite untrimmed claw.

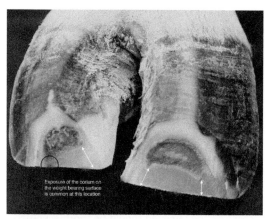

Fig. 14. The sole of the CSC is thinner adjacent to the white line in zones 1 and 2.

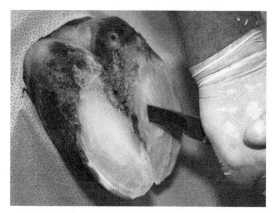

Fig. 15. Slope the overgrown sole at the interdigital space bearing surface.

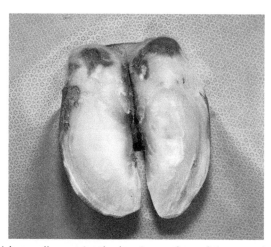

Fig. 16. If sole thickness allows, trim the bearing surface of the opposite claw to balance that of the CSC.

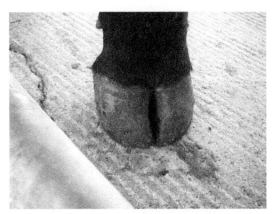

Fig. 17. Toes of both claws on the same leg should be short, even-sized, each with a good width.

of conformation traits, such as claw angles, that predispose to CSC is low and the genetic correlations between claw conformation and lesions is also low to moderate.[24] Despite this, sufficient genetic variation exists, as shown by large variability in sire estimated breeding value, for long-term genetic improvement through direct selection.[24] One study found the mean predictive correlation of genomic breeding values for CSC to be 0.29.[25]

However, heritability scores can be greatly influenced by environmental factors, particularly nutrition and body weight. This finding is particularly true in beef cattle, in which there seems to be a high correlation between lameness and phenotypic changes associated with CSC. Such claws usually also have signs of chronic laminitis.

Ideal claw conformation should include a short toe; have a good width, indicating a wide bearing surface; have a steep angle of 50° to 55° for front and 45° to 50° for rear feet; have high heels; and both claws on the same leg should be even-sized (**Fig. 17**).

It is reported that a visual scoring system of claws was reliable enough to rank progeny tested bulls with 70% or greater accuracy compared with actual measurements when based on 90 or more progenies.[26]

CONCLUSION

Environmental factors such as nutrition, body weight, and walking surface can have a major effect on claw horn growth and development.

These effects are exacerbated in the presence of preexisting conformational abnormalities such as claw size and length and claw angles.

A combination of these factors predisposes to the development of typical claw horn changes associated with CSC.

It is not recommended to include such animals in breeding herds because of negative effects on production and longevity.

REFERENCES

1. Bouckaert J. Lameness in cattle. Some diseases of the bovine foot – Tendon retraction in calves - Spastic paralysis. From Chirurgische Kliniek voor Grote Huisdieren van de Rijks-universiteit te Gent. Nord Vet Med 1964;(1):225–39.
2. Van Schaik P. Een veel voorkomend klauwgebrek bij ons zwartbonte rundvee. Tijdschr Dieregeneesk 1960; deel85:afl11659–l11663.

3. Greenough PR. Sand cracks, horizontal fissures, and other conditions affecting the wall of the bovine claw. Vet Clin North Am Food Anim Pract 2001;17(1): 93–110.

4. Gogoi SN, Nigam JM, Singh AP, et al. Incidence of foot disorders in cattle. Mod Vet Pract 1981;62(12):941–5.

5. Pijl R. Rotation of the medial claw in young heifers. Proceedings of the 10th International Symposium on Lameness in Ruminants, Lucerne, Switzerland, 1998. p. 18–9.

6. Shearer JK, van Amstel SR. Toe lesions in dairy cattle. Proceedings of the 46th Florida Dairy Production Conference, Gainesville, 2009. p. 47–55.

7. Van Amstel SR, Shearer JK. Application of functional trimming procedures to corkscrew claws. In: Manual for the Treatment and Control of Lameness in Cattle. Ames (IA): Blackwell Publishing Professional; 2006. p. 62–71.

8. Gogoi SN, Nigam JM, Singh AP. Angiographic evaluation of bovine foot abnormalities. Vet Radiol 1982;23(4):171–4.

9. Bouckaert J, Oyaert W, Deloddere F. De Kurketrekker Klauw. Vlaams Dieregeneeskundig Tijdschrift 1958;27(6):149–52.

10. Johansson H. Genotype by environment interactions of claw health in Swedish dairy cattle in tie-stalls and loose-housing. Degree project in animal science. Uppsala (Sweden): Swedish University of Agricultural Sciences, Faculty of Veterinary Medicine and Animal Science, Department of Animal Breeding and Genetics; 2012. p. 1–50.

11. Valencia GL, Renteria Evangelista TB, Jorquera AP, et al. Frequency and distribution of pathologies associated with lameness problems in commercial dairy herds in Baja California, Mexico. J Anim Vet Adv 2006;5(7):593–7.

12. Fjeldaas T, Sogstad AM, Osteras O. Locomotion and claw disorders in Norwegian dairy cows housed in freestalls with slatted concrete, solid concrete, or solid rubber flooring in alleys. J Dairy Sci 2011;94:1243–55.

13. Liinamo AE, Laakso M, Ojala M. Environmental and genetic effects on claw disorders in Finnish dairy cattle. In: Klopcic M, Reens R, Philipsson A, et al, editors. Breeding for robustness in cattle, vol. 126. Helsinki (Finland): EAAP publication; 2009. p. 169–79.

14. Greenough PR. An illustrated compendium of bovine lameness. Part 4. Corkscrew claw. Mod Vet Pract 1987; 216–20.

15. Huang YC, Shanks RD, McCoy GC. Evaluation of fixed factors affecting hoof health. Livestock Prod Sci 1995;44:115–24.

16. Prentice DE. Growth and wear rates of hoof horn in Ayrshire cattle. Res Vet Sci 1973;14:285–90.

17. Buydras KD, Horowitz A, Mulling CH. Rate of keratinization of the wall segment of the hoof and its relation to width and structure of the zona alba (white line) with respect to claw disease in cattle. Am J Vet Res 1996;57(4):444–55.

18. Toussaint RE. Trimming. Chapter 3. In: Toussaint Raven E, editor. Cattle foot care and claw trimming. Ipswich (United Kingdom): Farming Press; 1989. p. 75–94.

19. Van der Tol PP, Metz JH, Noordhuizen-Stassen EN, et al. The vertical ground reaction force and the pressure distribution on the claws of dairy cows while walking on a flat substrate. J Dairy Sci 2003;86:2875–83.

20. Van Amstel SR, Shearer JK. Application of functional trimming procedures to corkscrew claws. In: Manual for the Treatment and Control of Lameness in Cattle. Ames (IA): Blackwell Publishing Professional; 2006. p. 62–71.

21. Buda S, Mulling Ch. Innervation of the bovine hoof. International Symposium on Disorders of the Ruminant Digit & International Conference on Bovine Lameness, Parma, Italy, 2000. p. 100–101.
22. Somers JG, Schouten WG, Frankena K, et al. Development of claw traits and claw lesions in dairy cows kept on different floor systems. J Dairy Sci 2005;88:110–20.
23. Carvalho VCD, De Souza SRL, Venturi P, et al. Feed bunk height impact on dairy cow's front claws. BioEng. Campinas, Brazil 2009;3(1):1–8.
24. Chapinal N, Koeck A, Sewalem A, et al. Genetic parameters for hoof lesions and their relationship with feet and leg traits in Canadian Holstein cows. J Dairy Sci 2013;96:2596–604.
25. Odegard C, Svendsen M, Heringstsd B. Predictive ability of genomic breeding values for corkscrew claw in Norwegian red. Proceedings, 10th World Congress of Genetics Applied to Livestock Production. 2014.
26. Vermunt JJ, Greenough PR. Structural characteristics of the bovine claw: horn growth and wear, horn hardness and claw conformation. Br Vet J 1995;151: 157–79.

A Review of the Relationship Between Hoof Trimming and Dairy Cattle Welfare

CrossMark

Grant C. Stoddard, BS[a],*, Gerard Cramer, DVM, DVSc[b]

KEYWORDS

- Hoof trimming • Claw trimming • Dairy cattle • Welfare

KEY POINTS

- The evidence to support a specific hoof trimming (HT) technique is limited.
- The HT process creates a physiologic and behavioral response, but it is unclear if this is due to the removal of horn, the restraint, or change in a cow's time budget.
- More frequent HT seems to reduce lameness and hoof lesions in specific environmental conditions.
- There is a need for appropriately designed research on the appropriate technique, timing, and frequency of HT.
- Future HT studies should provide a clear description of the HT technique used.

INTRODUCTION

Lameness is an important concern for the dairy industry because of its high prevalence and the effect it has on the productivity and well-being of the animal. Worldwide estimates of lameness prevalence have varied from 20% to 55%.[1–3] Furthermore, the prevalence of hoof lesions at the time of HT has been shown to be even higher.[4–7] The effects of lameness results in a significant economic cost to producers and is estimated to range from $100 to $220 per cow.[8] These costs include decreases in milk production,[9–11] reproductive performance,[12–14] and increased culling.[14,15] Lameness also causes changes in behavior[16–18] as part of a pain response.[19,20]

Disclosure Statement: The authors have received funding from: AABP-HTA hoof health research funding opportunity, RK Anderson Fellowship, Rapid Agricultural Response Fund, established by the Minnesota Legislature and administered by the University of Minnesota, and Agricultural Experiment Station.

[a] Veterinary Population Medicine Department, University of Minnesota, 225 VMC, 1365 Gortner Avenue, St Paul, MN 55108, USA; [b] Dairy Production Medicine, Veterinary Population Medicine Department, University of Minnesota, 225 VMC, 1365 Gortner Avenue, St Paul, MN 55108, USA
* Corresponding author.
E-mail address: stodd038@umn.edu

Despite all the negative effects lameness has on the animal and the dairy industry, there has been limited research on evaluating preventative practices in clinical trials.[21] A variety of risk factors have been identified in observational studies[1,4,5] as potential targets for interventions. One commonly recommended practice is HT.[22] HT is a common practice in the US dairy industry with approximately 85% of herds HT a percentage of their herd at least once a year.[23]

HT is thought to prevent lameness by restoring a more upright foot angle by shortening dorsal wall length and excessive thickness of the sole at the toe, thereby distributing weight more evenly within the weight-bearing surface of each claw and balancing weight bearing between the 2 claws.[24] Several different HT techniques have been described in the peer reviewed literature,[25–28] text books,[22,24,29,30] or at HT conferences.[31,32] HT techniques can be split into categories based on how the technique leaves the angle of the sole relative to the metatarsals. A majority of methods[22,24,26,30] advocate a flat sole whereby the abaxial and axial walls are trimmed to be level and perpendicular to the axis of the metatarsals. The differences that exist between the flat HT methods are mainly procedural. This method advocated originally by Raven[24] focuses on using specific measurement to achieve proper dorsal wall length and toe thickness. Other methods prefer to use hoof angle[26] or sole reading methods[30] to achieve appropriate length and thickness. The measurements for proper dorsal wall length and corresponding sole thickness have recently been called into question.[33,34] Adaptations to the flat trimming method have been advocated and have focused on increasing the amount of horn removed underneath the flexor tuberosity to reduce pressure on the sole ulcer location.[25,35]

Alternative trimming methods to the flat trimming method encourage a sloped sole whereby the abaxial wall is higher than the axial wall.[31,36] Proponents of this method consider this a more natural sole angle and the procedures to achieve this angle focus on reading the sole and stopping when dehydrated horn disappears. A majority of hoof trimmers use either these methods as a basis for their own personalized trimming techniques.[32] Data from the authors' research groups show that of 44 hoof trimmers attending a 2014 HT conference, 55% used functional trimming (the method described by Raven[24]), 17% used the white line method (a sole reading method described by Blowey[30]), 12% used the Kansas method (the method described by Siebert[31]), and 15% used a combination of methods.[37]

Unfortunately, few data exist about the efficacy of these various HT methods. Because HT is a commonly recommend practice to prevent lameness, there is a need to evaluate the efficacy, frequency, and the physiologic and behavioral response of an animal to these different techniques. One method recently used to review current knowledge is to identify knowledge gaps and set directions for future research through a systematic evaluation of the current literature.[38] The objective of this method is to critically evaluate the evidence that exists for HT techniques as it relates to efficacy, frequency, and associations with behavior and physiologic parameters.

METHODS

To achieve our stated objective in the previous paragraph a narrative integrative review was carried out in June 2016 and bias was attempted to be reduced by incorporating aspects of a systematic review, as described by Sargeant and O'Connor[38] Databases searched included PubMed, AGRICOLA, Google Scholar, and Web of Science. The search terms used for all databases were "cattle HT" and "cattle claw trimming". All languages were included in the searches. A total of 613 articles were retrieved from the results of the 4 databases and stored in RefWorks software.[39] Of the 613 articles, 348 duplicates were removed, leaving 265 for further review. The abstracts of these 265 articles were retrieved and evaluated by the primary author (GCS) according to the inclusion criteria.

Inclusion criteria
1. Study animals were living adult dairy cows.
2. One group of cows underwent an HT procedure.
3. Study used either a before-and-after comparison or a separate control group.
4. Results were published in a peer reviewed journal and written in English.

A total of 16 articles met the inclusion criteria and were grouped into 4 categories, with one article fitting into 2 categories: behavior (4), physiology (7), efficacy (4), and frequency and timing (2).

ASSOCIATIONS WITH BEHAVIOR
Background

Behavior is used as a surrogate to indicate the effect a procedure has on an animal.[40] Common behavioral indicators used to evaluate lameness include locomotion scoring (LS), lying time, activity, and walking speed. LS is a subjective measure[41,42] that defines lameness based on an alteration in gait that develops due to pain. LS is commonly used to evaluate a herd's welfare status.[42,43] Unfortunately, a recent review[44] found 25 different manual LS systems and 15 different automatic LS systems described. This variation and the subjectivity of LS create difficulty when comparing studies that use LS as the outcome. Other behaviors that have been associated with lameness are lying time, activity, and walking speed. Changes to these parameters are hypothesized to be an indicator of a pain response.[42,45,46]

Review of the Literature

Chapinal and colleagues[18] evaluated the general effect of routine HT on LS, walking speed, lying time, and the distribution of weight between the rear legs while standing. This study consisted of 48 lame and nonlame lactating Holsteins with daily data collection 1 week prior to HT and for 5 weeks after. Results from this study showed that LS was impacted only in the 2 immediate days after HT with no long-term impact. Additionally, walking speed was decreased and lying time increased after HT and these change persisted for the entire study period. Finally, only lame cows showed a change in rear leg weight distribution after trimming. Unfortunately, this study failed to describe the HT methods or treatments used and housed cows in groups of 12, limiting its generalizability.

A follow-up study by Chapinal and colleagues[47] used a similar methodology and focused on the effect of using a nonsteroidal anti-inflammatory drug (NSAID), flunixin-meglumine (flunixinmeglumine [FLUMEG], Schering-Plough Animal Health, Union, NJ), before and 24 hours after HT. The study used 66 lactating Holstein cows allocated to 3 treatment groups. Group 1 (n = 10) underwent a sham HT. Group 2 (n = 28) cows were hoof trimmed and received Flumeg. Group 3 (n = 28) cows were hoof trimmed and received saline. Gait scores and weight distribution were monitored before HT, 2 hours after HT, and the day after HT. Lying time and frequency of steps were monitored in 3 time periods — 2 days before HT, 2 days after HT, and 3 days after HT. For both the Flumeg and saline groups, there was a tendency ($P<.10$) for an over 2-hour increase in lying time in the first 2 days post-HT. This increased lying time only persisted past 2 days in the saline group. The sham trimmed group did not show this increase in lying time. No biologically significant changes were found for the other outcomes measured in this study. Due to the inclusion of a sham trimming group, this study provides evidence that the HT process affects behavior. Unfortunately, the distribution of lame cows was not equal between groups because lame cows were not enrolled in the sham group. This makes it unclear if the relationships found in this study are due to the HT process, lameness, or treatment of the lameness. Similar to the first study, this study did not adequately describe the HT technique.

A small study by Tanida and colleagues[28] evaluated the gait components of 17 cows post-HT. The study measured vertical, lateral, and forward acceleration 1 month before HT and once monthly for the 2 months post-HT. Acceleration and direction were measured using a motion sensor on the final thoracic vertebrae of the cow and by analyzing video recordings of cow movements. Results suggested that the cows gait was smoother in the month post-HT because the variances of the lateral and vertical acceleration were lower than the baseline values. The utility of this study is limited due to a small sample size and a limited number of unclearly described measurement times. In addition, the lesion status of these cows was not described. Similar to the previous studies, HT method was not described clearly.

A more recent study by Van Hertem and colleagues[27] evaluated the relationships between HT and rumination, neck activity, and LS in a 1100 cow dairy. Cows in this study were evaluated at 19 different times for LS and had daily electronic rumination and activity data recorded. LSs were analyzed in several different manners, including long term (up to 70 days post-HT) and short term (1 week pre-HT and 1 week post-HT). Results from 152 cows with LS data from 6 different time periods ranging from 34 days before HT to 70 days post-HT showed that lameness prevalence doubled significantly, from 16% to 32% in the 2 weeks post-trimming, but returned to immediate pre-HT levels by 70 days. An analysis of 288 cows that had complete data on LS, rumination, activity, and milk yield for the week before and the week after HT was also completed. This analysis showed that LS increased in the week after HT, whereas neck activity decreased only on the first day post-HT. The effect of HT on rumination was dependent on parity. Due to the larger sample size, the investigators were able to explore potential confounders, such as lesion status, parity, and days in milk (DIM). This study provided adequate details about the HT equipment and technique used.

Summary

All 4 of the studies have several common experimental design issues that limit the conclusions that can be drawn about the association between HT and behavior. None of the studies fully describe the HT process, making it difficult to judge differences in techniques and limiting the external validity of each study. In addition, all 4 studies included lame cows, making it difficult to determine if the effect was due to the HT process or the lesion treatment process. Only 1 study had a large enough sample size to attempt to control for this confounding.[27] Based on these 4 studies, the HT process is associated with a change in animal behaviors, such as resting time and LS. The increase in LS from several studies[18,27] indicates this is a negative change in the welfare status of the animal[42,43] and supports the hypothesis that the increase in lying time is a compensatory response.[17,42,43,46] To truly evaluate the impact of preventative HT on animal behavior, however, there is a need for HT studies on cows without lesions.

ASSOCIATIONS WITH PHYSIOLOGIC CHANGES
Background

To assess the welfare impact of a procedure, it is important to evaluate the impact it has on the animal physiologically.[40,48] Exposure to stressors challenges the homeostasis of an animal, leading to the activation of the hypothalamic pituitary adrenal axis and the sympathetic nervous system. This subsequently leads to an increase in stress hormones in the blood stream[49] and can have an impact ton physiologic functions, such as heart and respiratory rate, milk production, and reproductive functions. The HT process has the potential to expose the animal to various stressors, including restraint, handling, isolation, and pain due to treatment.

Review of the Literature

Nishimori and colleagues[50] investigated the effect of HT on blood parameters, in addition to milk composition and production, using 11 Japanese Holstein cows. Samples were taken before and after HT at time points that were not clearly specified. This study showed that after HT, milk fat percentage, protein percentage, and some blood parameters changed. Due to limited sample size and sampling times, however, this study has limited value.

Pesenhofer and colleagues[51] compared the effect of different chute designs on fecal cortisol metabolites and milk yield before and after HT. This study consisted of 207 lame and nonlame animals randomly assigned to the different chute designs that underwent HT according to the functional HT method.[24] Milk yield was recorded 7 days before HT and until 13 days after HT. Fecal cortisol metabolites were sampled 12 hours before HT and until 7 days after HT. This study showed a significant decrease of 0.6 L in milk production on the day of HT and the day after. Fecal cortisol metabolites were significantly higher for up to 24 hours after HT for both chute designs. This study showed that HT caused a stress response and affected the productivity of the animal. The inclusion of lame animals, however, does not allow for evaluating if the physiologic changes are due to HT or lesion treatment.

A smaller study by Rizk and colleagues[52] evaluated the stress response to HT in lateral recumbency. This study used a paired 3-way crossover design with 6 Holstein cows. Treatment groups consisted of cows receiving either a saline or xylazine injection prior to HT. Sampling times started 15 minutes before HT and continued until 3.25 hours after HT. Changes in the cardiorespiratory system, stress hormones, and metabolism were measured and compared with status pre-HT. Results from this study showed that HT causes changes in blood diastolic blood pressure, mean arterial blood pressure, oxygen saturation, respiratory rate, cortisol, and lactate. Xylazine mitigated these effects but showed a depressive effect on respiratory parameters. Observed changes in this study indicate that the HT process resulted in a stress response in the animal. Caution must be used, however, when interpreting these results because the length of restraint in the HT chute was long (30 minutes).

Korkmaz and colleagues[53] completed a randomized clinical trial using 14 cows that evaluated the impact of dexketoprofen on cows that were trimmed in a squeeze chute. Outcomes evaluated included cortisol, nitric oxide, malondialdehyde, total antioxidant activity, and heart and respiratory rates. Data were collected 30 minutes before HT and again at 15 minutes and 30 minutes after HT. Results of the study showed an increase from baseline to 15 minutes post-HT for heart, respiratory rate, and cortisol. None of the other parameters were different compared with baseline. Similar to the previous studies, this study is limited by sample size and a short follow-up period; it supports the view that the HT process affects physiologic measures.

The study by Van Hertem and colleagues,[27] described previously, also investigated milk production in the week before and the week after HT. Unlike some of the behavioral parameters, no association with HT was found for milk production.

Using a randomized controlled trial, Maxwell and colleagues[54] evaluated the effect of an early lactation functional HT[24] compared with no trimming in 281 primiparous

Holstein cows. Outcomes in this study were 305-day adjusted milk yield and conception rate at 100 DIM. No significant difference between the HT and no HT group was found for either outcome. An interaction with LS existed, however, wherein HT lame animals resulted in higher milk production post-HT compared with untrimmed non-lame animals. Results of this study with limited sample size suggested that trimming all heifers would not provide an economic return. This is one of the few studies to provide a clear description of their HT method.

The most recent physiologic study investigated the claw temperature changes that occur at the coronary band after HT.[55] Skin temperature can be increased due to inflammation[56,57] or other metabolic activity.[58] This study consisted of 81 nonlame and lame cows that had infrared temperature readings at the coronary band taken pre-HT and 21 days post-HT. HT technique was not described. At 21 days after HT, the mean change in hind feet temperature was 0.25°C ($P = .08$) cooler. This temperature change was different, however, between medial and lateral claws and not present in the front feet. Although this study showed a trend for a change in coronary band temperature, the biological significance of this change after 21 days is unclear.

Summary

These studies provide evidence that the HT process changes physiologic parameters. Caution must be used when interpreting and comparing these studies because sample size was limited and HT technique was not adequately described in most of the studies. The design of the studies also makes it difficult to determine if it is the restraint or the actual removal of horn that is causing the change in physiologic measures. Even though effects on physiologic parameters can be found, there is still a knowledge gap on the exact cause and the biological significance of these changes.

EFFICACY OF HOOF TRIMMING
Background

In addition to knowing how HT affects an animal from behavioral and physiologic perspectives, it is important to know if HT is efficacious at preventing lameness and lesions. The goal of HT is to prevent lameness by restoring proper foot angle, removing excess horn growth, and redistributing the weight of an animal over the 2 claws.[24] As discussed previously, there are various HT methods and it is important to evaluate the efficacy of these methods in preventing lameness.

Review of the Literature

van der Tol and colleagues[59] evaluated the standing weight distribution and surface area between hind claws in 5 Holstein cows before and 2 weeks after functional HT[24] using force plates. Results from this study showed that the average pressure on the hind limbs decreased by 30% and improved the distribution of weight between the lateral and medial claws. The improvement in the weight distribution did not equalize weight bearing between the 2 claws. Additionally, HT did not show a significant change in the maximum pressure on the claws. Although this study showed an improvement in certain weight distribution parameters due to HT, the extent of the difference was much smaller than expected and left the investigators to speculate changes in HT techniques are necessary. This study had a small sample size and only used 1 follow-up sampling time period. This makes it possible that cow-level confounders could have influenced the result or that the follow-up period was inappropriate.

Using force plates in a different manner, Carvalho and colleagues[60] evaluated the weight distribution and pressure points on the sole between trimmed cows (14) and untrimmed cows (17). In this study, the untrimmed group had significantly more total pressure applied to heel of the lateral claw of the hind limb than trimmed cows. At the claw level, numeric differences were found for increased pressure on several other claw regions. Due to small sample size and the lack of descriptive data about the cows and HT technique, it is difficult to determine if these differences are due to confounding or HT.

As a follow-up study to the van der Tol and colleagues[59] study, Ouweltjes and colleagues[25] investigated the efficacy of functional HT[24] to an adaptation that decreases the pressure in the typical sole ulcer region on both claws. Nonlame cows were randomized to either the functional method (33) or the adaptation (32) and observed for 3 months. Outcome measures included claw health, claw conformation, LS activity, and floor contact pressures. Results of the study did not show any significant differences between the 2 HT methods. There are several possible reasons for the lack of differences between treatments, including a short follow-up observation period and limited sample size. Additionally, both the lateral and medial claws trimmed with the adaptation could have masked an effect. A similarly designed unpublished study[35] did show a difference in lesion prevalence when only the lateral claw was trimmed with the adaptation. The Ouweltjes and colleagues[25] study had a clearly described trimming method section and should be considered a model for how to describe HT techniques in future publications.

A study from New Zealand evaluated the efficacy of HT in New Zealand by randomly allocating 2695 cows to functional HT[24] or no HT.[61] Outcomes evaluated included incidence and time to lameness as identified by trained farm staff. In this study, HT did not change the cumulative incidence of lameness but did increase the median time to lameness in the 70 days post-HT. This well-designed study had several strengths, including accounting for confounders and the use of multiple farms with 1 hoof trimmer. Using farm staff to identify lameness leads to an underestimated level of lameness[2] but this is a nonselective bias.

Summary

These 4 studies evaluated HT efficacy from 2 different perspectives and 3 studies showed a benefit by reducing pressures in the claw or increasing time to lameness. All the studies used the functional HT[24] method, but several other methods have been described[22,24–32] that also need to be evaluated. In addition, several studies were small in size[25,59,60] or their findings are likely environment specific.[61] Therefore, more studies evaluating the efficacy of HT are necessary.

FREQUENCY AND TIMING OF HOOF TRIMMING
Background

Hoof growth can vary with breed and genetics, but the net growth of dorsal wall horn is approximately 1 mm/mo to 2 mm/mo.[62,63] Functional HT attempts to deal with this growth by restoring an upright foot angle and balancing the weight bearing between the 2 claws.[24] Some observational studies have found associations with more frequent HT and lower lameness prevalence.[64,65]

Review of the Literature

Manske and colleagues[26] conducted a 2-year study on 3444 dairy cattle on multiple Swedish dairy farms that were block randomized to a second HT in the autumn. Regardless of allocation, all cows were LS and trimmed at the spring trimming. Results indicated that the additional trimming in the autumn led to lower odds of lameness and horn-type lesions. This study was well designed and included a long observation period with block randomization to control confounding and used multiple hoof trimmers and farms to increase generalizability to other farms in Sweden.

Hernandez and colleagues[66] evaluated the efficacy of a hoof health examination and an HT at midlactation compared with no evaluation at midlactation in 313 randomly allocated cows in 1 herd. This study showed that cows in the nontrimmed group had a 25% higher ($P = .09$) lameness incidence and a 1.25 ($P = .12$) higher risk of becoming lame compared with the trimmed group. Some problems in study design limit the interpretation of this study because the study was done in only 1 herd, the study did not evaluate control cows for lesions on entry into the study, and there was inadequate detail of the HT method.

Summary

These 2 studies showed that an additional HT can be beneficial in the herds studied. Only 1 of the studies,[26] however, described the HT technique used enough detail that it could be repeated. From these studies it is still unclear what is the most efficacious time to trim animals for a second time during lactation and if the additional HT is beneficial in all situations.

SUMMARY

This review of 16 articles of HT as it relates to the efficacy, frequency, and associations with behavior and physiologic parameters found several common study design issues that limit generalizability and conclusions. A majority of studies use a small sample size and lack a clear description of the HT technique. In the reviewed studies, HT seems to initiate a stress response, change behavior, improve components of weight bearing, and reduce lameness in specific environmental conditions.

There are still multiple knowledge gaps that need to be answered to create a more complete picture of the impact HT has on cows and lameness. Primarily, it is necessary to determine the most efficacious HT technique from physiologic, behavioral, and productivity perspectives. Furthermore, it is necessary to understand what the change in physiologic parameters means to the animal and what is causing it — the restraint or the actual removal of horn. Additionally, to encompass all aspects of welfare,[48] it is necessary to understand the effect HT has on the behavior of a nonlame animal. Lastly, additional information is needed on appropriate timing and frequency of HT.

REFERENCES

1. Barker ZE, Leach KA, Whay HR, et al. Assessment of lameness prevalence and associated risk factors in dairy herds in England and Wales. J Dairy Sci 2010;93: 932–41.
2. Espejo LA, Endres MI, Salfer JA. Prevalence of lameness in high-producing holstein cows housed in freestall barns in Minnesota. J Dairy Sci 2006;89:3052–8.
3. Von Keyserlingk M, Barrientos A, Ito K, et al. Benchmarking cow comfort on North American freestall dairies: Lameness, leg injuries, lying time, facility design, and management for high-producing Holstein dairy cows. J Dairy Sci 2012;95: 7399–408.
4. Holzhauer M, Hardenberg C, Bartels CJ. Herd and cow-level prevalence of sole ulcers in The Netherlands and associated-risk factors. Prev Vet Med 2008;85: 125–35.
5. Solano L, Barkema HW, Mason S, et al. Prevalence and distribution of foot lesions in dairy cattle in Alberta, Canada. J Dairy Sci 2016;99:6828–41.

6. Cramer G, Lissemore KD, Guard CL, et al. Herd- and cow-level prevalence of foot lesions in Ontario dairy cattle. J Dairy Sci 2008;91:3888–95.

7. Becker J, Steiner A, Kohler S, et al. Lameness and foot lesions in Swiss dairy cows: I. Prevalence. Schweiz Arch Tierheilkd 2014;156:71–8.

8. Cha E, Hertl JA, Bar D, et al. The cost of different types of lameness in dairy cows calculated by dynamic programming. Prev Vet Med 2010;97:1–8.

9. Hernandez JA, Garbarino EJ, Shearer JK, et al. Comparison of milk yield in dairy cows with different degrees of lameness. J Am Vet Med Assoc 2005;227:1292–6.

10. Green LE, Hedges VJ, Schukken YH, et al. The impact of clinical lameness on the milk yield of dairy cows. J Dairy Sci 2002;85:2250–6.

11. Warnick LD, Janssen D, Guard CL, et al. The effect of lameness on milk production in dairy cows. J Dairy Sci 2001;84:1988–97.

12. Peake KA, Biggs AM, Argo CM, et al. Effects of lameness, subclinical mastitis and loss of body condition on the reproductive performance of dairy cows. Vet Rec 2011;168:301.

13. Hudson CD, Huxley JN, Green MJ. Using simulation to interpret a discrete time survival model in a complex biological system: fertility and lameness in dairy cows. PLoS One 2014;9:e103426.

14. Bicalho RC, Cheong SH, Cramer G, et al. Association between a visual and an automated locomotion score in lactating holstein cows. J Dairy Sci 2007;90:3294–300.

15. Booth CJ, Warnick LD, Grohn YT, et al. Effect of lameness on culling in dairy cows. J Dairy Sci 2004;87:4115–22.

16. Navarro G, Green LE, Tadich N. Effect of lameness and lesion specific causes of lameness on time budgets of dairy cows at pasture and when housed. Vet J 2013;197:788–93.

17. Gomez A, Cook NB. Time budgets of lactating dairy cattle in commercial freestall herds. J Dairy Sci 2010;93:5772–81.

18. Chapinal N, de Passille AM, Rushen J. Correlated changes in behavioral indicators of lameness in dairy cows following hoof trimming. J Dairy Sci 2010;93:5758–63.

19. Bustamante HA, Rodriguez AR, Herzberg DE, et al. Stress and pain response after oligofructose induced-lameness in dairy heifers. J Vet Sci 2015;16:405–11.

20. Tadich N, Tejeda C, Bastias S, et al. Nociceptive threshold, blood constituents and physiological values in 213 cows with locomotion scores ranging from normal to severely lame. Vet J 2013;197:401–5.

21. Potterton SL, Bell NJ, Whay HR, et al. A descriptive review of the peer and non-peer reviewed literature on the treatment and prevention of foot lameness in cattle published between 2000 and 2011. Vet J 2012;193:612–6.

22. Shearer JK, van Amstel SR. Functional and corrective claw trimming. Vet Clin North Am Food Anim Pract 2001;17:53–72.

23. NAHMS. Changes in dairy cattle health and management practices in the United States, 1996-2007: July 2009. Fort Collins (CO): US Department of Agriculture; Animal and Plant Health Inspection Service; Veterinary Services, National Animal Health Monitoring System; 2007.

24. Raven ET, Toussaint E. Cattle footcare and claw trimming. Ipswich (United Kingdom): Farming Press; 1985.

25. Ouweltjes W, Holzhauer M, van der Tol PPJ, et al. Effects of two trimming methods of dairy cattle on concrete or rubber-covered slatted floors. J Dairy Sci 2009;92:960–71.

26. Manske T, Hultgren J, Bergsten C. Prevalence and interrelationships of hoof lesions and lameness in Swedish dairy cows. Prev Vet Med 2002;54:247–63.

27. Van Hertem T, Parmet Y, Steensels M, et al. The effect of routine hoof trimming on locomotion score, ruminating time, activity, and milk yield of dairy cows. J Dairy Sci 2014;97:4852–63.

28. Tanida H, Koba Y, Rushen J, et al. Use of three-dimensional acceleration sensing to assess dairy cow gait and the effects of hoof trimming. Anim Sci J 2011;82:792–800.

29. Greenough PR. Bovine laminitis and lameness: a hands on approach. Philadelphia (PA): Elsevier Health Sciences; 2007.

30. Blowey RW. Cattle lameness and hoof care. 3rd edition. Sheffield England: 5m Publishing; 2015.

31. Siebert L. The Kansas adaptation to the Dutch hoof trimming method. Eureka (SD): Hoof Trimmers Assoc Inc; 2005.

32. Daniel V. Trimmers tool box: working diverse methods and options for hoof care into a common goal of attaining healthy feet and satisfied clients. Missoula (MT): Hoof Trimmers Assoc Inc; 2014.

33. Nuss K, Paulus N. Measurements of claw dimensions in cows before and after functional trimming: a post-mortem study. Vet J 2006;172:284–92.

34. Archer SC, Newsome R, Dibble H, et al. Claw length recommendations for dairy cow foot trimming. Vet Rec 2015;177:222.

35. Gomez A, Cook NB, Kopesky N, et al. Should we trim heifers before calving? American Association of Bovine Practitioners. Milwaukee (WI), September 19–21, 2013.

36. Amstutz H. Hoof trimming [Cattle, lameness]. Mod Vet Pract 1979;60:137–8.

37. Scherping M, Klehr K, Cramer G. A descritptive study on hoof trimming methods using cadaver feet. 18th International Symposium & 10th Conference on Lameness in Ruminants. Valdivia (Chile), November 22–25, 2015.

38. Sargeant J, O'Connor A. Introducing a special issue with a focus on systematic reviews. Anim Health Res Rev 2016;17:1–2.

39. ProQuest LLC. RefWorks software. Ann Arbor (MI): RefWorks; 2016. Available at: http://www.refworks.com/.

40. Dawkins MS. Behaviour as a tool in the assessment of animal welfare. Zoology (Jena) 2003;106:383–7.

41. Winckler C, Willen S. The reliability and repeatability of a lameness scoring system for use as an indicator of welfare in dairy cattle. Acta Agric Scand Sect A-Anim Sci 2001;51:103–7.

42. O Callaghan K, Cripps P, Downham D, et al. Subjective and objective assessment of pain and discomfort due to lameness in dairy cattle. Anim Welfare 2003;12:605–10.

43. Flower FC, Weary DM. Gait assessment in dairy cattle. Animal 2009;3:87–95.

44. Schlageter-Tello A, Bokkers EA, Koerkamp PW, et al. Manual and automatic locomotion scoring systems in dairy cows: a review. Prev Vet Med 2014;116:12–25.

45. Cook NB, Mentink RL, Bennett TB, et al. The effect of heat stress and lameness on time budgets of lactating dairy cows. J Dairy Sci 2007;90:1674–82.

46. Ito K, von Keyserlingk MA, Leblanc SJ, et al. Lying behavior as an indicator of lameness in dairy cows. J Dairy Sci 2010;93:3553–60.

47. Chapinal N, de Passille AM, Rushen J, et al. Effect of analgesia during hoof trimming on gait, weight distribution, and activity of dairy cattle. J Dairy Sci 2010;93:3039–46.

48. Frazer D. Assessing animal well-being: common sense, uncommon science. In: The Proceedings of the Conference on Food Animal Well-Being. USDA and

Purdue University, Office of Agriculture Research for Programs. West Lafayette (IN), 1993. p. 37–51.

49. Harris RB. Chronic and acute effects of stress on energy balance: are there appropriate animal models? Am J Physiol Regul Integr Comp Physiol 2015; 308:R250–65.

50. Nishimori K, Okada K, Ikuta K, et al. The effects of one-time hoof trimming on blood biochemical composition, milk yield, and milk composition in dairy cows. J Vet Med Sci 2006;68:267–70.

51. Pesenhofer G, Palme R, Pesenhofer R, et al. Stress reactions during claw trimming in cattle-comparison of a tilt table and a walk-in crush by measuring faecal cortisol metabolites. Veterinarska Fakulteta, Univerza v Ljubljani 2006;43:216–9.

52. Rizk A, Herdtweck S, Meyer H, et al. Effects of xylazine hydrochloride on hormonal, metabolic, and cardiorespiratory stress responses to lateral recumbency and claw trimming in dairy cows. J Am Vet Med Assoc 2012;240:1223–30.

53. Korkmaz M, Saritas ZK, Demirkan I, et al. Effects of dexketoprofen trometamol on stress and oxidative stress in cattle undergoing claw trimming. Acta Sci Vet 2014;42.

54. Maxwell OJ, Hudson CD, Huxley JN. Effect of early lactation foot trimming in lame and non-lame dairy heifers: a randomised controlled trial. Vet Rec 2015;177:100.

55. Alsaaod M, Syring C, Luternauer M, et al. Effect of routine claw trimming on claw temperature in dairy cows measured by infrared thermography. J Dairy Sci 2015; 98:2381–8.

56. Alsaaod M, Syring C, Dietrich J, et al. A field trial of infrared thermography as a non-invasive diagnostic tool for early detection of digital dermatitis in dairy cows. Vet J 2014;199:281–5.

57. Van hoogmoed LM, Snyder JR. Use of infrared thermography to detect injections and palmar digital neurectomy in horses. Vet J 2002;164:129–41.

58. Stewart M, Webster JR, Verkerk GA, et al. Non-invasive measurement of stress in dairy cows using infrared thermography. Physiol Behav 2007;92:520–5.

59. van der Tol PP, van der Beek SS, Metz JH, et al. The effect of preventive trimming on weight bearing and force balance on the claws of dairy cattle. J Dairy Sci 2004;87:1732–8.

60. Carvalho V, Naas I, Bucklin R, et al. Effects of trimming on dairy cattle hoof weight bearing and pressure distributions. Braz J Vet Res Anim Sci 2006;43:518–25.

61. Bryan M, Tacoma H, Hoekstra F. The effect of hindclaw height differential and subsequent trimming on lameness in large dairy cattle herds in Canterbury, New Zealand. N Z Vet J 2012;60:349–55.

62. Hahn MV, McDaniel BT, Wilk JC. Rates of hoof growth and wear in Holstein cattle. J Dairy Sci 1986;69:2148–56.

63. Vokey F, Guard C, Erb H, et al. Effects of alley and stall surfaces on indices of claw and leg health in dairy cattle housed in a free-stall barn. J Dairy Sci 2001; 84:2686–99.

64. Fjeldaas T, Sogstad Å, Østerås O. Claw trimming routines in relation to claw lesions, claw shape and lameness in Norwegian dairy herds housed in tie stalls and free stalls. Prev Vet Med 2006;73:255–71.

65. Espejo LA, Endres MI. Herd-level risk factors for lameness in high-producing Holstein cows housed in freestall barns. J Dairy Sci 2007;90:306–14.

66. Hernandez JA, Garbarino EJ, Shearer JK, et al. Evaluation of the efficacy of prophylactic hoof health examination and trimming during midlactation in reducing the incidence of lameness during late lactation in dairy cows. J Am Vet Med Assoc 2007;230:89–93.

Treatment Options for Lameness Disorders in Organic Dairies

Pablo Pinedo, DVM, PhD[a], Juan Velez, MS, DVM[b,*],
Diego Manriquez, DVM[a], Hans Bothe, DVM[b]

KEYWORDS

- Lameness • Dairy • Organic

KEY POINTS

- Due to limitations in the use of therapeutic resources, preventive management and early detection of lameness is critical in organic dairies.
- Organic regulation includes a strict rule of not withholding treatment with a prohibited substance to maintain organic status if it causes the animal to suffer.
- Prompt decision to cull or euthanize is an important component of treatment evaluation.
- Comprehensive lameness evaluation should include periodic locomotion scoring, adequate record keeping, and consideration of percentage of cull cows due to locomotion problems.

BACKGROUND

Animal welfare is an important aspect of both organic and conventional dairying. Because the dairy industry has a moral and ethical obligation to provide for animal well-being,[1] proper control of locomotion disorders is a fundamental area of health management in organic farming.

Certified organic dairy systems require that cows graze for at least 120 days during the growing season (National Organic Program regulations) and that they consume at least 30% of their dry matter intake demand from grazing. In many cases this is complemented with some type of housing that also requires outdoor access during the whole year. This management combination results in unique features determining the cows' feet and legs health condition because the mixture of walking surfaces and displacement efforts requires a continuous adaptation of the hoof, ligaments, muscles, and bones to different flooring, humidity, and waste levels on the floors.[2]

Disclosure Statement: The authors have nothing to disclose.
[a] Department of Animal Sciences, Colorado State University, 305 West Pitkin Street, Fort Collins, CO 80523-1171, USA; [b] Aurora Organic Farms, 7388 CO-66, Platteville, CO 80651, USA
* Corresponding author.
E-mail address: jvelez@aodmilk.com

As previously stated, an adequate health status of the feet and legs is a priority for organic dairies and, as a consequence, preventative strategies, adequate diagnostic protocols, and effective lameness treatment constitute key components of in-farm health maintenance programs.

Most disorders resulting in lameness originate in the feet.[3] In general terms, depending on causality, claw lesions can be categorized as infectious and noninfectious. Due to regulations that include strict prohibition against the use of antimicrobials and other synthetic substances in organic systems, infectious lesions constitute the largest challenge for this system, although in many cases traumatic injury will also result in bacterial infection. Main infectious entities include digital dermatitis (DD; commonly known as hairy heels warts), heel erosion, interdigital dermatitis, toe abscess, and foot rot.[4–6] Noninfectious lesions are associated with loss of tissue integrity due to traumatic events, excessive wear, nutritional deficiencies, or overtrimming that may be the primary entry for infections. Among noninfectious lesions are laminitis; white line disease (WLD); sole, toe, and heel ulcers (**Fig. 1**); sole bruising (sole hemorrhage); corkscrew claw; hardship groove (horizontal fissure); vertical fissure; interdigital hyperplasia; and thin sole.[4,5,7] Other noninfectious lesions can be observed in the hock and knees and are mainly related to traumatic events.

In addition to the need for pointing out treatment options for organic dairies due to specific therapy restrictions, it is important to compare the risk factors, epidemiology, and the magnitude of the locomotion problems between organic and conventional farms to evaluate whether some current approaches for lameness control are exchangeable between these systems or whether they are exclusively functional for a specific operation.

LAMENESS EPIDEMIOLOGY IN ORGANIC DAIRY FARMS

Organic farms in the United States often have characteristics that differ from conventional dairy farms. These include a smaller herd size, use of non-freestall housing, and grazing-based diets,[8,9] which are management factors that have been associated with different levels of various diseases. Therefore, a confounding effect of organic management on disease incidence may be expected[10] and these features may also affect traits, such as the level of fat reserves in the cow, which are related to proper feet and leg health. In a study comparing indicators of animal welfare in organic and conventional dairies, locomotion and body condition scores (BCSs) were analyzed using a database containing 42 dairy farms, 6 of which were organic dairies.[1] BCS was similar in both systems and was significantly associated with locomotion score, percentage

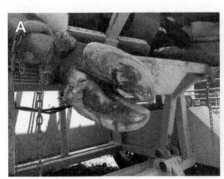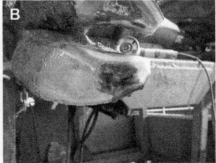

Fig. 1. Two cases of noninfectious disorders. (*A*) Sole ulcer exposing necrotic underlying tissue. (*B*) Toe ulcer as seen after removal of loose horn.

of swollen hocks or knees in the herd, and herd size. On a scale of 1 (normal) to 5 (severely lame), the average locomotion score of 1.04 for organic herds was statistically lower than the average score (1.28) of conventional herds.

In a large study, 292 dairy herds from conventional and organic farms were assessed for cow locomotion. The overall prevalence of lameness ranged from 0% to 54% (mean 8%) and did not differ between the 2 systems. Identified risk factors for lameness were prevalence of cows with BCS less than 2.5, prevalence of hock lesions, average hours that the cows spent outdoors in the 60 days before the herd visit, routine use of a footbath, and grazing system. The highest lameness prevalence was in conventional no-grazing systems.[11] Accordingly, a study performed in the United Kingdom found that organic farms had significantly lower lameness prevalence compared with conventional dairies.[2] However, it is necessary to account for differences in management standards for organic dairies in the United States compared with those of other regions of the world.

From the point of view of prevalence of locomotion disorders, DD is the most relevant cause of lameness in US dairy farms (USDA, 2009).[12] Data indicate that in conventional farms there is a wide range in the prevalence of limb disorders (15%–57%[5]); DD (40% of lame cows) is followed by sole ulcer (30%–40%) and WLD (29%).[5,11] Interestingly, sole ulcers have been found to be very relevant foot lesions on organic dairies.[4]

The main risk factors for DD include type of bedding, cubicle size, and cleanliness of the environment. Introduction of new animals to the herd and the proportion of concentrate supplementation in the diet have been also pointed out as potential risk factors.[13]

Some studies have reported that some diseases, such as DD, have lower prevalence in organic dairies than conventional farms. This is probably due to the increased time that cows spend pasturing in organic[4] compared with conventional dairies. Similarly, another report indicated that the prevalence of lame cows was higher on non-grazing conventional dairies compared with organic and grazing conventional farms.[5] Usually, grazing keeps cows cleaner and is associated with more exposure to solar radiation, limiting hoof moisture, and the microbial load.[4] However, information regarding the incidence of DD or other causes of lameness in US organic dairies is too limited to make a well-documented comparison.[5]

Data from an extensive assessment of DD that was recently performed in a large organic dairy in northern Colorado provide a reference on DD prevalence in an organic system (Brunson K, DVM, Aurora Organic Dairy, personal communication, 2016). Cows were evaluated using the Mortellaro (M) score,[14,15] which classifies the stages of DD as M0 (healthy skin), M1 (early stage, skin defect<2 cm diameter), M2 (acute active ulcerative lesion), M3 (healing stage, lesion covered with scab-like material), and M4 (chronic stage, that may contain mostly thickened or proliferative epithelium). The assessment included more than 8000 cows housed and milked in 4 different units within the same dairy operation. The results indicated that 90% of the cows were in the nonaffected category. The results also indicated that the most prevalent state of DD (7% of the cows) was M3–M4 (healing and chronic state), whereas 3% of the cows were in the M1 state (active and acute lesion; **Fig. 2**). In addition, farm records indicated that 1.4% of the culled cows left this herd due to feet and leg problems, and 0.6% of these cows were euthanized due to lameness that for welfare reasons precluded transport.

A critical factor limiting an adequate control of lameness in dairy herds is the lack of precise measurements for lameness incidence. This results in farmers underestimating the significance of this problem on their farms.[16] In agreement, some studies indicated

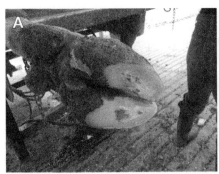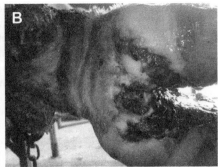

Fig. 2. Different DD states based on the Mortellaro scoring system. (M0 = no lesion to M4 = chronic stage). (*A*) M2, acute active ulcerative lesion. (*B*) Healing stage, lesion covered with scab-like material. (*Courtesy of* John Coatney, DVM, Veterinary Diagnostic and Production Animal Medicine, Iowa State University, Ames, IA, USA.)

that farmers' perception of the prevalence of lameness in a herd was lower than that of a researcher assessing cows individually.[5,17,18] Even though isolated data provide some references about the situation of lameness in organic farms in the United States (Brunson K, DVM, Aurora Organic Dairy, personal communication, 2016),[2,5] there is limited information about the dynamics of the disease, risk factors, duration, and cure rates. More scientific evidence would allow for comparisons between organic and conventional systems to address specific issues in this production system.

TREATMENT OPTIONS FOR LAMENESS
Preventive Management

The US regulations for production of organic milk include a strict prohibition against the use of antimicrobials and other synthetic substances, but the effect of these regulations on dairy animal health has not been previously reported.[10] In general terms, organic management principles aim to benefit cow health and welfare, with an emphasis on stress reduction, lower stocking density, less focus on intensive production, and better housing. Consequently, a basic concept in organic farming is based on the principle that animal health should be maintained through proactive husbandry measures rather than reactive treatments.[2] Interestingly, data from 192 organic farms, 64 conventional nongrazing farms, and 36 conventional grazing farms indicated that organic farmers were less likely to have regular veterinary visits (36%) than conventional nongrazing (77%) or conventional grazing farmers (56%).[18] This situation may preclude the implementation of adequate lameness prevention programs and may result in an underestimation of lameness prevalence.[5]

The interaction between cattle, facilities, and management are a determinant triangle to prevent lameness and these 3 elements should be considered to address locomotion problems in organic dairies. From the animal perspective, in recent years, genetic components for health traits have gained more attention.[19] The introduction of animals with genetic merit for suitable body, feet, and hoof conformations represent a valid option to improve the chances that the cows have to resist or recover from lameness diseases. Cow size and pigmentation of the hoof have been associated with the risk of hoof and leg lameness.[4] Therefore, small cows and cows with darker hooves tend to be more resistant to hoof lameness because they place less stress on their limbs and have harder horny material on their hooves.[4] The role of genetic variation in the susceptibility to specific feet disorders is now under scrutiny and DD has become an intensive subject of research.[19]

Facility design is a key component of the prevention of lameness. Flooring surfaces should be designed to diminish their abrasive effect by using smooth concrete floors with proper grooving preferably three-fourths inch wide and three-fourths inch deep for alleys surrounding the free stalls, and diagonal grooving for high traffic areas, which will increase the traction.[5,7] Nonetheless, concrete has a negative effect on the health of the hoof independently of its shape and composition. Consequently, placing rubber flooring in transit lanes or rest areas may help to mitigate the concrete's abrasive effects.[4,5] It is important to avoid narrow walking alleys and pens, such as the holding pen, to prevent crowded moving groups, which may increase the risk of trauma between cows and might affect cow vison for possible obstacles[20] Moreover, it is important to provide soft resting floors, such as straw or sand for cows that have suffered leg of feet injuries.[5] Finally, hygienic maintenance and moisture control will help improve foot health. Therefore, cleaning protocols should be applied routinely. Heat abatement strategies are also important components of lameness control because under hot conditions cows will stand longer to dissipate heat. In addition, hyperventilation in response to heat may lead to metabolic acidosis, which is a significant risk factor for lameness.

Management plays an important role in prevention of lameness, especially nutritional management. Consequently, continuous evaluation of diets directed to avoid subacute and acute acidosis will have a significant impact on the control of laminitis.[6,7,20] Supplemental feeds can also promote and prevent some hoof disorders. For example, supplementation of 20 mg per day of biotin has been shown to reduce the incidence of WLD in conventional multiparous cows by 45%[4,21] and could be applied in organic dairies. Preventative management, such as functional trimming, is fundamental in organic dairies. Routine claw trimming 2 times per year is recommended to restore proper function balance weightbearing between claws, to correct foot overgrowth that might lead to overburdening of the claws, and to identify and correct claw lesions at early stages.[22]

Footbaths with disinfectant are used as preventive management of infectious lameness lesions.[5] In organic dairies, stationary or walk-through footbaths are commonly set up using copper sulfate (as approved for use in organic herds by the NOP). Baths 6 inches deep, with 5% copper sulfate solutions are common and acceptable in organic farms.[4] Copper sulfate is allowed in organic dairy farms, whereas zinc sulfate and formaldehyde are not.[23] Location of the footbaths should permit good cow flow and be followed by appropriate cleaning and replacement of the disinfectant agent as needed. Copper sulfate is quickly deactivated in combination with organic matter[5] and, if excessively contaminated, it could facilitate the transmission of infectious pathogens.[4]

In agreement with the previous statements, researchers in the United Kingdom who monitored cow locomotion in 67 organic dairies for 1 year, determined that the main interventions that resulted in reductions of lameness prevalence were improvement of tracks, better cubicle comfort, more frequent foot bathing, increased foot trimming, and higher frequency or effectiveness of removing slurry and manure.[16,24]

Treatment of Noninfectious Lameness

As a general concept, claw lesions affecting the dermal–epidermal tissues of the claw heal by second intention with granulation tissue. The process includes 4 phases: hemostasis, inflammation, proliferation, and maturation.[3] Main events during the initial clotting phase are the recruitment of platelets and the release of cytokines and vasoactive mediators, such as epinephrine, norepinephrine, and prostaglandins, that cause vasoconstriction to reduce blood loss and also activate inflammatory cells. The inflammatory phase is characterized by the influx of white blood cells that phagocytize bacteria and cellular debris within the site of injury. Angiogenesis, fibroplasia, and granulation tissue formation, epithelialization, and tissue contraction are the main events during the proliferative phase, followed by the formation of a scar.[3] Consequently, the strategies for treating noninfectious claw lesions are centered on allowing an unimpeded succession of these events.

As in conventional dairies, a central component in managing this group of disorders in organic dairies is the use of corrective trimming and the application of claw blocks to relieve weightbearing on the affected hooves.

In the case of WLD, the detached wall is removed by paring or sloping the horn material of the sole in the abaxial direction over the lesion at a 45° or greater angle.[5] In the case of concurrent infection, lesion removal would allow for pus drainage and would help to prevent the entrance of mud or stones that might worsen the lame condition or trigger a new infection (**Fig. 3**). As the lesion is exposed, abundant flushing with water and iodine should be applied. Hygiene and soft flooring conditions are advised for cows during the convalescent period. The attachment of an orthopedic foot block helps to relieve pain and weightbearing of the affected claw, accelerating the recovery. Depending on the magnitude of the wound, 4 to 5 weeks are expected for recovery and daily reexamination should be performed throughout the first week.[5]

The treatment of sole and toe ulcers is designated to provide high hygiene and to relieve weightbearing of the affected claw. Placement of a block on the healthy claw will provide elevation and rest to the claw with the ulcer (**Fig. 4**). Cleaning and disinfection of ulcers should be done every other day, if not more often when possible.[5] The progression of the ulcer recovery is very variable but frequently requires a minimum of 20 to 30 days.[3] Follow-up should be accompanied by cleaning and disinfection. The only possible treatment of bruising is rest, offering the cow open areas well-bedded with straw or sand, along with block on the unaffected claw.[20]

Fissures on the hoof wall are treated in a similar way independent of its location and direction (axial or abaxial, horizontal or vertical). The use of corrective trimming, the relief of the weightbearing in the affected claw, and the housing of lame cows in on softer flooring surfaces, such as rubber mats or pastures, are the key points to consider when handling fissures. Like all noninfectious lesions, fissures on the hoof

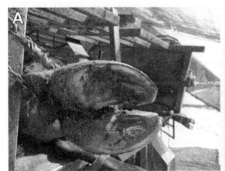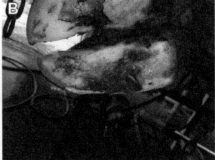

Fig. 3. (*A, B*) Two cases of WLD evidencing an extensive lesion after removal of loose and undermined claw horn.

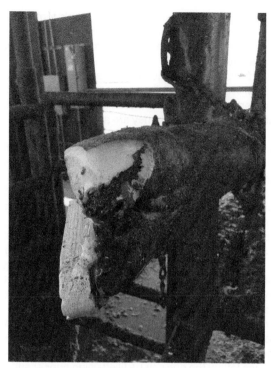

Fig. 4. Application of an orthopedic block to release the pressure in the affected digit after therapeutic trimming in 2 severe cases of WLD.

wall are produced by mechanical forces that break the integrity of the hoof due to the weakness of the wall and sole that may be related to nutritional deficiencies.[5]

Finally, appropriate nutritional management designated to avoid rumen acidosis, plus the supplementation of biotin and zinc, the reduction of abrasive flooring, and appropriate cattle handling, should be done to control the incidence of traumatic events that may progress to lameness. After healing, especially for lesions that require orthopedic shoes or blocks, a corrective trimming is fundamental to restore balanced weightbearing on all hooves.[3–5,11]

Treatments of Infectious Lameness

As indicated previously, DD is the main infectious entity resulting in lameness. Topical application of antibiotic solutions have been shown to be an effective therapy[3,4]; however, this is not available for organic dairies. Therefore, the focus is directed toward the use of natural components that reduce bacterial growth.

The usage of topical treatment under a bandage is the main option to treat DD and interdigital dermatitis in organic dairies. Several poultices or emulsions are used on DD, including copper sulfate powder, powdered aspirin, tea tree oil, aloe vera, oregano oil, and iodine, which are mixed using a base oil or honey to create an ointment.[4] A successful treatment of DD includes a thorough cleaning of the affected area, followed by the application of an emulsion of copper sulfate and iodine that is applied directly to the lesion. The lesion is subsequently bandaged and scheduled for removal and recheck at day 3 following treatment.

Some investigators propose the use of stand-in portable footbath with a copper sulfate solution (5% is well-tolerated by the skin) in which the feet are soaked from 5 to 10 minutes.[5] However, because it is time-consuming, this strategy may be impractical if the prevalence of acute DD is high.

The application of botanic sprays based on organic oils (Skin Joy, foot fix spray) to help skin cells to improve their immunity and also to confer antimicrobial, antifungal and antioxidant properties to the wounded area has been reported and anecdotal reports suggest that granular sugar and honey are also used as topical wound dressings on claw lesions.[3] The idea is that sugar's high osmolarity draws moisture from the wound, inhibiting bacterial growth. Sugar has also been used in infected lesions for the debridement of necrotic tissue. Honey's antibacterial benefits are likely related to its low pH, high osmolarity, and peroxide activity.[3]

In general, lesions should be reexamined within 3 days after the bandage is applied.[4] After bandage removal, the lesion must be cleaned with water and carefully reexamined to determine if more time with a bandage is needed.

The treatment of interdigital dermatitis follows a similar procedure. The foot should be thoroughly cleaned before the ointment (as previously described) is applied to the lesion. Next, the claw is bandaged for a maximum of 3 days. Subsequently, the foot is soaked and disinfected in iodine (Povidone) with special attention to the interdigital space twice a day, ideally at the parlor, for 1 week.

Toe abscesses have multiple causes and are often chronic conditions. The approach to treatment of toe abscesses includes the removal of all loose and necrotic horn, which will permit the drainage of purulent material. Subsequent cleaning with abundant water and disinfection of the foot with a dilute iodine solution is recommended. Finally, the space left by the pus can be filled using copper sulfate ointment, honey, or the aspirin and copper sulfate emulsion. A daily examination during the first 3 days is encouraged to remove contamination with organic matter and for treatment as necessary.

Foot rot cases represent an important challenge if not detected in early stages, especially when complication leads to deep digital sepsis because of its poor prognosis. This can compromise the overall health of the cow.[5] Regarding the necrotic lesion on the foot, the first approach begins with a careful debridement of necrotic tissue, avoiding healthy areas, and considering the reactions of the cow to painful debridement procedures. After necrotic tissue removal, the hoof must be thoroughly cleaned with copious amounts of water and iodine followed by the use of topical treatment under a bandage.[4,5] The bandage should be changed daily and the feet must be cleaned and soaked in iodine every time. Systemic treatment includes oral aspirin, intravenous iodide, and supplementation of zinc and biotin (40 g per day) for several weeks. This has shown to accelerate the healing process and improve the quality of the hoof horn.[4]

Pharmacologic Management of Pain in Lameness Lesions for Organic Dairies

Pain management in lame cows is crucial to improve cure rates and is important due to animal welfare considerations. The presence and location of pain is also critical for adequate diagnosis of lameness (**Fig. 5**). Additionally, the use of local anesthesia may be needed for nerve blocking to help in the diagnosis of lame pathologic conditions or to assist in painful corrective trimming procedures. Analgesic and anti-inflammatory drugs allowed in organic dairies include aspirin and flunixin meglumine.[23] Oral aspirin boluses provide mild analgesia for musculoskeletal lesions but can also be used in the case of septic foot rot to relieve fever.[4] The dosage is 2 to 4

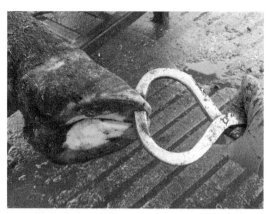

Fig. 5. Proper determination of the presence and location of pain is critical for adequate diagnosis of lameness.

boluses twice daily. The manufacturers or distributors approved for use in organic dairies are Bimeda, IBA, Merrick's Inc., Vet One, and Leedstone Animal Health.[23]

Flunixin Meglumine has a more potent analgesic and anti-inflammatory effect. This drug has demonstrated substantial acute analgesia in induced lameness models as illustrated through modifications of gait and improved pressures placed on the affected foot and claw.[25] The indicated dosage is 1 to 2 mL per 100 lb, administered intravenously at a slow rate. If administered in organic settings, the withdrawal period must be twice that indicated by the US Food and Drug Administration.[23] The manufacturers or distributors approved for use in organic dairies are AgrilLabs, Schering-Plough/Merck Animal Health, and Norbrook. Nerve blocking can be performed using lidocaine 2% (Vet One/MWI)[12] under veterinary supervision. The restrictions in organic dairies include 7-day milk withdrawal and a 90-day withdrawal period for animals going to slaughter.[23]

FINAL COMMENTS

Lameness is a significant multifactorial disorder affecting both organic and conventional dairy farms. In addition to detrimental effects on production, pain and distress associated with lameness are well-documented. Furthermore, the evaluation and prevalence of lame cattle is among the primary factors in third-party welfare audit programs.[12]

A significant proportion of the treatments used in organic dairies regarding the use of alternative medicine, minerals, and oils lack scientific evidence to support their therapeutic benefit. Therefore, the authors highly encourage the development of controlled trials in organic dairies to produce information regarding the usefulness, methodologies, and cure rates of the strategies presented here as well as others currently used by organic dairy farmers.

Although critical for both conventional and organic systems, due to limited therapeutic resources, early detection of lameness to improve cure rates is even more important in organic farms. It is critical that organic regulation includes a strict rule of not withholding treatment with a prohibited substance to maintain organic status if it causes the animal to suffer. In addition, a prompt decision to cull or euthanize is also an important component of treatment evaluation. Finally, a comprehensive lameness evaluation protocol should include periodic locomotion scoring of the complete cow population, determination of DD prevalence, consideration of percentage of cull and dead cows due to locomotion problems, and adequate record keeping, including counts of clinical cases.

REFERENCES

1. Goff SS, Dhuyvetter KC, Velez JS, et al. Measurable Indicators of Animal Welfare in Organic and Conventional Dairies in the United States. 16th IFOAM 2008 Organic World Congress, Modena, Italy. Available at: http://orgprints.org/view/projects/conference.html. Accessed April 26, 2017.

2. Rutherford K, Langford FM, Jack MC, et al. Lameness prevalence and risk factors in organic and non-organic dairy herds in the United Kingdom. Vet J 2009;180: 95–105.

3. Shearer JK, Plummer PJ, Schleining JA. Perspectives on the treatment of claw lesions in cattle. Vet Med 2015;6:273–92.

4. Biagiotti P. Practical organic dairy farming. Fort Atkinson (WI): WD Hoard &Sons Company; 2016.

5. Richert RM, Cicconi KM, Gamroth MJ, et al. Perceptions and risk factors for lameness on organic and small conventional dairy farms. J Dairy Sci 2013;96: 5018–26.

6. Guard C. Investigating herds with lameness problems. Vet Clin North Am Food Anim Pract 2001;17:175–87.

7. McNamara JP, Gay JM. Non-infectious diseases: acidosis/laminitis. In: Fuquay JW, editor. Encyclopedia of dairy sciences. 2nd edition. Elsevier Ltd; 2011. p. 199–205. Available at: http://doi.org/10.1016/B978-0-12-374407-4.00139-4. Accessed April 26, 2017.

8. Zwald AG, Ruegg PL, Kaneene JB, et al. Management practices and reported antimicrobial usage on conventional and organic dairy farms. J Dairy Sci 2004; 87:191–201.

9. Pol M, Ruegg PL. Treatment practices and quantification of antimicrobial drug usage in conventional and organic dairy farms in Wisconsin. J Dairy Sci 2007;90: 249–61.

10. Richert RM, Cicconi KM, Gamroth MJ, et al. Risk factors for clinical mastitis, ketosis, and pneumonia in dairy cattle on organic and small conventional farms in the United States. J Dairy Sci 2013;96:4269–85.

11. Shearer JK, Van Amstel SR, Brodersen BW. Clinical diagnosis of foot and leg lameness in cattle. Vet Clin North Am Food Anim Pract 2012;28(3):535–56.

12. USDA. Dairy 2007, Part IV: reference of dairy cattle health and management practices in the United States. Fort Collins (CO): USDA: APHIS: VS, CEAH; 2009.

13. Palmer MA, O'Connell NE. Digital dermatitis in dairy cows: a review of risk factors and potential sources of between-animal variation in susceptibility. Animals (Basel) 2015;5:512–35.

14. Relun A, Guatteo R, Roussel P, et al. A simple method to score digital dermatitis in dairy cows in the milking parlor. J Dairy Sci 2011;94:5424–34.

15. Döpfer D. The dynamics of digital dermatitis in dairy cattle and the manageable state of disease. In Proc. CanWest Veterinary Conference Banff, AB, Canada. Available at: http://www.hoofhealth.ca/Dopfer.pdf. Accessed April 26, 2017.

16. Leach KA, Whay HR, Maggs CM, et al. Working towards a reduction in cattle lameness: 1. Understanding barriers to lameness control on dairy farms. Res Vet Sci 2010;89:311–7.

17. Wells SJ, Trent AM, Marsh WE, et al. Prevalence and severity of lameness in lactating dairy cows in a sample of Minnesota and Wisconsin herds. J Am Vet Med Assoc 1993;202:78–82.
18. Stiglbauer KE, Cicconi-Hogan KM, Richert R, et al. Assessment of herd management on organic and conventional dairy farms in the United States. J Dairy Sci 2013;96:1290–300.
19. Schöpke K, Gomez A, Dunbar KA, et al. Investigating the genetic background of bovine digital dermatitis using improved definitions of clinical status. J Dairy Sci 2015;98:8164–74.
20. ODPG. Organic Management of lameness in Dairy Cows. Organic Dairy & Pastoral Group Inc. New Zealand. Avalilable at: http://www.organicpastoral.co.nz/Resources/Animal+Health/Lameness.html. Accessed April 26, 2017.
21. Pötzsch CJ, Hedges VJ, Blowey RW, et al. The impact of parity and duration of biotin supplementation on white line disease lameness in dairy cattle. J Dairy Sci 2003;86:2577–82.
22. Shearer JK, van Amstel SR. Functional and corrective claw trimming. Vet Clin North Am Food Anim Pract 2001;17:53–72.
23. OEFFA Certification. OEFFA approved products list for producers. Columbus (OH): OEFFA Certified Organic; 2016.
24. Leach K, Barker Z, Maggs C, et al. Activities of organic farmers succeeding in reducing lameness in dairy cows. Agric and Forest Res 2012;365:143–6. Available at: http://orgprints.org/21760/1/Leach_lameness_2OAHC_2012.pdf. Accessed April 26, 2017.
25. Shearer JK, Stock ML, Van Amstel SR, et al. Assessment and management of pain associated with lameness in cattle. Vet Clin North Am Food Anim Pract 2013;29:135–56.

An Update on the Assessment and Management of Pain Associated with Lameness in Cattle

Johann F. Coetzee, BVSc, Cert CHP, PhD[a],*, J.K. Shearer, DVM, MS[b],
Matthew L. Stock, VMD, PhD[b,c], Michael D. Kleinhenz, DVM[b,c],
Sarel R. van Amstel, BVSc, MMedVet[d]

KEYWORDS

• Cattle • Lameness • Analgesics • Corrective trimming

Lameness affects the cattle industry via both economic losses and welfare consider-ations. In addition to production deficits, the pain and distress associated with lame-ness have been documented.[1] Furthermore, the evaluation and prevalence of lame cattle are among the primary factors in third-party welfare audit programs, including the National Dairy FARM (Farmers Assuring Responsible Management) Program, Val-idus, and the New York State Cattle Health Assurance Program (NYSCHAP).[2–4] Invol-untary culling of lame cattle continues to be an important reason for losses in both the dairy and beef industries.[5,6] Mean lameness prevalence in herds has been reported to be as high as 33.7% and 36.8% in Wisconsin and the United Kingdom, respectively; however, in other survey studies, a less than 10% prevalence of lame cattle was re-ported by producers.[7–9] Note that lameness is usually underreported by producers compared with independent observers, potentially because of a decreased sensitivity in detecting lame cattle.[10,11]

This article originally appeared in *Veterinary Clinics of North America: Food Animal Practice*, Volume 29, Issue 1, March 2013. It has been updated to reflect new developments.
Disclosure: Dr J.F. Coetzee is supported by Agriculture and Food Research Initiative Competitive grant no. 2013-67015-21332 from the USDA National Institute of Food and Agriculture. Drs J.K. Shearer, M.L. Stock, M.D. Kleinhenz, and S.R. van Amstel have nothing to disclose.
^a Department of Anatomy and Physiology, College of Veterinary Medicine, Kansas State Uni-versity, 228 Coles Hall, 1710 Denison Ave, Manhattan, KS 66506, USA; ^b Department of Veter-inary Diagnostic and Production Animal Medicine, College of Veterinary Medicine, Iowa State University, 2203 Lloyd Vet Med Center, 1800 Christensen Drive, Ames, IA 50011, USA; ^c Department of Biomedical Science, College of Veterinary Medicine, Iowa State University, 2008 Vet Med, 1800 Christensen Drive, Ames, IA 50011, USA; ^d Department of Large Animal Clinical Sciences, College of Veterinary Medicine, The University of Tennessee, 2407 River Drive, Knoxville, TN 37996, USA
* Corresponding author.
E-mail address: jcoetzee@vet.k-state.edu

In efforts to improve earlier detection and treatment of lameness, locomotion scoring systems have been developed for routine use by farm employees.[12,13] It has been suggested that earlier analgesia treatment may aid in the alleviation of acute pain perception or in the mitigation of wind-up, which can lead to central sensitization.[14] Central sensitization is responsible for the observed pain-related behavioral changes through increased sensitivity of pain (hyperalgesia) and pain from nonpainful stimuli (allodynia).[14] Whay and colleagues[1] reported hyperalgesia in lame cattle compared with sound animals through significant decreases in nociceptive thresholds at the time of lameness detection and 28 days later, suggesting prolonged chronicity. Analgesic treatment difficulties in chronic lame cattle may be best explained through the aforementioned central sensitization based on current pain models. As a result, preemptive analgesia that is usually advocated is difficult, if not impossible, to implement in lame cattle.[14] Recommendations for pain management often include a multimodal approach. In lame cattle, pain can be best alleviated following a multimodal approach, including primarily corrective claw trimming and placement of foot blocks with additional benefits provided by analgesic compounds. Excerpts of this article were published in a previous edition of *Veterinary Clinics of North America Food Animal Practice*, but data were updated to include current research.[15]

ASSESSMENT OF PAIN IN LAME CATTLE
Locomotion or Lameness Scoring Systems

Behavioral changes associated with lameness indicate attempts by the animal to protect the affected limb from further injury.[16] Although these may vary between individual animals, signs such as head bobbing, an arching of the spine, or changes in stride length allow rapid identification of lame individuals.[16] Changes in posture associated with lameness have been summarized in an excellent review article by Whay[16] and form the basis of most locomotion scoring systems. An arched back is frequently associated with lameness and is the key behavioral change evaluated in the Sprecher lameness scoring system (1997) (**Table 1**).[12] Other behavioral changes associated with lameness that can be visually scored include[16]:

1. Hanging or bobbing of the head during locomotion
2. Shortening or lengthening of the stride
3. Changes in the degree of abduction or adduction of the limbs with an increased deviation from the vertical seen in 1 hind limb
4. Changes in claw placement (overextension or underextension of the stride) resulting in the hind claw not being placed in the same location as the front claw after initiation of the stride

Table 1	
Sprecher lameness scoring system	
LS	**Clinical Description**
1	Normal: stands and walks normally, with all feet placed with purpose
2	Mildly lame: stands with flat back, but arches when walks; gait is slightly abnormal
3	Moderately lame: stands and walks with an arched back, and short strides with 1 or more legs
4	Lame: arched back standing and walking, with 1 or more limbs favored but at least partially weight bearing
5	Severely lame: arched back, refuses to bear weight on 1 limb, may refuse or have great difficulty moving from lying position

5. Changes in the alignment of the pin bones (tuber coxae) when walking, which results in deviations from a hypothetical horizontal line when viewed from behind
6. Changes in the animal's willingness to walk, with a reluctance to move being frequently associated with lameness affecting multiple claws
7. Changes in the stance phase of the stride resulting in the animal maintaining its weight on the sound limb for as long as possible in order to minimize weight-bearing time on the lame limb

The extent to which the aforementioned changes occur can be assigned a score ranging from a simple binomial score (present or absent) to an ordinal scale based on the presence and perceived severity of 1 or more of these behavioral signs in the same animal. Ordinal data should be analyzed using appropriate statistical methods and should not be subjected to analysis using methods reserved for continuous data, such as paired t-tests.

In the future, visual analog scales (VASs) may become more widely used as an alternative to ordinal locomotion scoring methods in a research setting because these generate continuous data. This information is considered to provide more robust outcomes when analyzed statistically because traditional methods of assessment for continuous data, such as t-tests, can be used. The VAS is a 100-mm (10-cm) line anchored at either end by descriptors, typically "normal" or "lame" or, in humans, "no pain" or "worst pain imaginable."[13,17] The scorer marks the line between the 2 descriptors to indicate the lameness or pain intensity. A millimeter scale is used to measure the score from the zero anchor point to the scorer's mark. This system therefore potentially provides 101 levels of intensity that are considered more sensitive for assessing the effects of an analgesic compound than an ordinal scale. Lame cattle have been successfully identified using overall VAS scores with VAS assessment possessing reasonable intraobserver and interobserver reliability; however, a 5-point numeric rating score (NRS) provided a better estimate of hoof lesions.[13] Additional research is necessary for further evaluation and its potential application.

A deficiency of locomotion scoring systems creates the potential for a lack of reproducibility between scorers. This has limited the utility of locomotion scoring as a validated outcome measure for assessing analgesic efficacy during the drug approval process. In the author's experience (JFC), there is typically a 70% agreement between 2 masked scorers evaluating lameness using the Sprecher system. Furthermore, male scorers tend to assign lower pain scores compared with female scorers. These factors have necessitated the development of more objective methods of pain assessment involving the use of force plates or pressure mats.

VISUAL LAMENESS SCORING ALTERNATIVES

Researchers have investigated alternative lameness detection methods that allow convenient sampling to be performed by trained farm personnel. Hoffman and colleagues[18] described a method to detect lameness while cows are restrained in headlock stanchions. This system uses the cow's posture while restrained to detect cows that need to visit the hoof trimmer. Specific postures studied include arch back, cow-hocked, wide stance, and favoring limbs.[18] Additional researchers have further investigated this method as well as adapting these methods so they can be used by cow pushers in the milking parlor.[19] When these methods were tested against lesions found at trimming, they lacked sensitivity as lameness diagnostic tests.[19]

PRESSURE MATS

A commercially available floor mat–based pressure/force measurement system (MatScan, Tekscan, Inc, South Boston, MA) can be used to record and analyze naturally occurring or experimentally induced lameness. The pressure mat is calibrated daily and each time the computer software is engaged using a known mass to ensure accuracy of the measurements at each time point. Another benefit of this system is that video synchronization can be used to ensure consistent gait between and within calves for each time point and to correlate lameness scores (LSs) with pressure mat data. Research-grade software (HUGEMAT Research 5.83, Tekscan, Inc, South Boston, MA) is used to determine the contact pressure, contact area, and stance phase duration in the affected claws. Surface area is calculated by area only of the loaded or contact-sensing elements inside a measurement box. Contact pressure is calculated as force on the loaded sensing elements inside a measurement box divided by the contact area.[20]

Kotschwar and colleagues[20] found that contact surface area by Sprecher LS was different (P = .018) in calves subjected to induced lameness using amphotericin B. Calves with LS 1 had a greater surface area compared with LS 3 and 4 calves (**Fig. 1**). Furthermore, contact pressure was different across Sprecher LSs (P = .02), with calving classified as having an LS of 3 exerting greater ground contact pressure compared with that of LS 1 calves (**Fig. 2**). This finding was likely caused by the smaller contact surface area in calves with a higher LS.

Weighing Platform

Much like the difference detected in pressure mats for lame cattle, weight distributions of individual limbs have also been calculated using a weighing platform (Pacific

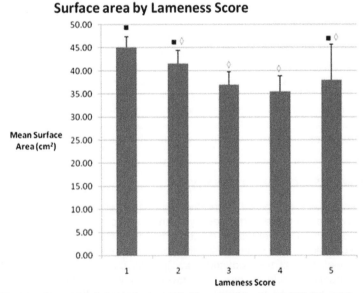

Fig. 1. Mean surface area plus or minus standard error of the mean (SEM) by LS for all treatment groups. Data points with different symbols indicate $P<.05$. (*From* Kotschwar JL, Coetzee JF, Anderson DE, et al. Analgesic efficacy of sodium salicylate in an amphotericin B-induced bovine synovitis-arthritis model. J Dairy Sci 2009;92:3740; with permission.)

Contact Pressure by Lameness Score

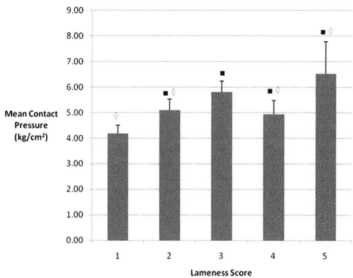

Fig. 2. Mean contact pressure plus or minus SEM by LS for all treatment groups. Data points with different symbols indicate *P*<.05. (*From* Kotschwar JL, Coetzee JF, Anderson DE, et al. Analgesic efficacy of sodium salicylate in an amphotericin B-induced bovine synovitis-arthritis model. J Dairy Sci 2009;92:3740; with permission.)

Industrial Scale Co Ltd, Richmond, British Columbia, Canada) containing 4 stainless steel load cells (3-mV Shear Beam Load cells, Anyload LLC, Santa Rosa, CA; maximum capacity = 454 kg/load cell).[21–25] Neveux and colleagues[21] first described the use of this weight platform to measure the redistributions of weight to cattle limbs that occurs in response to pain associated with lameness. These platforms indicate that cattle redistribute weight to avoid uncomfortable surfaces as well to distribute weight away from a limb with discomfort primarily toward the contralateral limb.[21] Following studies involving the use of this assessment technique, variations in weight distributions in lame animals were mildly attenuated through the use of analgesia, such as nonsteroidal antiinflammatory drugs (NSAIDs) or a local anesthetic.[23–25]

NOCICEPTIVE THRESHOLD

Because of a hyperalgesic state, it has been suggested lame cattle have a more sensitive and exaggerated reaction to noxious stimuli compared with sound animals.[1] Using a mechanical pneumatic blunt pin (2 mm in diameter) pressed on the dorsal aspect of the metatarsus with gradually increasing pressure, a reaction from the animal can be observed.[26,27] The pressure at which the reaction occurs has been recorded as the nociceptive threshold, thus presumably quantifying regional sensitivity and potentially pain. The results of this test may be related to other sensory perception rather than pain but Whay and colleagues[27] described the use of nociceptive threshold as a more sensitive measure of pain associated with lameness compared with a visual locomotion scoring technique. Increased nociceptive thresholds have been reported in cattle over a 28-day period following 3 days of ketoprofen administered at the detection of lameness[27]; however, this suggested long-term attenuation of the hyperalgesic state caused by the administration of NSAIDs was not observed in another study using nociceptive thresholds.[28]

Heart Rate

Heart rate data can be recorded and analyzed using commercially available heart rate monitors and the associated research software (RS800 and Polar Pro Trainer Equine Edition, Polar Electro, Inc, Lake Success, NY). The heart rate monitor consists of a transmitter placed over the heart in the left foreflank attached to a girth strap placed around the heart girth of the calves. A wrist unit attached to the elastic strap receives and records the signal from the transmitter. Appropriate conductance for the electrodes on the strap, 1 positioned on the sternum and 1 over the right scapula, is facilitated by use of ultrasonography gel. The transmitter measures the electric signal (electrocardiogram) of the heart every 15 seconds. Kotschwar and colleagues[20] found that mean heart rate was less in LS 1 calves compared with that of LS 2, 3, and 4 calves (**Fig. 3**).

Cortisol Response

Serum cortisol level can be determined using a solid-phase competitive chemiluminescent enzyme immunoassay and an automated analyzer system (Immulite 1000 Cortisol, Siemens Medical Solutions Diagnostics, Los Angeles, CA) or a radiolabeled immunoassay. Kotschwar and colleagues[20] reported that mean serum cortisol concentrations were less in LS 1 calves compared with LS 3 calves ($P = .004$) (**Fig. 4**).

Accelerometers

Accelerometers are devices that continuously measure gravitational force in multiple axes, and these values can be processed to determine activity and postural behaviors. Schulz and colleagues[29] reported that flunixin-treated steers spent a significantly

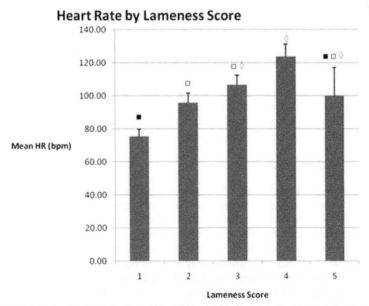

Fig. 3. Mean heart rate (HR) plus or minus SEM by LS for all treatment groups. Data points with different symbols indicate $P<.05$. (*From* Kotschwar JL, Coetzee JF, Anderson DE, et al. Analgesic efficacy of sodium salicylate in an amphotericin B-induced bovine synovitis-arthritis model. J Dairy Sci 2009;92:3739; with permission.)

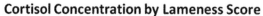

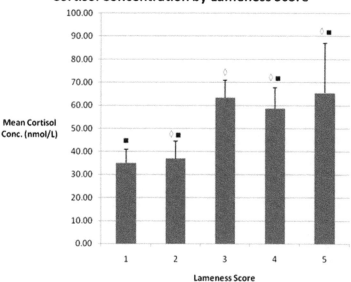

Fig. 4. Mean cortisol concentration (Conc.) plus or minus SEM by LS for all treatment groups. Data points with different symbols indicate $P<.05$. (*From* Kotschwar JL, Coetzee JF, Anderson DE, et al. Analgesic efficacy of sodium salicylate in an amphotericin B-induced bovine synovitis-arthritis model. J Dairy Sci 2009;92:3739; with permission.)

greater percentage of time standing after lameness induction with amphotericin B than the control calves in the initial postinduction period.

Pain Management Using Corrective Claw Trimming and Foot Blocks

Most people assume that the management of pain associated with lameness requires the use of some form of antiinflammatory therapy, whereas the discomfort caused by claw lesions can be dramatically reduced by corrective trimming techniques and the application of a foot block to the healthy claw. Beyond corrective trimming and the relief of weight bearing on injured claws are housing considerations whereby moving animals to pastures or special needs areas can increase the comfort of uncomfortable cows.

Pathogenesis of Claw Lesions

Ulcers and white line disease are largely consequences of metabolic disorders and the mechanical loading that contributes to injury of the solar and perioplic (corium of the heel) corium.[30] The metabolic conditions predisposing to claw lesions include rumen acidosis and laminitis; activation of metalloproteinases; and hormonal changes, specifically relaxin and estrogen in the peripartum period.[31–34] The mechanical loading occurs from the overgrowth of claw horn that leads to unbalanced weight bearing whereby the damage associated with metabolic disease disorders is compounded by excessive weight load.[35]

Traumatic lesions of the sole associated with penetration of the sole by foreign bodies such as a nail, stone, or other sharp object are a common cause of subsolar abscess formation. Depending on the depth of penetration, these types of lesions can have serious consequences. For example, when the foreign body is able to penetrate sufficiently deep to make contact with the third phalanx, a severe osteitis is likely to develop. In cases in which the foreign object penetrates only the more superficial tissues of the corium and digital cushion, the prognosis is more favorable.

Complicated lesions of the claw and/or foot that result in deep digital sepsis cause severe lameness and extreme discomfort for affected animals. The options for management of deep digital sepsis conditions include surgery and euthanasia. The key to minimizing pain is early recognition of the condition and prompt application of the most appropriate of these options, taking into consideration the likely prognosis, costs, and welfare of the animal.

Corrective Trimming to Relieve Pain and Promote Recovery from Claw Lesions

Cows with lameness disorders involving the claw capsule of the digit or claw generally require some degree of corrective trimming. This trimming consists of the removal of all necrotic and loose or undermined horn to create an aerobic microenvironment that reduces the possibility of further complication associated with abscess formation. When these procedures are conducted carefully to avoid damage to peripheral tissues of the corium, postprocedural pain is minimized and the rate of recovery is more rapid.[35–38]

A second step in the corrective trimming of claw lesions is to adjust weight bearing on diseased or damaged claws. This adjustment may be accomplished by trimming the weight-bearing surface of the injured claw lower and further by applying a foot block to the healthy claw.[35–38] By adjusting weight bearing on injured claws, pain is relieved and healing may proceed without interruption.

Although frequently used, topical treatment and the application of a bandage or wrap are generally not advised.[35–38] Exceptions to this include conditions in which corrective trimming has resulted in severe bleeding (should occur rarely) or the exposure of a large area of the corium for which protection of these delicate tissues is desired. Good restraint, local anesthesia as needed, and a sharp knife are the primary tools required for corrective trimming procedures.

Anesthesia of the Lower Limb and Foot

Whenever it is necessary to perform procedures that may be uncomfortable, anesthesia is indicated. There are at least 2 methods that may be used: intravenous regional anesthesia and ring block. Both procedures are easy to perform under field conditions. In addition to alleviating discomfort for the cow, anesthesia lessens movement of the foot associated with corrective trimming adjacent to sensitive tissues of the corium, which eases trimming procedures and reduces the potential for inadvertent movement by the cow that might lead to accidental damage of healthy tissues.

Intravenous regional and ring block anesthesia of the lower limb

Anesthesia of the foot is indicated for corrective trimming and surgical conditions that are likely to be uncomfortable. All that is required are a tourniquet, 20 to 30 mL of 2% lidocaine, and a 25-mm (1-inch) 19-gauge butterfly catheter. Veins used most commonly are those on the medial or lateral aspect of the digits (ie, medial and lateral digital veins, respectively) approximately 25 mm (1 inch) anterior to the dewclaws or the common digital vein, which lies on the dorsal aspect on the midline below the fetlock and between the digits.[36,38]

Intravenous regional anesthesia For anesthesia of the foot, begin by applying a tourniquet approximately 75 to 100 mm (3 to 4 inches) above the fetlock joint. Next, prepare the injection site by doing a light surgical scrub to clean the injection site areas.

Some clinicians prefer to shave these areas to improve asepsis. It is a good idea to prepare 2 sites (eg, the front and lateral or medial aspects) just in case a second site is needed. Once the site is prepared, remove the butterfly catheter from its package, along with the needle guard and end cap on the extension tube. Pick the desired site for introduction of the needle (note that the vein may not be visible, so the needle is often paced where the vein is likely to be). The needle is inserted rapidly and straight into the desired area (perpendicular to the skin, do not try to thread the needle into the vein) (**Fig. 5**). The cow may jerk or move her leg slightly as the needle is inserted. Next, slowly move the needle outward until blood flows into the catheter. As soon as there is a good flow of blood into the catheter, attach the syringe of lidocaine to the extension tube and administer it into the vein. It is best to inject the lidocaine over a period of 30 to 60 seconds to avoid damage to the vein. Complete anesthesia is usually accomplished within 3 to 5 minutes. In chronic cases in which there is extreme inflammation; anesthesia may require a larger dose of lidocaine (30 mL) and a little longer for complete anesthesia. The tourniquet should not be left in place longer than 45 minutes, and less if possible. Anesthesia is short-lived once the tourniquet is removed.

On release from the trimming chute, the cow will have immediate use of the foot and will walk noticeably better (ie, without lameness, assuming the problem was in the foot), making it tempting to think the problem has been remedied by the treatment just performed. Although some of the improvement may be a result of the treatment, anesthesia masks much of the discomfort until its effects have worn off, which usually occurs over a period of 30 to 60 minutes beyond removal of the tourniquet.

Ring block anesthesia The ring block generally requires more lidocaine and a little more time for complete anesthesia. There are 4 sites for injection of the lidocaine. First, on the midline of the dorsal aspect of the digit below the fetlock joint; place a 38-mm (1.5-inch) needle directly (anterior to posterior) into this region to the hub and inject approximately 15 to 20 mL as the needle is withdrawn, being sure to deposit approximately 2 mL subcutaneously. Do the same on the posterior or ventral aspect by placement of a 38-mm needle into the skin fold or crease (between the digits) and inject 15 to 20 mL of lidocaine as the needle is withdrawn. The final 2 injections are on the medial and lateral aspects of the lower leg just above the dewclaws: inject 10 to

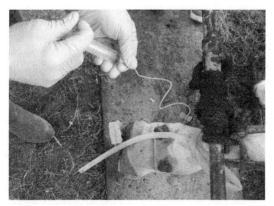

Fig. 5. Intravenous regional anesthesia with a tourniquet and 20 mL of lidocaine administered using 19-gauge butterfly catheter. (*From* Shearer JK, Stock ML, van Amstel SR, et al. Assessment and management of pain associated with lameness in cattle. Vet Clin North Amer Food Animal Practice 2013;29(1):135–56; with permission.)

15 mL of lidocaine subcutaneously going from anterior to posterior, beginning approximately 50 mm (2 inches) dorsal to the dewclaws.[36,38] Complete anesthesia may require a little longer than that achieved by the intravenous route, depending on how much the blood supply to the affected areas has been compromised by the inflammatory response. A tourniquet is unnecessary for this procedure.

Application of Corrective Trimming Procedures

In Toussaint Raven's[35] book, *Cattle Footcare and Claw Trimming*, he describes the principles of corrective hoof trimming as:

1. The removal of all loose and/or undermined, necrotic horn tissue without causing damage to adjacent healthy tissues
2. Adjustment of weight bearing within and between the claws by raising the affected area of the injured or diseased claw so that it does not bear weight

The primary claw lesions are ulcers, white line disease, and traumatic lesions of the sole. Regardless of cause, they are all treated by the application of these principles of corrective trimming.

Removal of loose and undermined claw horn

Whenever claw horn lesions are encountered, the first step is removal of all loose horn, irrespective of how extensive it might be. Pare away hard ridges to create smooth surfaces to reduce the tendency for the collection or entrapment of organic matter in horn lesions. Only healthy hoof horn should be left in place.

Always slope horn away from the lesion; never dig holes in the sole, because these are quickly filled by organic matter that prevents or delays healing. For example, trim the area around sole ulcers and slope the sole axially. When trimming white line lesions, slope the lesion abaxially and remove portions of the lateral wall, white line, and sole that are defective. Trim carefully and try not to damage new healthy horn. In all cases, avoid damage to the corium (ie, stop when trimming leads to bleeding of the corium).

Adjust weight bearing on damaged claws

When confronted with claw lesions, pare the damaged claw lower to increase weight bearing on the healthy claw. In most cases the diseased claw is the outside claw of the rear feet and medial claw of the front feet. Specific indications for this trimming procedure include conditions in which overgrowth has led to overloading or excessive weight bearing on the claw. Lowering the damaged claw reduces weight bearing and thus pain, and permits recovery and eventual return to normal function and health. In many cases it is necessary to apply a claw block to the healthy claw in order to achieve reduced weight bearing in the damaged claw. The details of claw block application are described later.

Foot Blocks for Relief of Weight Bearing in Diseased or Injured Claws

The application of corrective trimming procedures as described earlier often provides a sufficient difference in height between the two claws to relieve weight bearing and promote recovery of claw lesions. However, when pain is severe or it is not possible to create sufficient difference in height between the two claws, additional elevation of the diseased claw can be achieved by means of a block attached to the sound claw. Proper application of claw blocks requires attention to the following[35–38]:

1. Before attaching a block to the healthy claw, the claw must be pared flat and in the same plane as the corresponding injured claw. When claws have been trimmed by

the functional trimming method, claws are already flat, ready (or nearly ready) for the application of a foot block. This flat surface provides a bearing surface that is perpendicular to the long axis of the leg.

2. Prepare the claw with a rasp or angle grinder fitted with a grinding wheel or sandpaper-type disc so that the block adhesive properly adheres to the wall and sole of the claw.
3. Mix the adhesive to the proper consistency and apply to the block and claw as needed. Follow the manufacturer's directions for proper use of adhesives.
4. Apply the block and position it so that it lies flat on the sole and provides proper support of the heel. This is one of the most common mistakes made in applying blocks. Blocks should be even with the back of the heel bulb in order to provide sufficient support.
5. Always ensure that adhesive is cleared away from the area between the block and the heel. Heel horn is soft and can easily be damaged by the hard and sometimes sharp edges of fully cured adhesive material.
6. Remove blocks after a period of 3 to 4 weeks. Blocks that are wearing abnormally or cause discomfort before then should be removed sooner. Encourage owners, managers, and/or employees to pull cows that are not walking correctly on blocked claws. Note that foot blocks generally wear faster at the heel. Furthermore, as the claw grows, the block tends to gradually move forward. The wear at the heel and continued claw horn growth result in upward rotation of the toe of the blocked claw. Excess weight bearing and continued trauma to the heel may lead to the formation of a sole or heel ulcer. It is for this reason that readers are advised to monitor claw blocks and recheck no later than 30 days after application (sooner in conditions in which block wear is more rapid).
7. After removing a block, always retrim the foot and adjust weight bearing as needed. Foot blocks are a critical adjunct to the therapy for claw lesions; however, they require management by observation and changing as necessary. One scenario is to use a foot block to treat acute claw lesions that result in lameness during the first 30 days. After this time, recheck the foot and remove the claw block, retrim the claws, and adjust weight bearing in the damaged claw by lowering the damaged portion.

The Application of Bandages or Wraps to Lesions of the Claw Capsule

Correction of horn lesions often results in small to moderate exposure of the corium. In general, minor lesions or injuries to the corium are best left untreated and without a bandage. Severe lesions in which large areas of the corium may be exposed may benefit from topical treatment with a mild antiseptic or nonirritating antibiotic under a bandage with the proviso that it be removed within 3 to 5 days. If it is the practice of the dairy to allow bandages to fall off on their own, they should probably be left off from the start. Results from a Cornell study comparing cows with claw lesions with a wrap versus no wrap indicate no advantage to the application of bandage.[39]

The environment of most dairy cows is such that bandages become very contaminated within a day or so of application. It is doubtful that they offer significant therapeutic benefit beyond this point. A second problem with bandages in herds using footbaths is that after 1 or 2 trips through the footbath, the bandage becomes soaked with footbath solutions. These solutions are generally very irritating types of formulations (eg, formaldehyde and copper sulfate) and prone to causing increased irritation to raw corium tissues.

In contrast, antibiotics under a loose wrap are very effective for treatment of infectious skin disorders such as digital dermatitis.[36–38] Lesions treated with topical oxytetracycline under a bandage seem to respond rapidly, with cows showing improved gait and pain relief within 24 hours of treatment. The improvement following treatment of digital dermatitis with topical antibiotics shows the value of properly directed therapy whereby antibiotics are used to treat an infectious skin disease. Claw lesions in cows are unlikely to respond to topical antibiotic therapy because their pathogenesis is related to metabolic and mechanical factors rather than infectious agents.

Topical Therapy for Claw Lesions: Why or Why Not?

Claw lesions are very painful conditions that generally cause clinicians to conclude that some form of topical treatment and a bandage are essential parts of therapy. In reality, as described earlier, it is likely that treatment beyond corrective trimming and a foot block is counterproductive.

The best way to understand why it may not be beneficial to aggressively treat claw lesions is to consider their pathogenesis. For example, sole ulcers are lesions that develop as a consequence of the sinking of the third phalanx (P3) within the claw horn capsule after laminitis, activated metalloproteinase enzymes, or hormonal changes. Regardless of cause, the sinking of P3 results in compression of the solar corium and digital cushion immediately beneath P3, which is exacerbated by claw horn overgrowth, particularly of the outside claw of the rear foot. After a period of time and with continued trauma to these tissues, the formation of horn at the heel-sole junction (described as the typical site for sole ulcers) is interrupted. This interruption is the start of the development of a sole ulcer. Eventually, the ulcer becomes sufficiently inflamed to cause pain and lameness, which prompts the evaluation and discovery of the lesion during the course of trimming. The point is that ulcers are not caused by infectious organisms; they are caused by conditions (such as laminitis) that predispose to the sinking of P3 and physical trauma to the corium, complicated by excessive weight bearing.

White line disease frequently results in abscess formation, so it is reasonable to ask why antibiotics are not an essential part of therapy in this instance. There are essentially 2 types of bacteria responsible for lesions in dairy cows: anaerobic (bacteria that require little or no oxygen for life) and aerobic (bacteria that require oxygen for life). The bacteria that commonly cause abscesses in cattle claw disorders are anaerobes. They require, and thrive, in those conditions (inside the abscess) in which they become sealed off from exposure to air, and particularly oxygen. As long as they are able to maintain themselves within this microenvironment they continue to multiply and in the process expand the size of their environment (continue to undermine claw horn). The abscess capsule in which they reside continues to enlarge and in the process does more and more damage as long as it remains enclosed. The single most important factor in managing abscesses caused by white line disease or sole ulcers is to remove all loose and damaged horn; this changes the microenvironment from an oxygen-deprived to an oxygen-rich environment, thereby eliminating anaerobic bacteria and preventing further abscess development.

When topical treatment under a wrap is deemed necessary, readers are encouraged to read label directions on guidance for such applications. Avoid using topical medications that are not intended for use under a bandage or wrap. If necessary, only nonirritating types of antibiotics or other compounds should be used. In summary, when considering treatment of claw lesions, the best rule is, quite logically: do not do anything to a cow's foot that you would not do to your own.

Housing Considerations for Cows with Lameness Disorders

In deciding on follow-up care for a lame animal it is important to consider the severity of the animal's condition, its mobility, distance from the trim chute and hospital, and possible complications for the animal if returned to its pen of origin. For example, for a lactating cow it is important to consider the distance and number of times per day it must walk to and from the milking parlor. If returned to the pen of origin, will the animal be able to comfortably use a stall? Will it be able to lie down and rise without complication? Is it likely to become the victim of bullying by others within the group? Care during the convalescence period has a significant influence on treatment outcome.

Some of the obstacles presented by stalls can be overcome by moving animals to areas, such as pasture (when weather permits), dry lot, or a bedded pack, where natural behaviors associated with lying down and rising are unrestricted. Canadian researchers found that lame cows offered a 4-week period on pasture had improved gait scores, despite spending less time lying down.[40] These results indicate that moving lame cows to pasture can help lame cattle recover, in part because it provides them a more comfortable surface for recovery from hoof and leg injuries. Barberg and colleagues[41] reported improved foot and leg health whereby the prevalence of lameness in compost barns was 7.8% (locomotion score, ≥ 3), with 2 herds having no lame cows.

Behavioral observations by Endres and Barberg[42] of 147 cows in 12 compost barns included that cows moved freely on the bedded pack and assumed all natural lying positions. Observations of social interactions from a total of 96 continuous hourly observations included that chasing and pushing behaviors occurred 0.94 times per hour and head butting 1.4 times per hour. Positive interactions such as grooming and social licking occurred 2.3 times per hour. Researchers concluded that these interactions were very similar to the kind of behaviors they expected to observe on pasture.

In either case, lame cow areas or pens should be within close proximity to the milking parlor to reduce the distance animals are required to walk each day. Flooring surfaces should be clean and secure to prevent slipping. Properly textured surfaces or rubber flooring may improve comfort and also footing. It is also advantageous to house lame cows near the hospital, where animals can be observed and treated more conveniently by health and foot care personnel. A trim chute should also be located near these areas so that animals may be examined or retreated as needed.

PAIN MANAGEMENT OF LAMENESS USING ANALGESIA

In addition to the management of pain associated with lameness through corrective trimming and foot blocks, a multimodal approach using analgesics such as local anesthetics, NSAIDs, and sedative-analgesics may be beneficial to lame cattle. As observed with the management of other painful procedures, a multimodal approach provides the best pain management strategy. In the case of lame cattle, this approach includes the use of pharmaceuticals together with the use of corrective foot trimming with foot blocks as detailed earlier.

A review of publications revealed a scant number of controlled studies investigating the effects of analgesic compounds on cattle lameness. The literature was identified on PubMed or Web of Science databases using the search terms "Lame" and "Bovine" and "Analgesia." Two types of studies emerged following examination of the published material. The first type of study involved mostly field trials with animal recruitment occurring via lameness detected by the use of a visual locomotion scoring system (NRS) in lactating adult dairy cattle (**Table 2**).[23–25,27,28,43,44] Additional studies induced lameness in cattle via an intra-articular injection of amphotericin B in the distal interphalangeal joint, resulting in a transient lameness (**Table 3**).[20,29] Amphotericin B is a polyene antimicrobial that is primarily used as an antifungal but following an intra-articular injection causes an aseptic synovitis as a result of disrupting lysosomes

Table 2
Summary of the scientific literature examining the effect of analgesic drug administration on cattle lameness detected by a visual locomotion score

Reference	Lameness Recruitment	Study Population	Analgesic Regimen	Outcome Parameter	Change (%)	Significance
Whay et al,[27] 2005	Detected by a visual locomotion score	Adult cattle dairy	Ketoprofen 3 mg/kg IM administered for 3d, 1 h before locomotion score and nociception threshold testing	Locomotion score (1 d)	-14.29	NS
				Locomotion score (3 d)	-20.00	NS
				Locomotion score (8 d)	100.00	NS
				Locomotion score (28 d)	50.00	NS
				Nociceptive threshold (1 d)	0.00	NS
				Nociceptive threshold (3 d)	13.64	NS
				Nociceptive threshold (8 d)	14.44	NS
				Nociceptive threshold (28 d)	15.22	NS
Rushen et al,[25] 2006	Detected by a visual locomotion score	Adult cattle dairy	Lidocaine local anesthetic (palmar digital nerves medial and lateral; 2 mL each site)	Locomotion score	-7.75	NR
				Weight distribution (SD)	-55.56	<0.05
Flower et al,[43] 2008	Detected by a visual locomotion score	Adult cattle dairy	Ketoprofen 0.3 mg/kg IM administered 1 h before gait assessment	Locomotion score	-128.57	NS
				Gait attributes (VAS) (ie, back arch, tracking up, joint flexion, asymmetric steps, head bob, reluctance to bear weight)	3.00	NS
			Ketoprofen 1.5 mg/kg administered 1 h (IM) or 15 min (IV) before gait assessment	Locomotion score	-185.71	NS
				Gait attributes (VAS) (ie, back arch, tracking up, joint flexion, asymmetric steps, head bob, reluctance to bear weight)	-17.98	NS
			Ketoprofen 3.0 mg/kg IM administered 1 h (IM) and 15 min (IV) before gait assessment	Locomotion score	-357.14	<0.05
				Gait attributes (VAS) (ie, back arch, tracking up, joint flexion, asymmetric steps, head bob, reluctance to bear weight)	149.86	NS

Study	Detection	Animal	Intervention	Outcome measure	Value	Significance
Laven et al,[28] 2008	Detected by a visual locomotion score and confirmed by veterinarian to have only noninfectious foot disease	Adult cattle dairy	Corrective trimming and tolfenamic acid 2 mg/kg	Nociceptive threshold (3 d)	25.00	NS
				Nociceptive threshold (8 d)	0.00	NS
				Nociceptive threshold (28 d)	0.00	NS
				Nociceptive threshold (100 d)	0.00	NS
				Locomotion score (3 d)	20.00	NS
				Locomotion score (8 d)	0.00	NS
				Locomotion score (28 d)	0.00	NS
				Locomotion score (100 d)	−11.11	NS
			Corrective trimming & tolfenamic acid 2 mg/kg & plastic shoe placed on the contralateral claw of the affected foot to elevate lesion from weight bearing	Nociceptive threshold (3 d)	0.00	NS
				Nociceptive threshold (8 d)	0.00	NS
				Nociceptive threshold (28 d)	0.00	NS
				Nociceptive threshold (100 d)	0.00	NS
				Locomotion score (3 d)	20.00	NS
				Locomotion score (8 d)	0.00	NS
				Locomotion score (28 d)	0.00	NS
				Locomotion score (100 d)	0.00	NS
Chapinal et al,[23] 2010	Detected by a visual locomotion score	Adult cattle dairy	Ketoprofen 3.0 mg/kg IM once daily for 2 d administered 2 h before gait scoring and measures of weight distributions	Locomotion score	NR	NS
				Weight distribution (SD)	18.00	<0.01
				Activity (ie, lying %, frequency of lying bouts, frequency of steps)	NR	NS
Chapinal et al,[24] 2010	Detected by a visual locomotion score	Adult cattle dairy	Flunixin meglumine 2.2 mg/kg IV once daily for 2 d administered immediately before hoof trimming on the first day and 2 h before gait scoring and measures of weight distributions	Locomotion score (VAS) (analgesia: 24 h)	1030.00	NS
				Locomotion score (VAS) (analgesia: 48 h)	−167.28	NS
				Weight distribution of rear legs (SD) (analgesia: 24 h)	47,200.00	<0.10
				Weight distribution of rear legs (SD) (analgesia: 48 h)	215.46	NS
				Rear leg weight ratio (analgesia: 24 h)	−166.67	NS
				Rear leg weight ratio (analgesia: 48 h)	1030.00	NS
				Daily lying time (analgesia: 48 h)	2.09	NS
				Daily lying time (24 h postanalgesia)	−113.69	<0.10
				Frequency of steps (analgesia: 48 h)	−80.30	NS
				Frequency of steps (24 h postanalgesia)	−140.62	NS

(continued on next page)

Table 2
(continued)

Reference	Lameness Recruitment	Study Population	Analgesic Regimen	Outcome Parameter	Change (%)	Significance
Rizk et al,[44] 2012	Lame cattle diagnosed with a sole ulcer referred to tertiary referral hospital for surgical claw treatment	Adult cattle dairy	Xylazine (0.05 mg/kg) IM 15 min before placement in lateral recumbency and 20 min before local anesthesia of 20 mL of 2% procaine at the start of claw surgery	Heart rate (15 min)	−27.91	<0.001
				Heart rate (lateral recumbency)	−20.00	<0.001
				Heart rate (1 h postoperative)	−2.50	NS
				Heart rate (3 h postoperative)	3.75	NS
				Respiratory rate (15 min)	−57.45	<0.01
				Respiratory rate (lateral recumbency)	−38.00	0.01
				Respiratory rate (1 h postoperative)	−21.43	NS
				Respiratory rate (3 h postoperative)	−26.53	NS
				Cortisol (15 min)	−57.72	<0.01
				Cortisol (lateral recumbency)	4.16	NS
				Cortisol (1 h postoperative)	6.40	NS
				Cortisol (3 h postoperative)	11.76	NS
				Locomotion score (1 h)	−25.00	<0.05
				Locomotion score (2 h)	−6.25	NS
				Locomotion score (3 h)	−3.23	NS
				Pedometer standing (1 h)	106.78	<0.01
				Pedometer standing (2 h)	63.52	NS
				Pedometer standing (3 h)	34.45	NS

Percentage change was calculated using the formula [(mean of analgesic group/mean of control group) − 1] × 100. The outcome parameter Locomotion Score was determined by a 5-point NRS unless otherwise noted as VAS, indicating the use of a 100-unit VAS.

Abbreviations: IM, intramuscularly; IV, intravenously; NR, values were not reported; NS, not significant; SD, standard deviation.

Table 3
Summary of the scientific literature examining the effect of analgesic drug administration following an amphotericin B–induced lameness model

Reference	Lameness Recruitment	Study Population	Analgesic Regimen	Outcome Parameter	Change (%)	Significance
Kotschwar et al,[20] 2009	Induced: amphotericin B (20 mg) injected lateral distal interphalangeal joint of hind limb	4–6 mo beef	Sodium salicylate 50 mg/kg IV administered 4 min after arthritis induction model	Cortisol (AUEC)	9.35	NS
				Surface area (cm²) (AUEC)	3.51	NS
				Contact pressure (AUEC)	−1.17	NS
				Stance phase duration (AUEC)	−0.88	NS
				Heart rate (AUEC)	20.30	NS
				Electrodermal activity (AUEC)	0.53	NS
			Sodium salicylate 50 mg/kg IV administered 4 min and 24 h after arthritis induction model	Cortisol (AUEC)	3.93	NS
				Surface area (cm²) (AUEC)	8.67	NS
				Contact pressure (AUEC)	−5.47	NS
				Stance phase duration (AUEC)	4.07	NS
				Heart rate (AUEC)	11.25	NS
				Electrodermal activity (AUEC)	−1.23	NS
Schulz et al,[29] 2011	Induced: amphotericin B (20 mg) injected lateral distal interphalangeal joint of hind limb	Adult cattle beef	Flunixin meglumine 1 mg/kg IV administered immediately and 12 h after synovitis-arthritis induction	Cortisol	NR	P = .13
				Visual lameness score (probability of having a score >0)	−55.86	<0.05
				Lying % (days 0 and 1)*	−18.42	<0.01
				Lying % (days 2 and 3)*	−0.79	NS
				Pressure Mat Analysis		
				Arthritis-synovitis induced limb: maximum force	24.54	P = .03
				Arthritis-synovitis induced limb: mean force	28.38	P = .05
				Arthritis-synovitis induced limb: mean area	25.42	P = .04
				Arthritis-synovitis induced limb: impulse	51.28	P = .06
				Arthritis-synovitis induced claw: maximum force	26.27	P = .02
				Arthritis-synovitis induced claw: mean force	48.51	P = .01
				Arthritis-synovitis induced claw: mean area	39.41	P = .01
				Arthritis-synovitis induced claw: impulse	73.66	P = .03

* Percentage change was calculated using the formula [(Mean of analgesic group/Mean of control group) − 1] × 100.
Abbreviation: AUEC, area under the effect curve.

and release of inflammatory mediators within the synovial tissue.[45] This model for lameness has historical reference in studies involving equine lameness.[45]

Behavioral, physiologic, and neuroendocrine changes have been reported in the studies evaluating the pain associated with lameness. In general, antiinflammatories such as flunixin meglumine have shown substantial acute analgesia in induced lameness models shown through modifications of gait and improved pressures placed on the affected foot and claw; however, in field trials, antiinflammatories have yielded variable results, with mild improvement to locomotion score and nociceptive thresholds. An inconsistent translation from induced lameness models to clinical field trials may be a result of clinical heterogeneity present in different cases of clinical lameness, the sensitivity of experiments to detect differences in analgesic-treated animals, or the potential for the central sensitization from pain noted to occur in lame cattle resulting in animals being more refractory to pain management.[1,14] Additional studies are necessary to further evaluate pharmacologic analgesia in mitigating the pain associated with lameness using both induced lameness models and field studies. The evaluation of additional analgesic compounds and the development of methods with improved sensitivity to detecting changes associated with the provision of analgesia are paramount to further pain management in lame cattle.

Local Anesthetics

Lidocaine
Rushen and colleagues[25] evaluated the analgesic effects of lidocaine in adult lactating cattle following lameness detection via a 5-point locomotion score. Following the administration of local anesthesia, gait scores were reduced (0.3) but significance was not reported. The variance (standard deviation) observed in weight bearing between the affected limb and the contralateral limb was significantly reduced following the administration of lidocaine. Therefore, the use of a local anesthetic such as lidocaine reduces gait scores and affects the distribution of weight acutely.

Nonsteroidal Antiinflammatory

Ketoprofen
The NSAID ketoprofen has been evaluated in multiple clinical field trials to determine its analgesia effectiveness on the pain mitigation of lameness in cattle.[23,27,43] In all studies, adult lactating dairy cattle were detected as lame using a locomotion scoring technique before enrollment into the study.[13] Following ketoprofen administration of a gradually increasing dose with a maximum dose of 3 mg/kg, mild improvements were observed in gait attributes, including an increased number of symmetric steps and a more even weight distribution among all 4 limbs.[43] Moreover, a reduced variation in weight distribution has also been reported following administration of ketoprofen analgesia.[23] Based on the results of a numerical rating scale, locomotion score mildly improved (0.25 ± 0.05); however, this improvement should be interpreted with caution because this value is similar to the reported resolution of the scoring system used.[43] Nociceptive threshold was tested 4 times over 28 days, indicating acute and chronic improvements following ketoprofen administration for the first 3 days; however, this increase was not significantly different than placebo-treated controls on each nociceptive threshold test day.[27] Ketoprofen was also shown to result in a sound LS 35 days after an acute lameness episode when given as part of a trim and block treatment regimen.[46] However, when given as a preemptive analgesic to acutely lame cattle before corrective trimming, ketoprofen failed to alleviate stress results.[47]

Flunixin meglumine

The analgesic efficacy of intravenously administered flunixin meglumine (1 mg/kg) in an amphotericin B–induced lameness model was evaluated.[29] Compared with untreated controls, animals receiving flunixin meglumine at the time of lameness induction and 12 hours following were less likely to be lame as determined by a locomotion score, and placed more pressure and surface area contact on pressure mats with the affected foot as well as the contralateral claw of the affected foot. In addition, treated cattle were recumbent less than untreated controls on the day of induction and the following day; however, lying percentage was not different after the first day. Although cortisol levels were not significantly different ($P = .13$), the investigators state that untreated control cattle generally had increased cortisol concentrations compared with those treated with flunixin meglumine. Results from this study suggest the acute analgesic properties of flunixin meglumine in a lameness model in cattle.

In addition, analgesic properties of flunixin meglumine were evaluated in a clinical trial using lame cattle detected by locomotion scoring.[24] Lame cattle were administered flunixin meglumine (2.2 mg/kg) immediately before corrective hoof trimming and 24 hours following the first treatment. Gait scores as determined by a VAS and weight distribution were not significantly affected by the provision of analgesia; however, a prolonged increase in daily lying time was observed in untreated controls compared with those administered flunixin meglumine. In addition, a mild significant reduction in variation (standard deviation [SD]) of weight distribution of the rear legs was observed following analgesia administration, as observed acutely with lidocaine or ketoprofen administration.[23,25]

Salicylic acid derivatives

In an amphotericin B–induced lameness model of steers 4 to 6 months old, sodium salicylate (50 mg/kg) administered intravenously was investigated for its potential analgesic efficacy.[20] Following analgesic treatment at the time of lameness induction and 24 hours postinduction, cortisol concentrations and pressure mat measurements, including contact pressure and surface area, percentage standing, heart rate, electrodermal activity, and LS, were examined for analgesic effects. Analyses of the data indicate no overall differences between salicylate-treated and placebo-treated animals, indicating its ineffectiveness at providing analgesia to a lameness model in cattle.

Tolfenamic acid

Although not approved for use in the United States, tolfenamic acid, an NSAID in the anthranilic acid class, was evaluated for analgesic potential in lame cattle in a New Zealand field study.[28] Cattle were enrolled into the study by farm staff detection of lameness and confirmation by a veterinarian. Only animals with noninfectious foot disease were included (ie, white line disease and sole penetration) and corrective trimming was performed on all cattle. Evaluations of nociceptive threshold and gait scores were recorded on days 1, 3, 8, 28, and 100, with treated cows receiving tolfenamic acid (2 mg/kg) and/or a foot block. All cows showed improvement over time in nociceptive threshold and gait scores; however, no significant differences were reported in either the acute or chronic period following treatment with tolfenamic acid compared with the untreated controls. All cattle had access to pasture following treatment, which may have resulted in an improved response in the control cattle.

Meloxicam

Meloxicam is an NSAID that is not approved in the United States but has approval in Canada and Europe. The pharmacokinetics of oral meloxicam have been investigated, including tissue residue profiling.[48] Meloxicam has been shown to improve LSs when given orally at doses between 0.5 and 1 mg/kg.[49,50] Cattle undergoing resection of the distal interphalangeal joint had improved LSs and lower cortisol levels compared with control cattle.[48]

Sedative-Analgesic Drugs

Xylazine

The analgesic effect of xylazine was examined in one study evaluating adult cattle referred to a university hospital for claw surgery.[44] Animals were administered either xylazine (0.05 mg/kg, intramuscularly) or a placebo treatment. Following placement into lateral recumbency on a surgery tipping table, regional anesthesia was performed of the affected limb using procaine 2%, and surgery of the affected claw was initiated. As expected with administration of an α_2-adrenergic agonist, heart rate and respiratory rate were reduced in the acute period. In addition, cortisol level was significantly decreased for xylazine-treated cattle compared with placebo-treated cattle during the initial 15 minutes following xylazine administration; however, no differences were observed at later time points. Modifications were observed acutely to gait and behavior as well. Xylazine-treated animals stood longer and had reduced gait scores in the first hour compared with placebo-treated animals, suggesting the provision of acute analgesia. This change was not observed after 2 or more hours.

Gabapentin

Gabapentin [1-(aminomethyl) cyclohexane acetic acid] is a gamma-aminobutyric acid (GABA) analogue originally developed for the treatment of spastic disorders and epilepsy.[51] Studies have reported that gabapentin is also effective for the management of chronic pain of inflammatory of neuropathic origin.[52] It has also been reported that gabapentin can interact synergistically with NSAIDs to produce antihyperalgesic effects.[52] The pharmacokinetics of gabapentin suggest that this compound may be useful in mitigating chronic neuropathic and inflammatory pain in ruminant cattle.[53] In a study conducted by our research group, administration of gabapentin at 15 mg/kg combined with meloxicam at 0.5 mg/kg once daily for 4 days increased the amount of force applied on the lame claw in calves subjected to an experimental lameness model. Stride length was also improved in calves that received gabapentin combined with meloxicam compared with placebo-treated controls. Further studies are needed to investigate the utility of gabapentin as an adjunctive therapy in the treatment of pain associated with lameness.

REFERENCES

1. Whay HR, Waterman AE, Webster AJF, et al. The influence of lesions type on the duration of hyperalgesia associated with hindlimb lameness in dairy cattle. Vet J 1998;156:23–9.
2. National Dairy FARM Program: farmers assuring responsible management. 2012. Available at: http://www.nationaldairyfarm.com/. Accessed December 27, 2016.
3. Validus Ventures, LLC. 2012. Available at: http://www.validusservices.com/. Accessed September 13, 2012.
4. NYS Department of Agriculture and Markets, New York State Cattle Health Assurance Program (NYSCHAP). 2002. Available at: http://nyschap.vet.cornell.edu/. Accessed December 27, 2016.
5. Cattle and calves non-predator death loss in the United States, 2010. USDA-APHIS National Animal Health Monitoring System; 2011.

6. Dairy 2007: facility characteristics and cow comfort on U.S. dairy operations, 2007. USDA-APHIS National Animal Health Monitoring System; 2010.

7. Cook NB. Prevalence of lameness among dairy cattle in Wisconsin as a function of housing type and stall surface. J Am Vet Med Assoc 2003;223:1324–8.

8. Barker ZE, Leach KA, Whay HR, et al. Assessment of lameness prevalence and associated risk factors in dairy herds in England and Wales. J Dairy Sci 2010;93: 932–41.

9. Fulwider WK, Grandin T, Rollin BE, et al. Survey of dairy management practices on one hundred thirteen North Central and Northeastern United States dairies. J Dairy Sci 2008;91:1686–92.

10. Wells SJ, Trent AM, Marsh WE, et al. Prevalence and severity of lameness in lactating dairy cows in a sample of Minnesota and Wisconsin herds. J Am Vet Med Assoc 1993;202:78–82.

11. Whay HR, Main DCJ, Green LE, et al. Assessment of the welfare of dairy cattle using animal-based measurements: direct observations and investigation of farm records. Vet Rec 2003;153:197–202.

12. Sprecher DJ, Hostetler DE, Kaneene JB. A lameness scoring system that uses posture and gait to predict dairy cattle reproductive performance. Theriogenology 1997;47:1179–87.

13. Flower FC, Weary DM. Effect of hoof pathologies on subjective assessments of dairy cow gait. J Dairy Sci 2006;89:139–46.

14. Anderson DE, Muir WM. Pain management in cattle. Vet Clin North Am Food Anim Pract 2005;21:623–35.

15. Shearer JK, Stock ML, Van Amstel SR, et al. Assessment and management of pain associated with lameness in cattle. Vet Clin North Am Food Anim Pract 2013;29(1):135–56.

16. Whay HR. Locomotion scoring and lameness detection in dairy cattle. In Practice 2002;24:444–9.

17. Williamson A, Hoggart B. Pain: a review of three commonly used pain rating scales. J Clin Nurs 2005;14:798–804.

18. Hoffman AC, Moore DA, Vanegas J, et al. Association of abnormal hind-limb postures and back arch with gait abnormality in dairy cattle. J Dairy Sci 2014;97: 2178–85.

19. Garcia-Munoz A, Vidal G, Singh N, et al. Evaluation of two methodologies for lameness detection in dairy cows based on postural and gait abnormalities observed during milking and while restrained at headlock stanchions. Prev Vet Med 2016;128:33–40.

20. Kotschwar JL, Coetzee JF, Anderson DE, et al. Analgesic efficacy of sodium salicylate in an amphotericin B-induced bovine synovitis-arthritis model. J Dairy Sci 2009;92:3731–43.

21. Neveus S, Weary DM, Rushen J, et al. Hoof discomfort changes how dairy cattle distribute their body weight. J Dairy Sci 2006;89:2503–9.

22. Chapinal N, de Passillé AM, Rushen J. Weight distribution and gait in dairy cattle are affected by milking and late pregnancy. J Dairy Sci 2009;92:581–8.

23. Chapinal N, de Passillé AM, Rushen J, et al. Automated methods for detecting lameness and measuring analgesia in dairy cattle. J Dairy Sci 2010;93:2007–13.

24. Chapinal N, de Passillé AM, Rushen J, et al. Effect of analgesia during hoof trimming on gait, weight distribution, and activity of dairy cattle. J Dairy Sci 2010;93: 3039–46.

25. Rushen J, Pombourcq E, de Passillé AM. Validation of two measures of lameness in dairy cows. Appl Anim Behav Sci 2006;106:173–7.

26. Chambers JP, Waterman AE, Livingston A. Further development of equipment to measure nociceptive thresholds in large animals. J Vet Anaesth 1994;21:66–72.

27. Whay HR, Webster AJF, Waterman-Pearson AE. Role of ketoprofen in the modulation of hyperalgesia associated with lameness in dairy cattle. Vet Rec 2005;157: 729–33.

28. Laven RA, Lawrence KE, Weston JF, et al. Assessment of the duration of the pain response associated with lameness in dairy cows, and the influence of treatment. N Z Vet J 2008;56:210–7.

29. Schulz KL, Anderson DE, Coetzee JF, et al. Effect of flunixin meglumine on the amelioration of lameness in dairy steers with amphotericin B-induced transient synovitis-arthritis. Am J Vet Res 2011;72:1431–8.

30. Ossent P, Lischer CJ. Bovine laminitis: the lesions and their pathogenesis. In Practice 1998;20:415–27.

31. Lischer CJ, Ossent P, Raber M, et al. The suspensory structures and supporting tissues of the bovine 3rd phalanx and their relevance in the development of sole ulcers at the typical site. Vet Rec 2002;151(23):694–8.

32. Mulling CKW, Lischer CJ. New aspects on etiology and pathogenesis of laminitis in cattle. Proc of the XXII World Buiatrics Congress (keynote lectures). 2002, Hanover (Germany). p. 236–47. Accessed August 23, 2002.

33. Tarleton JF, Holah DE, Evans KM, et al. Biomechanical and histopathological changes in the support structures of bovine hooves around the time of first calving. Vet J 2002;163:196–204.

34. Webster J. Effect of environment and management on the development of claw and leg diseases. Proc of the XXII World Buiatrics Congress (keynote lectures). 2002, Hanover (Germany). p. 248–56.

35. Raven T. Cattle footcare and claw trimming. Ipswich (United Kingdom): Farming Press; 1989.

36. Shearer JK, van Amstel SR. Functional and corrective claw trimming. Vet Clin North Am Food Anim Pract 2001;17(1):53–72.

37. Shearer JK, van Amstel SR. Manual of foot care in cattle. Fort Atkinson (WI): WD Hoard & Sons; 2005.

38. Van Amstel SR, Shearer JK. Manual for the treatment and control of lameness in cattle. Ames (IA): Blackwell Publishing Professional; 2006.

39. White EM, Glickman LT, Embree C. A randomized field trial for evaluation of bandaging sole abscesses in cattle. J Am Vet Med Assoc 1981;178:375–7.

40. Hernandez-Mendo O, von Keyserlingk MA, Veira DM, et al. Effects of pasture on lameness in dairy cows. J Dairy Sci 2007;90(3):1209–14.

41. Barberg AE, Endres MI, Salfer JA, et al. Performance, health and well-being of dairy cows in an alternative housing system in Minnesota. J Dairy Sci 2007;90: 1575–83.

42. Endres MI, Barberg AE. Behavior of dairy cows in an alternative bedded-pack housing system. J Dairy Sci 2007;90:4192–200.

43. Flower FC, Sedlbauer M, Carter E, et al. Analgesics improve the gait of lame dairy cattle. J Dairy Sci 2008;91:3010–4.

44. Rizk A, Herdtweck S, Offinger J, et al. The use of xylazine hydrochloride in an analgesic protocol for claw treatment of lame dairy cows in lateral recumbency on a surgical tipping table. Vet J 2012;192:193–8.

45. McIlwraith CW, Fessler JF, Blevins WE, et al. Experimentally induced arthritis of the equine carpus: clinical determinations. Am J Vet Res 1979;40:11–20.

46. Thomas HJ, Miguel-Pacheco GG, Bollard NJ, et al. Evaluation of treatments for claw horn lesions in dairy cows in a randomized controlled trial. J Dairy Sci 2015;98(7):4477–86.
47. Janssen S, Wunderlich C, Heppelmann M, et al. Short communication: pilot study on hormonal, metabolic, and behavioral stress response to treatment of claw horn lesions in acutely lame dairy cows. J Dairy Sci 2016;99(9):7481–8.
48. Coetzee JF, Mosher RA, Griffith GR, et al. Pharmacokinetics and tissue disposition of meloxicam in beef calves after repeated oral administration. J Vet Pharmacol Ther 2015;38(6):556–62.
49. Nagel D, Wieringa R, Ireland J, et al. The use of meloxicam oral suspension to treat musculoskeletal lameness in cattle. Vet Medicine Research Rep 2016;7: 149–55.
50. Offinger J, Herdtweck S, Rizk A, et al. Postoperative analgesic efficacy of meloxicam in lame dairy cows undergoing resection of the distal interphalangeal joint. J Dairy Sci 2013;96(2):866–76.
51. Cheng JK, Chiou LC. Mechanisms of the antinociceptive action of gabapentin. J Pharm Sci 2006;100:471–86.
52. Hurley RW, Chatterjea D, Rose Feng M, et al. Gabapentin and pregabalin can interact synergistically with naproxen to produce antihyperalgesia. Anesthesiology 2002;97:1263–73.
53. Coetzee JF, Mosher RA, Kohake LE, et al. Pharmacokinetics of oral gabapentin alone or co-administered with meloxicam in ruminant beef calves. Vet J 2011; 190:98–102.

Index

Note: Page numbers of article titles are in **boldface** type.

A

Abscess(es)
    bulbar
        sepsis in cattle and, 344–345
    retroarticular
        sepsis in cattle and, 345–347
    toe
        sepsis in cattle and, 338–339
        trauma-induced
            in feedlot cattle, 278–279
Accelerometers
    in assessment of lameness-related pain in cattle, 394–395
Age
    as factor in CSC, 355–356
Anesthesia/anesthetics
    local
        in management of lameness-related pain in cattle, 406
    of lower limb and foot
        in management of lameness-related pain in cattle, 396–398
Animal welfare
    freedoms associated with
        in understanding impact of lameness in dairy cattle, **153–164** *See also*
            Lameness, in dairy cattle, welfare implications of
Ankylosis
    DIJ, 330–338
Antibacterial agents
    in footbaths for dairy cattle, 196
Antibiotics
    sepsis in cattle related to, 347–348
Anti-inflammatory agents
    sepsis in cattle related to, 347–348
Arthritis
    septic
        of proximal limb, 265–266

B

Beef cattle
    DD in, **165–181** *See also* Digital dermatitis (DD), in dairy and beef cattle
Behavior(s)
    estrous
        lameness in dairy cattle effects on, 159–160

Vet Clin Food Anim 33 (2017) 413–425
http://dx.doi.org/10.1016/S0749-0720(17)30040-3
0749-0720/17

Printed and bound by CPI Group (UK) Ltd, Croydon, CR0 4YY

03/10/2024

01040392-0012